Study Guide for

Understanding Pathophysiology

Study Guide for

Understanding Pathophysiology

Sue E. Huether, MSN, PhD
Professor Emeritus
College of Nursing
University of Utah
Salt Lake City, Utah

Kathryn L. McCance, MSN, PhD
Professor
College of Nursing
University of Utah
Salt Lake City, Utah

Section Editors
Valentina L. Brashers, MD
Professor Nursing and Attending Physician in Internal Medicine
University of Virginia Health System
Charlottesville, Virginia

Neal S. Rote, PhD
Academic Vice-Chair and Director of Research
Department of Obstetrics and Gynecology
University Hospitals of Cleveland;
Professor of Reproductive Biology and Pathology
Case School of Medicine
Case Western Reserve University
Cleveland, Ohio

Prepared by
Clayton F. Parkinson, PhD
Professor Emeritus
College of Health Sciences
Weber State University
Ogden, Utah

ELSEVIER

ELSEVIER
MOSBY

3251 Riverport Lane
St. Louis, Missouri 63043

STUDY GUIDE FOR UNDERSTANDING PATHOPHYSIOLOGY, 5TH EDITION

ISBN: 978-0-323-08489-5

Vice President and Publisher: Loren S. Wilson
Senior Editor: Sandra Clark
Senior Developmental Editor: Charlene Ketchum
Editorial Assistant: Brooke Kannady
Publishing Services Managers: Jeffrey Patterson and Hemamalini Rajendrababu
Senior Project Managers: Jeanne Genz and Srikumar Narayanan
Designer: Paula Catalano
Multimedia Producer: Lisa Godoski

Printed in the United States of America

Last digit is the print number: 9 8 7 6 5 4

Reviewers

Mandi Counters, RN, MSN, CNRN
Assistant Professor
Nursing Department
Mercy College of Health Sciences
Des Moines, Iowa

Bradley R Harrell, DNP, ACNP-BC, CCRN
Assistant Professor of Nursing
School of Nursing
Union University-Germantown
Germantown, Tennessee

Jane Cross Norman, Ph.D., R.N., CNE
Professor of Nursing
MSN Program Director
Tennessee State University
Nashville, Tennessee

Marylou Virginia Robinson, PhD, FNP-C
Assistant Professor
College of Nursing
University of Colorado
Aurora, Colorado

Preface

The study of pathophysiology is complex, ever expanding, and challenging. It requires correlations between normal and abnormal anatomy and physiology as well as the processes resulting in the manifestations of disease.

This Study Guide is designed for students as an adjunct to Understanding Pathophysiology, fifth edition, by Sue E. Huether and Kathryn L. McCance. It is intended to facilitate an understanding of the consequences of pathologic processes on the structure and function of the human body.

The Study Guide contains 40 chapters, each following the organization of the textbook. The Guide's chapters have two different formats—one for *normal anatomy and physiology* and another for *anatomic and physiologic alterations*.

For the normal anatomy and physiology chapters, it is assumed that the student possesses foundational knowledge of anatomy and physiology; therefore, no supplemental narrative is provided.

- These chapters have *foundational objectives* that direct *review* of the information, principles, and concepts that are essential for understanding the specific diseases that follow in the next chapter. Chapters five and six depart from the usual normal anatomy and physiology chapter's format. This departure is because inflammation and immunity concepts are frequently referenced throughout the following text and study guide chapters.
- Each chapter has a practice examination to give students an opportunity to assess their understanding of normality.

The chapters on *alterations* direct the learner's study of abnormal anatomy and physiology.

- These chapters include 1) *foundational objectives* for *review* and 2) *learning objectives* for *study* with narrative, charts, and tables.
- Each chapter has a practice examination requiring factual and conceptual knowledge related to disease mechanisms.
- Each chapter includes one or two case studies linking fact and concept to reality that require analysis and application.

The objectives for all chapters are referenced to corresponding pages in the fifth edition of Understanding Pathophysiology. Huether and McCance's philosophy that students need to grasp basic laws and principles to understand how alterations occur led them to develop an understandable and conceptually integrated textbook.

I enjoyed working with Mosby, particularly with Charlene Kechum and Jeanne Genz. All of Mosby's staff ensured that my efforts were developed into a creative, professional, and pleasing style for student learners. I wish to dedicate my efforts during the preparation of this Study Guide to students who inspired me to search for a better way to convey information to them.

Clayton F. Parkinson

Contents

1 Cellular Biology

FOUNDATIONAL OBJECTIVES

After reviewing this chapter, the learner will be able to do the following:

1. **State the functions of a typical eukaryotic cell.**
   Review pages 2-3.

2. **Describe the structure and function of the nucleus and identify the cytoplasmic organelles.**
   Review page 3; refer to Figures 1-1 and 1-2 and Table 1-1.

3. **Describe the structure and function of the plasma membrane.**
   Review pages 3 and 5-7; refer to Figures 1-3 through 1-5 and Tables 1-2 and 1-3.

4. **Describe cellular receptors.**
   Review pages 7-8; refer to Figure 1-6.

5. **Identify the three mechanisms that bind cells together.**
   Review pages 8-9; refer to Figures 1-7 and 1-8.

6. **Describe the primary modes of chemical signaling.**
   Review pages 9, 11, and 13 refer to Figures 1-9 through 1-12 and Table 1-3.

7. **Describe cellular catabolism and the transfer of energy to accomplish other cellular processes.**
   Refer to Figures 1-13 through 1-15.

8. **Differentiate between passive and active transport, between endocytosis and exocytosis, and between phagocytosis and pinocytosis.**
   Refer to Figures 1-16 through 1-24 and Table 1-4.

9. **Describe the changes in the plasma membrane that result in an action potential.**
   Review pages 21-22; refer to Figure 1-25.

10. **Identify the phases of mitosis and cytokinesis.**
    Review pages 22-23; refer to Figure 1-26.

11. **Describe the stimulation of cell proliferation by growth factors.**
    Review pages 23-24; refer to Figure 1-27 and Table 1-5.

12. **Characterize pattern formation.**
    Review page 24.

13. **Identify the location and a major function for each type of tissue: epithelial, connective, muscle, and nervous.**
    Refer to Boxes 1-3 through 1-5.

PRACTICE EXAMINATION

Multiple Choice

Circle the correct answer for each question:

1. Which are principal parts of a eukaryotic cell?
   a. fat, carbohydrate, and protein
   b. minerals and water
   c. organelles
   d. phospholipids and protein
   e. protoplasm and nucleus

2. The cell membrane is described as a fluid mosaic. Some proteins have a degree of mobility within the lipid bilayer. (More than one answer may be correct.)
   a. The first sentence is true.
   b. The first sentence is false.
   c. The second sentence is true.
   d. The second sentence is false.
   e. The second sentence is relevant to the first.
   f. The second sentence is irrelevant to the first.

3. Which particle can penetrate cell membranes most easily?
   a. lipid soluble, transport protein present
   b. neutral charge, water soluble
   c. smaller, water soluble
   d. uncharged, larger

4. For a cell to engage in active transport processes, it requires:
   a. mitochondria.
   b. appropriate fuel.
   c. ATP.
   d. enzymes.
   e. All of the above are correct.

5. Which is *inconsistent* with the others?
   a. diffusion
   b. osmosis
   c. filtration
   d. phagocytosis
   e. facilitated diffusion

6. Which can transport substances uphill against the concentration gradient?
   a. active transport
   b. osmosis
   c. dialysis
   d. facilitated diffusion
   e. None of the above is correct.

7. Caveolae:
   a. serve as repositories for some receptors.
   b. provide a route for transport into a cell.
   c. relay signals into cells.
   d. All of the above are correct.

8. Which statement is true for cytoplasm?
   a. It is located outside the nucleus.
   b. It provides support for organelles.
   c. It is mostly water.
   d. a, b, and c
   e. a and b

9. The retinoblastoma (Rb) protein:
   a. is a brake on the progress of the cell cycle.
   b. binds to gene regulatory proteins.
   c. slows cell proliferation.
   d. a and c
   e. a, b, and c

10. A major function of connective tissue is:
   a. to form glands.
   b. support and binding.
   c. covering and lining.
   d. movement.
   e. to conduct nerve impulses.

11. Which are characteristic of epithelial tissue? (More than one answer may be correct.)
   a. elasticity
   b. protection
   c. fills spaces between organs
   d. secretion

12. Signaling molecules cause all of the following *except*:
   a. acceleration/initiative of intracellular protein kinases.
   b. arrest of cellular growth.
   c. apoptosis.
   d. conversion of an intracellular signal into an extracellular response.

13. Ligands that bind with membrane receptors include which of the following? (More than one answer may be correct.)
   a. hormones
   b. antigens
   c. neurotransmitters
   d. drugs
   e. infectious agents

14. The products from the metabolism of glucose include which of the following? (More than one answer may be correct.)
   a. kilocalories
   b. CO_2
   c. H_2O
   d. ATP

15. Identify the correct sequence of events for initiation and conduction of a nerve impulse.
   1. Sodium moves inside.
   2. Potassium leaves cell.
   3. Sodium permeability changes.
   4. Resting potential is reestablished.
   5. Potassium permeability changes.
      a. 1, 3, 2, 5, 4
      b. 3, 1, 5, 2, 4
      c. 5, 2, 3, 1, 4
      d. 4, 5, 2, 3, 1

16. Increased cytoplasmic calcium:
   a. causes one cell to adhere to another.
   b. increases permeability at the junctional complex.
   c. decreases permeability at the junctional complex.
   d. None of the above is correct.

17. Cell junctions:
   a. coordinate activities of cells within tissues.
   b. are an impermeable part of the plasma membrane.
   c. hold cells together.
   d. Both a and c are correct.
   e. Both b and c are correct.

Matching

Match the term with its descriptor:

_______ 18. Anaphase
_______ 19. Chromatin
_______ 20. Metaphase
_______ 21. Mitochondria
_______ 22. Prophase
_______ 23. Ribosome

a. 75% to 90% H_2O, lipids, and protein
b. within the nucleus, stored RNA
c. compartmentalizes cellular activity
d. single strand of DNA, nondividing cell
e. "generation plant" for ATP
f. centriole migration
g. chromatid pair alignment
h. chromatid migration
i. daughter nuclei
j. protein synthesis site

Match the location with the tissue type found:

_______ 24. Lining of the kidney tubules
_______ 25. Lining of the upper respiratory tract

a. simple squamous
b. simple cuboidal
c. simple columnar, ciliated
d. stratified squamous
e. transitional

Fill in the Blank

Complete the following table identifying membrane transport of cellular intake or output:

Membrane Transport

Transport Mechanism	Description
Diffusion	
Filtration	
Osmosis	
Mediated transport	Two molecules move simultaneously in one direction (symport) or in opposite direction (antiport) or a single molecule moves in one direction (uniport)
Passive mediated transport/facilitated diffusion	Does not require the expenditure of metabolic energy (ATP)
Active mediated transport	Requires the expenditure of metabolic energy (ATP)
Endocytosis	
Pinocytosis	
Phagocytosis	

2 Genes and Genetic Diseases

FOUNDATIONAL OBJECTIVES

a. Describe the interrelationships of DNA, RNA, and proteins.

Review pages 35-39; refer to Figures 2-1 through 2-8.

MEMORY CHECK!

- The *gene* consists of a particular sequence of *nucleotides* in the deoxyribonucleic acid (DNA) of the *chromosome*. The sequence of nucleotides in a gene determines which proteins are found in a cell, and these *proteins determine both the form and the function of the cell.*
- Genetic information flows from *DNA to RNA to proteins*. Three major processes are involved in the preservation and transmission of genetic information. The first is *replication*, or the copying of DNA to form identical daughter molecules. The second is *transcription*, in which the genetic message encoded within DNA is transcribed into RNA and is carried to the ribosomes, the sites of protein synthesis. The third is *translation*, in which the genetic message is decoded and converted into the 20-letter alphabet of protein structure. Because the sequence of nucleotides in the DNA bears a linear correspondence to the sequence of amino acids in the formed proteins, genetic information is preserved and transmitted to progeny.

b. Define general genetic terms.

MEMORY CHECK!

Genetic Term	Definition
Progeny	Offspring
Chromosomes	Structures in the nucleus that contain DNA, which transmits genetic information; each chromosome is composed of many genes arranged in linear order
Gene	DNA, the basic unit of heredity, located at a particular locus on the chromosome
Locus	The position each gene occupies along a chromosome
Allele	One of two or more alternative genes that contain specific inheritable characteristics (such as eye color) and occupy corresponding positions on paired, homologous chromosomes—one gene from each parent; a different version of the same paired gene
Homozygous	A trait of an organism produced by identical or nearly identical alleles
Heterozygous	Possessing different alleles at a given chromosomal location
Karyotype/karyogram	A display of human chromosomes based on their lengths and the locations of their centromeres
Genotype	The basic combination of genes of an organism
Phenotype	The expression of the gene or trait in an individual (e.g., physical appearance, such as eye color)
Carrier	An individual who has a gene for disease but is phenotypically normal
Dominant traits	Traits for which one of a pair of alleles is necessary for expression (e.g., brown eyes)
Recessive traits	Traits for which two alleles of a pair are necessary for expression (e.g., blue eyes, a recessive gene on the male's X chromosome, will be expressed because the gene is not matched by a corresponding gene on the Y chromosome)
Pedigree chart	A schematic method for classifying genetic data
Penetrance	The percentage of individuals with a specific genotype who exhibit the expected phenotype
Expressivity	The extent of variation in phenotype for a particular genotype
Genetic imprinting	Different expression of a disease gene depending on which parent transmits the gene; it is associated with methylation

Single-gene disorders are known to be caused by mutation in a single gene. The mutated gene may be present on one or both chromosomes of a gene pair.

Multifactorial disorders result when small variations in genes combine with environmental factors to produce serious defects. Multifactorial disorders tend to cluster in families.

LEARNING OBJECTIVES

After studying this chapter, the learner will be able to do the following:

1. Characterize the chromosome and its aberrations.
Study pages 40-46; refer to Figures 2-9 through 2-18.

In **chromosome disorders**, the defect is due to an abnormality in chromosome *number* or *structure*. The structure of the genes in chromosome disorders may be normal, but the genes may be present in multiple copies or may be situated on a different chromosome.

Normal somatic cells that have two sets of 23 chromosomes are **diploid** (double), or 2N. Gametes with a single set of 23 chromosomes are **haploid** (single), or N. A cell with an exact multiple of the haploid number is **euploid**. Euploid numbers may be 2N, 3N (triploid), or 4N (tetraploid). Chromosome numbers that are exact multiples of N, but greater than 2N, are called **triploid or polyploid.** **Aneuploidy** refers to a chromosome complement that is abnormal in number but is not an exact multiple of N. An aneuploid cell may be **trisomic** (2N + 1 chromosome) or **monosomic** (2N – 1 chromosome).

Disjunction is the normal separation and migration of chromosomes during cell division. Failure of the process, or **nondisjunction**, in a meiotic division results in one daughter cell receiving both homologous chromosomes and the other receiving neither. It is the primary cause of aneuploidy. If this deviation in normal processes occurs during the first meiotic division, half of the gametes will contain 22 chromosomes and half will contain 24. If joined with a normal gamete, a gamete produced in this manner will produce either a monosomic (2N – 1) or trisomic (2N + 1) zygote.

Deviations in the normal structure of chromosomes result when the chromosome material breaks and reassembles in an abnormal arrangement. Structural abnormalities include deletion, duplication, inversion, and translocation.

In **deletion**, or loss of a portion of a chromosome, usually the zygote has one normal chromosome united with a chromosome with some missing genes. **Cri-du-chat** ("cry of the cat") **syndrome** is such a deletion and is manifested by the high-pitched cat-like cry of an affected child.

Duplication is the presence of a repeated gene or gene sequence. A deleted segment of one chromosome may become incorporated into its homologous chromosome.

Inversion is the reversal of gene order. The linear arrangement of genes on a chromosome is broken, and the order of a portion of the gene complement is reversed in the process of reattachment.

Translocation is the transfer of part of one chromosome to a nonhomologous chromosome. This occurs when two chromosomes break and the segments are rejoined in an abnormal arrangement.

2. Cite examples of chromosome disorders.
Refer to Figures 2-13 through 2-16 and Table 2-1.

A common example of an autosomal aneuploidy disorder that results from an abnormality of chromosome number is *trisomy 21*, or **Down syndrome**. This disorder can result when nondisjunction of chromosome 21 occurs at meiosis, producing one gamete with an extra chromosome 21 and one gamete with no chromosome 21. Union of the extra chromosome female gamete with a normal sperm produces a 47-chromosome zygote, or trisomy 21.

The overall incidence of Down syndrome is 1 per 800 live births. The incidence rises with increasing maternal age. Clinical diagnosis of trisomy 21 is often based on *facial appearance*. A low nasal bridge, epicanthal folds, protruding tongue, and low-set ears are common. Mental retardation is consistent in children with Down syndrome, but its degree may vary. The average IQ is approximately 50.

Two sex chromosome aneuploidy disorders are **Turner syndrome** (female) and **Klinefelter syndrome** (male). The most common karyotype showing female phenotype is 45,X or the absence of one X chromosome; the male karyotype is 47,XXY or an extra X chromosome.

The diagnosis of Turner syndrome is suggested in the newborn by the presence of redundant neck skin and peripheral lymphedema. Later, the presence of short stature is suggestive.

Klinefelter syndrome is a common cause of infertility in men. Other manifestations are long lower extremities, sparse body hair with female distribution, and female breast development in about 50% of cases. A moderate degree of mental impairment may be present.

3. Characterize single-gene disorders.
Study pages 47-54; refer to Figures 2-19 through 2-31.

An inherited gene may be present on one or both chromosomes of a pair. The pedigree patterns of inherited traits depend on whether the gene is located on an autosomal chromosome, any chromosome other than a sex chromosome, or the X chromosome and whether the gene is dominant or recessive. These factors allow four basic patterns of inheritance for single-gene traits, whether normal or abnormal: autosomal dominant, autosomal recessive, X-linked dominant, and X-linked recessive.

In **autosomal dominant** inheritance of genetic defects, the abnormal allele is dominant and the normal allele is recessive. The phenotype is the same whether the allele is present in either a homozygous or a heterozygous state.

Characteristics of autosomal dominant inheritance are (1) affected persons have an affected parent; (2) affected persons mating with normal persons have affected and unaffected offspring in equal proportion; and (3) males and females are equally affected.

In **autosomal recessive** disorders, the abnormal allele is recessive. For the trait to be expressed, a person must be homozygous for the abnormal allele. Because the dominant or normal allele masks the trait, most persons who are heterozygous for an autosomal recessive allele are phenotypically normal. When two heterozygous individuals mate and an offspring receives the recessive allele from each parent, the trait is expressed.

Characteristics of autosomal recessive inheritance are: (1) the trait usually appears in siblings only, not in the parents; (2) males and females are equally likely to be affected; (3) for parents of one affected child, the recurrence risk is one in four for every subsequent birth; (4) both parents of an affected child carry the recessive allele; and (5) the parents of the affected child may be blood relatives, for example, first cousins.

Unlike the 44 autosomes that can be arranged in 22 homologous pairs, the two sex chromosomes in the female are XX and in the male are XY. The ovum must contain an X chromosome, so if it is fertilized by a sperm containing an X chromosome, the progeny will be a female (XX). If the sperm contributes a Y chromosome, the progeny will be male (XY).

Traits determined by either dominant or recessive **X-linked genes** are expressed in the male. The genes on the X chromosome cannot be transmitted from father to son (fathers contribute a Y chromosome to sons) but are transmitted from father to all daughters through one X chromosome. Recessive abnormal genes on the X chromosome of a female may not be expressed because they are matched by normal genes inherited with the other X chromosome.

X-linked dominant disorders are rare. The main characteristic of this inheritance pattern is that an affected male transmits the gene to all of his daughters and to none of his sons. The affected female may transmit the gene to offspring of either sex.

In **X-linked recessive** disorders, the recessive gene located on the one X chromosome of the male is not balanced by the dominant allele on the Y chromosome and is thus expressed. Only matings between an affected male and a carrier or affected female should result in an affected female.

Males affected with an X-linked recessive disorder cannot transmit the gene to sons, but transmit it to all daughters. An unaffected female who is heterozygous (a carrier) for the recessive gene transmits it to 50% of her sons and daughters.

Principles of the X-linked recessive inheritance are: (1) males are predominantly affected; (2) affected males cannot transmit the gene to sons, but do transmit the gene to all daughters; (3) sons of female carriers have a 50% risk of being affected; and (4) daughters of female carriers have a 50% risk of being carriers.

4. Cite examples of single-gene disorders.
Refer to Figures 2-23 and 2-31.

One of the best-known autosomal dominant diseases is **Huntington disease**, a neurologic disorder that exhibits progressive dementia and increasingly uncontrollable movements of the limbs. A key feature of this disease is that *symptoms* are not usually evident *until after age 40 years*. Thus, those in whom the disease develops often have had children before they are aware that they have the gene.

The severity of an autosomal dominant disease can vary greatly. An example of variable expressivity in an autosomal dominant disease is type 1 **neurofibromatosis**, or von Recklinghausen disease, which has been mapped to the long arm of chromosome 17. The expression of this gene can vary from a *few harmless café au lait–colored spots* on the skin to numerous malignant neurofibromas, scoliosis, seizures, gliomas, neuromas, hypertension, and mental retardation.

The **cystic fibrosis** gene, the cause of an autosomal recessive disease, has been mapped to the long arm of chromosome 7. In this disease, *defective transport of chloride ion* leads to a salt imbalance that results in secretions of abnormally *thick, dehydrated mucus.* Some of the digestive organs, particularly the pancreas, become obstructed with mucus, resulting in malnutrition. The lung airways tend to become clogged with mucus, making them highly susceptible to bacterial infections.

The most common and severe of all X-linked recessive disorders is **Duchenne muscular dystrophy**, which affects males. This disorder is characterized by progressive muscle degeneration; individuals are usually unable to walk by age 10 or 12. The disease also affects the heart and respiratory muscles, and death due to respiratory or cardiac failure may occur before age 20 years. These cases result from an *absence of dystrophin*, without which the muscle cell cannot survive, and muscle deterioration follows.

5. Characterize multifactorial inheritance, and cite examples.
Study pages 55 and 56; refer to Figures 2-30 and 2-31.

Not all traits are produced by single genes; some traits are the result of several genes acting together. When several genes act together, the trait is referred to as **polygenic traits**. When environmental factors also influence the expression of the trait, the term **multifactorial inheritance** is used. Both genes and environment contribute to variation in traits. Multifactorial disorders tend to cluster in families.

Although genes determine both height and IQ, the environment also influences these traits. Also, IQ scores can be improved by exposing children to enriched learning environments.

A number of diseases do not follow the bell-shaped distribution of polygenic and multifactorial traits. Instead, a certain *threshold of liability* must be crossed before the disease is expressed. A well-known example of a threshold trait is *pyloric stenosis*, a disorder characterized by narrowing or obstruction of the pylorus. Chronic vomiting, constipation, weight loss, and electrolyte imbalance can result from this condition. Pyloric stenosis is much more common in males than in females. The reason for this difference is that the *threshold of liability* is much lower in males than in females. Thus, fewer defective alleles are required to generate the disorder in males. This situation also means that the offspring of affected females are more likely to have pyloric stenosis because affected females carry more disease-causing alleles than do most affected males.

Other multifactorial diseases include cleft lip and cleft palate, neural tube defects, clubfoot, and some forms of congenital heart disease. Hypertensive heart disease and diabetes mellitus likely can be grouped in the category of multifactorial disorders.

PRACTICE EXAMINATION

Multiple Choice

Circle the correct answer for each question:

1. Which genetic disease is caused by an abnormal karyotype?
   a. Down syndrome
   b. Huntington disease
   c. phenylketonuria (PKU)
   d. neurofibromatosis
   e. cystic fibrosis

2. Which is *not* characteristic of Down syndrome?
   a. It is an autosomal aneuploidy.
   b. It is a genetic error of metabolism.
   c. Mental retardation is consistently expressed.
   d. Clinical diagnosis can be suggested by facial appearance.
   e. The karyotype is 47,XY + 21.

3. Cri-du-chat syndrome is an abnormality of chromosomal structure involving:
   a. translocation.
   b. inversion.
   c. duplication.
   d. deletion.

4. An individual's karyotype lacks a homologous X chromosome and has only a single X chromosome present. Which statement is *not* true?
   a. The karyotype is 45,X.
   b. Features include ribbed neck and short stature.
   c. The karyotype is 46,XY.
   d. The disorder is a sex chromosome aneuploidy.

5. If homologous chromosomes fail to separate during meiosis, the disorder is:
   a. polyploidy.
   b. aneuploidy.
   c. disjunction.
   d. nondisjunction.
   e. translocation.

6. Cystic fibrosis has been mapped to chromosome:
   a. 17.
   b. 7.
   c. X.
   d. 16.

7. In autosomal dominant inherited disorders:
   a. affected individuals do not have an affected parent.
   b. affected persons mating with normal persons have a 50% risk of having an affected offspring.
   c. male offspring are most often affected.
   d. unaffected children born to affected parents will have affected children.

8. Indentify the characteristic(s) of X-linked recessive inherited disorders:
   a. affected males have normal sons.
   b. affected males have affected daughters.
   c. sons of female carriers have a 50% risk of being affected.
   d. the affected female may transmit the gene to both sons and daughters.

9. Which is/are *not* autosomal dominant disease(s)?
   a. Huntington disease
   b. neurofibromatosis
   c. Duchenne muscular dystrophy
   d. von Recklinghausen disease
   e. pyloric stenosis

10. When environmental influences cause varied phenotypic expressions of genotypes, the result is:
    a. a multifactorial trait.
    b. a threshold liability.
    c. an autosomal dominant trait.
    d. an X-linked recessive trait.

11. Which likely is *not* a multifactorial inherited disorder?
    a. cleft palate
    b. hypertension
    c. diabetes mellitus
    d. cystic fibrosis
    e. heart disease

Matching

Match the term with the circumstance:

_______ 12. Recessive disorder

_______ 13. Multifactorial inheritance

_______ 14. Aneuploidy

_______ 15. Chromosomal aberration

_______ 16. Phenotype

_______ 17. Pedigree

_______ 18. Autosomal recessive inheritance

a. results from numerical or structural aberrations
b. many genes are common
c. two or more cell lines with different karyotypes
d. individual is homozygous for a gene
e. failure of homologous chromosomes to separate during meiosis or mitosis
f. outward appearance of an individual
g. a probability of .25
h. summarizes family relationships

Match the term with the circumstance:

_______ 19. Expressivity

_______ 20. X-linked

_______ 21. Inversion

_______ 22. Dominant trait

_______ 23. Allele

_______ 24. 47,XXY

_______ 25. Karyotype

a. a probability of 0.5
b. females are unlikely to be affected
c. species chromosomal morphology
d. expressed by one allele
e. Turner syndrome
f. different version of the same paired gene
g. Klinefelter syndrome
h. no loss or gain of genetic material, reversed order
i. extent of phenotypic variation of a particular genotype

Complete the following table comparing the transmission patterns of single-gene and multifactorial diseases:

Transmission Patterns for Genetic Diseases		
	Single-Gene Diseases	Multifactorial Diseases
Inheritance pattern		

CASE STUDY

Mrs. S.J., a 42-year-old woman who is pregnant for the first time, was admitted to the labor and delivery unit. She appeared to be in excellent health, and this anticipated delivery would be the culmination of an uneventful pregnancy. Eight hours later, she delivered a 7-pound, 3-ounce baby boy. The infant had low-set ears, a flat facial profile with a small nose, wide epicanthal folds, and simian creases. The parents were told that the baby's features were the result of a genetic aberration and that he had Down syndrome. The father asked, "Why did this happen, and what does the future hold?"

How would you answer the father's questions?

3 Altered Cellular and Tissue Biology

FOUNDATIONAL OBJECTIVES

a. Describe processes of cellular intake and output.
Review pages 13-18 and 20.

MEMORY CHECK!

- The intact, normally functioning plasma membrane is *selectively* or *differentially permeable* to substances; that is, it allows some substances to pass while excluding others. Water and small, uncharged substances move through pores of the lipid bilayer by *passive transport*, which requires *no* expenditure of energy. This process is driven by the forces of osmosis, hydrostatic pressure, and diffusion. Larger molecules and molecular complexes are moved into the cell by *active transport*, which requires the expenditure of energy or *ATP* by the cell. In active transport, materials move from low concentrations to high concentrations. The largest molecules and fluids are ingested by endocytosis (from the extracellular medium) and expelled by exocytosis (into the extracellular medium) after cellular synthesis of smaller building blocks. When the plasma membrane is injured, it becomes permeable to virtually everything, and substances move into and out of the cells in an unrestricted manner. Notably, such substances may affect: (1) the nucleus and its genetic information or (2) the cytoplasmic organelles and their varied functions. Then, there is altered cellular physiology and pathology.

LEARNING OBJECTIVES

After studying this chapter, the learner will be able to do the following:

1. Describe the cellular adaptations occurring in atrophy, hypertrophy, hyperplasia, dysplasia, and metaplasia. Identify the conditions under which each can occur.
Study pages 59-62; refer to Figures 3-1 through 3-5.

When confronted with environmental stresses that disrupt normal structure and function, the cell undergoes adaptive changes that permit survival and maintain function. The adaptation is a reversible, structural, or functional response to normal or adverse conditions; it enables the cell to maintain a steady state called *homeostasis*. These changes may lead to atrophy, hypertrophy, hyperplasia, dysplasia, or metaplasia.

Cellular atrophy decreases the cell substance and results in cell shrinkage. Causes of atrophy may be *physiologic* (associated with normal development), *pathologic* (accompanying disease), or *disuse* (because of lack of stimulation). All three causes may result in decreased protein synthesis, increased protein catabolism, or both. A **ubiquitin-proteosome pathway** degrades proteins to ubiquitin, a smaller protein, and then proteosomes in the cytoplasm complete the proteolysis.

Hypertrophy increases cell size. Hypertrophy is commonly seen in cardiac and skeletal muscle tissue. The increase in cell components is related to an *increased* rate of *protein synthesis*. Mechanical signals, such as stretch, and trophic signals, such as growth factors, hormones, and vasoactive agents, are triggers for hypertrophy. Physiologic hypertrophy is observed in uterine tissue and mammary glands during pregnancy.

Hyperplasia is an increase in the number of cells of a tissue or organ. It occurs in tissues where cells are capable of *mitotic division*. Breast and uterine enlargement during pregnancy are examples of *physiologic hyperplasia* and hypertrophy that are hormonally regulated. A *pathologic hyperplasia* occurs when the endometrium enlarges because of excessive estrogen production. Then, the abnormally thickened uterine layer may bleed excessively and frequently. *Compensatory hyperplasia* enables certain organs, such as the liver, to regenerate after loss of substance. Hyperplasia and hypertrophy often occur together if cells can synthesize DNA; however, in nondividing cells, only hypertrophy occurs.

Dysplasia is deranged cell growth that results in cells that vary in size, shape, and appearance in comparison with mature cells and is related to hyperplasia. Dysplasia occurs in association with chronic irritation or inflammation in the uterine cervix, oral cavity, gallbladder, and respiratory passages. Dysplasia is *potentially reversible* once the irritating cause has been removed. Dysplastic changes *do not indicate cancer* and may not progress to neoplastic disease.

Metaplasia is a *reversible conversion* from one adult cell type to another adult cell type. It allows for replacement with cells that are *better able to tolerate environmental stresses*. In metaplasia, one type of cell may be converted to another type of cell within its tissue class.

An example of metaplasia is the substitution of stratified squamous epithelial cells for ciliated columnar epithelial cells in the airways of an individual who is a habitual cigarette smoker.

2. **Identify the mechanism of cellular injury from hypoxia, free radicals, chemicals, unintentional and intentional injuries, infectious agents, immunologic and inflammatory responses, and genetic factors.**
   Study pages 62-66, 68-75, and 78-80; refer to Figures 3-6 through 3-16 and Tables 3-1 through 3-10.

Hypoxia *deprives* the cell of *oxygen* and interrupts oxidative metabolism and the generation of ATP. As oxygen tension within the cell falls, oxidative metabolism ceases and the cell reverts to anaerobic metabolism. One of the earliest effects of reduced ATP is acute cellular swelling caused by failure of the sodium-potassium membrane pump. With impaired function of this pump, intracellular potassium levels decrease and sodium and water accumulate within the cell. As fluid and ions move into the cell, there is dilation of the endoplasmic reticulum, increased membrane permeability, and decreased mitochondrial function as extracellular calcium accumulates in the mitochondria. If the oxygen supply is not restored, loss of essential enzymes, proteins, and ribonucleic acid continues through the permeable membrane of the cell. Hypoxia can result from inadequate oxygen in the air, respiratory disease, decreased blood flow due to circulatory disease, anemia, or inability of the cells to utilize oxygen. Restoration of oxygen, however, can cause **reperfusion injury**. Reperfusion injury results from the generation of highly reactive oxygen intermediates, including hydroxyl radical, superoxide, and hydrogen peroxide (free radicals; see next paragraph).

An important mechanism of *membrane damage* is caused by *reactive oxygen species (ROS),* especially by activated oxygen species. A free radical is an atom or group of atoms with an unpaired electron. The unpaired electron makes the atom or group unstable. To gain stability, the radical gives up an electron to another molecule or steals an electron. These highly reactive radicals have low chemical specificity and can bond with key molecules in membranes and nucleic acids. These reactive species cause injury by: (1) lipid peroxidation, which destroys unsaturated fatty acids; (2) fragmentation of polypeptide chains within proteins; and (3) alteration of DNA by breakage of single strands. Free radicals may be initiated within cells by the absorption of ultraviolet light or x-rays, oxidative reactions that occur during normal metabolism, and enzymatic metabolism of exogenous chemicals or drugs.

Toxic chemical agents can injure the cell membrane and cell structures, block enzymatic pathways, coagulate cell proteins, and disrupt the osmotic and ionic balance of cells. Chemicals may injure cells during the process of metabolism or elimination. Carbon tetrachloride, for example, causes little damage until it is metabolized by liver enzymes to highly reactive free radicals, and then it is extremely toxic to liver cells. Carbon monoxide has a special affinity for the hemoglobin molecule and reduces hemoglobin's ability to carry oxygen.

Liver disease, nutritional disorders, and CNS impairment are serious consequences of **alcohol** abuse. The hepatic changes, initiated by ethanol conversion to acetaldehyde, include deposition of fat, enlargement of the liver, interruption of transport of proteins and their secretion, increase in intracellular water, depression of fatty acid oxidation, greater membrane rigidity, and acute liver cell necrosis. In the CNS, alcohol is a depressant, initially affecting subcortical structures. Consequently, motor and intellectual activity becomes disoriented. At high blood alcohol levels, respiratory medullary centers become depressed.

Unintentional and intentional injuries affect more men than women and more blacks than whites or other racial groups. Injuries by blunt force result from mechanical energy applied to the body. *Contusion* (bleeding in skin or underlying tissue) and *abrasion* (removal of skin) are consequences of blunt blows. Contusions and abrasions exhibit a patterned appearance that mirrors the shape and features of an injuring object. *Asphyxial injuries* are caused by a failure of cells to receive or use oxygen; these injuries can be categorized as suffocation, strangulation, chemical, and drowning.

Infectious agents that survive and proliferate in the body may produce toxic substances and hypersensitivity reactions that injure cells and tissues.

Immunologic and inflammatory injuries are important causes of cellular injury. Cellular membranes are injured by direct contact with cellular and chemical components of the innate and adaptive immune responses. Such mediators are lymphocytes and macrophages and chemicals such as histamine, antibodies, lymphokines, complement, and proteases. Complement, a serum protein, is responsible for many of the membrane alterations that occur during immunologic injury. Membrane alterations are associated with rapid *leakage of potassium* out of the cell and rapid *influx of water*. Antibodies can interfere with membrane function by binding to and occupying receptor molecules on the plasma membrane. (Later chapters deal with these injurious consequences, as well as with hypersensitivity and autoimmune disease.)

Genetic disorders may alter the cell's nucleus and the plasma membrane's structure, shape, receptors, or transport mechanisms. (Mechanisms causing genetic abnormalities are discussed in Chapter 2.)

Errors in health care are unintended events that harm individuals. Such errors involve medications, surgery, diagnosis, equipment, and laboratory reports. They can occur in hospitals, clinics, outpatient surgery centers, health provider offices, pharmacies, and individuals' homes.

3. **Identify various cellular accumulations occurring in response to injury and the subsequent manifestations of cellular damage.**
Study pages 80-84; refer to Figures 3-17 through 3-22 and Table 3-11.

Cellular accumulations or infiltrations occur whenever *normal substances* are produced in excess, normal and *abnormal substances* are ineffectively catabolized, or harmful *exogenous materials* accumulate intracellularly.

4. **Identify the major types of cellular necrosis and cite examples of the tissues involved in each type. Compare necrosis with apoptosis and describe autophagy.**
Study pages 84-88 and 90; refer to Figures 3-23 through 3-31 and Table 3-12.

Cellular death leads to cellular dissolution, or **necrosis**. It is likely that under certain conditions, such as activation of proteases, necrosis is *regulated or programmed* in a well-orchestrated way. Hence, it is termed **programmed necrosis** or **necroptosis**. Necrosis is local cell death and involves the process of cellular self-digestion known as *autodigestion* or *autolysis*. As necrosis progresses, most organelles are disrupted and *karyolysis*, nuclear dissolution from the action of hydrolytic enzymes, becomes evident. In some cells, the nucleus shrinks and is termed *pyknosis*. The process of the fragmentation of nucleus into nuclear dust is known as *karyorrhexis*. There are four major types of necrosis: coagulative, liquefactive, caseous, and fatty. Gangrenous necrosis is not a distinctive type of cell death, but instead refers to large areas of tissue death.

Coagulative necrosis occurs primarily in the kidneys, heart, and adrenal glands and usually results from hypoxia caused by severe ischemia. *Protein denaturation* causes coagulation.

Liquefactive necrosis is common following ischemic injury to neurons and glial cells in the brain. Because brain cells are rich in digestive hydrolytic enzymes and lipids, the brain cells are digested by their own hydrolases. The brain tissue becomes soft, liquefies, and is walled off from healthy tissue to form cysts. *Bacterial infections* are causes of liquefactive necrosis.

Caseous necrosis, which is commonly seen in tuberculous pulmonary infection, is a combination of *liquefactive* necrosis and *coagulative* necrosis. The necrotic debris is not digested completely by hydrolases, so tissues appear soft and granular and resemble clumped cheese. A granulomatous inflammatory wall may enclose the central areas of caseous necrosis.

The **fatty necrosis** found in the breast, pancreas, and other abdominal structures is a specific cellular dissolution caused by *lipases*. Lipases break down triglycerides and release free fatty acids, which then combine with calcium, magnesium, and sodium ions to create soaps, in a process known as *saponification*. The necrotic tissue appears opaque and chalk white.

Gangrenous necrosis refers to death of tissue, usually in considerable mass and with putrefaction. It results from severe hypoxic injury subsequent to arteriosclerosis or blockage of major arteries followed by bacterial invasion. *Dry gangrene* is usually caused by a coagulative necrosis, whereas *wet gangrene* develops when neutrophils

Cellular Accumulations

Accumulation	Causes	Consequence of Cellular Damage
H_2O	Shift of extracellular H_2O into cell, reduced ATP and ATPase, sodium accumulates in cell	Cellular swelling, vacuolation, oncosis cell, reduced ATP and ATPase, accumulation of sodium in cell
Lipids, carbohydrates	Imbalance in production, utilization, or mobilization of lipids or carbohydrates	Vacuolation, displacement of nucleus and organelles leading to fibrosis and scarring
Glycogen	Genetic disorders, diabetes mellitus	Cytoplasmic vacuolation
Proteins	Enzyme digestion of cellular organelles, renal disorders, plasma cell tumors	Disrupted function and intracellular communication, displaced cellular organelles
Pigments	Exogenous particle ingestion, UV light stimulates melanin production malignancy, loss of hormonal feedback, genetic defects, hemosiderin increase due to bruising and hemorrhage, liver dysfunction	Membrane injury, disruption of cellular metabolism
Calcium	Altered membrane permeability, influx of extracellular calcium excretion of H^+ leading to more OH^-, which precipitates Ca^{++}, endocrine disturbances	Hardening of cellular structure, interference with function
Urate	Absence of enzymes	Crystal deposition, inflammation

invade the site and cause liquefactive necrosis. Gas gangrene, a special type of gangrene, results from bacterial infection of injured tissue by species of *Clostridium.* These anaerobic bacteria produce hydrolytic enzymes and toxins that destroy connective tissue and cellular membrane; bubbles of gas likely form in muscle cells.

Apoptosis is an important, distinct type of cell death that differs from necrosis. It is a regulated or programmed cell program characterized by "dropping off" cellular fragments known as *apoptotic bodies.* It is an active process of cellular *self-destruction* in both *normal* and *pathologic* tissue changes. Apoptosis likely plays a role in deletion of cells during embryonic development and in endocrine-dependent tissues that are undergoing atrophic change. It may occur spontaneously in malignant tumors and in normal, rapidly proliferating cells treated with cancer chemotherapeutic agents and ionizing radiation. Defective apoptosis may not eliminate lymphocytes that react to self-antigens, leading to autoimmune disorders. Increased apoptosis occurs in neurodegenerative diseases, myocardial infarction and stroke, and death in virus-infected host cells. Apoptosis affects scattered, single cells and results in *shrinkage of a cell*, whereas in necrosis, cells swell and lyse.

Autophagy, which literally means *"eating of self,"* is a self-destructive and a survival mechanism. When cells are nutrient deprived, autophagy cannibalizes and recycles the digested contents. Autophagy may be an immune defense against infectious microbes that penetrate intracellularly.

5. Describe the biology of aging; characterize frailty.
Study pages 90-93; refer to Figures 3-32 and 3-33, and Tables 3-13 and 3-14.

Three mechanisms of aging have emerged, as follows: (1) cellular changes produced by genetic, environmental, and behavioral factors; (2) changes in regulatory mechanisms, especially in the cells of the endocrine, immune, and central nervous systems, that are responsible for aging; and (3) degenerative extracellular and vascular alterations.

Alterations of *cellular control mechanisms* include increased hormonal degradations, decreased hormonal synthesis and secretion, and a reduction in receptors for hormones and neuromodulators.

Immune function declines with age, and the number of autoantibodies that attack body tissues increases with age. These observations implicate the immune system in the aging process.

A *degenerative extracellular change* that affects the aging process is *collagen cross-linking*, which makes collagen more rigid and results in *decreased cell permeability* to nutrients. It is believed that free radicals of oxygen damage tissues as they age. These reactive species not only permanently damage cells, but also may lead to cell death. Damage accumulates over time and reduces the body's ability to maintain a steady state. There is new support for the theory that reactive species damage to the DNA in mitochondria is greater than that occurring in nuclear DNA. *Superoxide radicals* react with mitochondrial nitric oxide to produce damaging peroxynitrite.

Reduced insulin signaling likely causes glucose intolerance and hyperinsulinemia; type 2 diabetes mellitus shortens life. *Oxidative stress* damages DNA and could lead to altered gene expression by *modifying chromatin*, which dictates nuclear structure, to promote aging. Aging might be associated with *declining stem cells* because of accumulating DNA damage. *Telomeres*, the ends of chromosomes, shorten with age, causing cell cycle arrest, so fewer new cells develop to replace damaged cells. Reactive oxygen species (ROS) cause modification of proteins, lipids, and nucleic acids. Autophagy may slow down, allowing harmful agents to accumulate in cells, damage cells, and increase aging.

Frailty is a wasting syndrome of aging. Changes in the musculoskeletal system are determinates of frailty. Endocrine-immune dysregulation occurs in aging as hormones decline and proinflammatory cytokines increase.

6. Characterize somatic death and its manifestations.
Study pages 93 and 94.

Somatic death is death of the entire organism. Unlike the changes that follow cellular death in a viable body, somatic death is diffuse and *does not involve* components of the *inflammatory response*, a vascular response to injury. The most notable manifestations of somatic death are that there is *complete cessation of respiration and circulation*, the surface of the skin usually becomes pale and yellowish, and body temperature falls gradually until, after 24 hours, it equals the temperature of the environment.

Within 6 hours after death, depletion of ATP interferes with ATP-dependent detachment of the contractile proteins, and muscle stiffening or *rigor mortis* develops. Within 12 to 14 hours, rigor mortis usually affects the entire body. Rigor mortis gradually diminishes as the body becomes *flaccid* because of the release of enzymes and lytic dissolution.

PRACTICE EXAMINATION

Multiple Choice

Circle the correct answer for each question:

1. A cellular adaptation observable in uterine cervical epithelium is:
   a. atrophy.
   b. hyperplasia.
   c. hypertrophy.
   d. dysplasia.
   e. metaplasia.

2. What are the consequences when a cell is forced into anaerobic glycolysis? (More than one answer may be correct.)
   a. insufficient glucose production
   b. excessive pyruvic acid retention
   c. increased lactic acid
   d. inadequate ATP production
   e. excessive CO_2 production

3. What is the probable cause of cellular swelling in the early stages of cell injury?
   a. fat inclusion
   b. loss of genetic integrity
   c. hydrolytic enzyme activation
   d. Na-K pump fails to remove intracellular Na+.
   e. None of the above is correct.

4. Dystrophic calcification:
   a. occurs in dying or dead tissues.
   b. is the result of excess calcium in the blood.
   c. is observed in chronic lesions.
   d. Both a and c are correct.
   e. a, b, and c are correct.

5. Cellular swelling is:
   a. irreversible.
   b. evident early in all types of cellular injury.
   c. manifested by decreased intracellular sodium.
   d. None of the above is correct.
   e. Both b and c are correct.

6. Which is *not* reversible?
   a. karyolysis
   b. fatty infiltration
   c. oncosis
   d. All of the above are reversible.

7. Aging:
   a. is easy to distinguish from pathology.
   b. does not have a genetic relationship.
   c. is more advanced in primitive societies.
   d. is caused by declining stem cell numbers.
   e. a, b, and c are correct.

8. In aging, cross-linking implies that:
   a. the life span and number of times a cell can replicate are programmed.
   b. the number of cell doublings is limited.
   c. there is oxygen toxicity.
   d. cell permeability decreases.
   e. Both a and b are correct.

Match the descriptor with the term:

_______ 9. Reduced oxygen tension

_______ 10. Bleeding in skin or underlying tissue

a. anoxia
b. melanin
c. lipids
d. hypoxia
e. contusion

Match the process with its cause:

_______ 11. Autophagy

_______ 12. Necroptosis

_______ 13. Asphyxiation

_______ 14. Depressed fatty acid oxidation

_______ 15. Depressed protein synthesis

a. carbon monoxide
b. cannibalizes stressed cells
c. ethanol
d. regulated and programmed
e. detached ribosomes
f. increased lactate
g. lysosomal edema

Match the manifestation with the condition:

_______ 16. Necrosis caused by *Clostridium*
_______ 17. Rigidity of muscles after somatic death
_______ 18. Increased cell numbers
_______ 19. Necrosis resulting from lysosomal release
_______ 20. Replacement of one cell type with another, more suitable type

a. liquefactive
b. rigor mortis
c. gas gangrene
d. hyperplasia
e. metaplasia
f. cloudy swelling
g. coagulation

Match the circumstance with the condition:

_______ 21. Activated ubiquitin-proteosome pathway
_______ 22. Pancreatic necrosis
_______ 23. Coagulative and liquefactive necrosis
_______ 24. Tissue death
_______ 25. Normal and pathologic cellular self-destruction

a. fatty necrosis
b. gangrene
c. proteolysis
d. caseous necrosis
e. apoptosis
f. algor mortis
g. hypertrophy

Complete the following table distinguishing among the types of cellular necrosis:

Cellular Necrosis		
Type	**Cause**	**Sites**

4 Fluids and Electrolytes, Acids and Bases

FOUNDATIONAL OBJECTIVES

a. Describe the different compartments for body fluids and identify the fluid distribution changes occurring with age.
Review pages 98 and 99; refer to Tables 4-1 and 4-2.

> **MEMORY CHECK!**
>
> - Intracellular fluid (ICF) is 40% of body weight and measures 28 L. Extracellular fluid (ECF) consists of: (1) interstitial fluid, at 15% and 11 L, and (2) intravascular fluid, at 5% and 3 L. The total body water as a percentage of body weight for normal adult males, adult females, and infants is 60%, 50%, and 70%, respectively.

b. Describe the factors that affect water and electrolyte movement.
Review pages 99 and 100; refer to Figure 4-1.

> **MEMORY CHECK!**
>
> - Sodium and water balance are closely related; if sodium levels change, chloride levels change proportionally (chloride follows sodium). Sodium balance is regulated by *aldosterone,* which increases sodium reabsorption from the urine into the blood at the distal tubule of the kidney. *Antidiuretic hormone (ADH)* is secreted in response to increases plasma osmolality or decreased circulating blood volume, thus regulating water balance. *Renin and angiotensin* are enzymes that promote secretion of aldosterone and thus regulate sodium and water balance. *Atrial natriuretic hormone* is involved in decreasing tubular reabsorption and promoting urinary excretion of sodium. *Aquaporins* are water channel proteins within the lipid bilayer of cell membranes that provide permeability to water.

c. Identify body mechanisms to buffer excessive hydrogen ion/acid.
Review pages 109-111; refer to Figure 4-9 and Table 4-9. (See the following Memory Check!)

> **MEMORY CHECK!**
>
> - *Pulmonary* acid/base regulation of blood involves *CO_2* and is *rapid*:
>
> $$CO_2 + H_2O \leftrightarrow H_2CO_3 \leftrightarrow H^+ + HCO_3^-$$
>
> An increase in CO_2 tension liberates hydrogen ions; thus, the pH decreases. A decrease in CO_2 tension results in fewer hydrogen ions; thus, the pH increases.
> - *Renal* acid/base regulation of blood is *slow* and involves *Hco_3^-* conservation with H^+ and NH_4^+ excretion. This process essentially secretes H^+ into the urine and returns Hco_3^- to the blood plasma.

LEARNING OBJECTIVES

After studying this chapter, the learner will be able to do the following:

1. Identify the mechanisms causing edema.
Study pages 100 and 101; refer to Figures 4-2 and 4-3.

Edema is the accumulation of fluid within *interstitial spaces*. It may be excess or sequestered fluid. Edema may be localized or generalized. Localized edema appears confined to traumatized tissues or within organ systems. Generalized edema exhibits a uniform distribution of fluid in the interstitial spaces. As edematous fluid accumulates, it is trapped in the interstitial spaces or *"third space"* and is unavailable for perfusion and metabolic activity.

Fluid movement can be explained by the following formula:

$$Q = \underset{\text{[from vessel]}}{(CHP + IFOP)} - \underset{\text{[to vessel]}}{(IFPH + COP)}$$

where Q = net filtration, CHP = capillary hydrostatic pressure (blood pressure), IFOP = interstitial fluid oncotic pressure, IFHP = interstitial fluid hydrostatic pressure, and COP = capillary (plasma) oncotic pressure.

Fluids either *move from where there is more fluid to where there is less fluid* (in this way *fluids* can *dilute* the *solutes*) or remain where there are solutes.

2. Define isotonic, hypertonic, and hypotonic water and solute alterations and imbalances.
Study pages 104-106; refer to Table 4-5 and Figure 4-7.

Isotonic imbalances: Extracellular fluid loss or gain is accompanied by proportional changes of electrolytes in these alterations. Losses (isotonic dehydration) are seen in hemorrhage or excessive sweating. Gains occur in administration of intravenous normal saline or renal retention of sodium and water. Cells *do not shrink* nor swell in isotonic fluids.

Hypertonic imbalances: *Water loss or solute gain* occurs in these changes. These alterations are seen in administration of hypertonic saline solutions, hyperaldosteronism, Cushing syndrome, diabetes, diarrhea, or insufficient water intake. Cells *shrink* in hypertonic fluids.

Hypotonic imbalances: *Water gain or solute loss* occurs in these changes. These alterations may be caused by vomiting, diarrhea, burns, diuretics, excessive sweating, renal failure, or failure to excrete water. Cells *swell* in hypotonic fluids.

3. Identify the major manifestations of abnormal levels of sodium, potassium, calcium, phosphate, and magnesium.
Study pages 106-109; refer to Figure 4-8 and Tables 4-6 and 4-7 (see the following table).

Clinical Manifestations of Excess and Deficit States of Major Electrolytes

Excess	Deficit
Sodium	
***Hypernatremia* > 147 mEq/L** Cellular shrinking because of hypertonic extracellular fluid; may cause central nervous system irritability, convulsions, tachycardia, dry and flushed skin, hypervolemia, hypertension, thirst, elevated temperature, rapid pulse, weight loss, oliguria, anuria	***Hyponatremia* < 135 mEq/L** Cellular swelling; may cause cerebral edema, headache, stupor, coma, peripheral edema, polyuria, absence of thirst, decreased body, hypovolemia, hypotension, temperature, rapid pulse, nausea, vomiting, decreased urination
Potassium	
***Hyperkalemia* > 5.5 mEq/L** Depressed conductivity in heart, muscle cramping, paresthesias, oliguria, nausea, diarrhea; associated with metabolic acidosis	***Hypokalemia* < 3.5 mEq/L** Cardiac irritability, dysrhythmias, vomiting, paralytic ileus, constipation, thirst, inability to concentrate urine; associated with metabolic alkalosis
Calcium	
***Hypercalcemia* > 10 mg/dL** Decreased neuromuscular excitability, muscle weakness, central nervous system depression, stupor to coma, increased risk of bone fracture, vomiting, constipation, kidney stones	***Hypocalcemia* < 8.5 mg/dL** Increased neuromuscular excitability, skeletal muscle cramps, tetany, laryngospasm, asphyxiation, cardiac arrest

Excess	Deficit
Phosphate	
***Hyperphosphatemia* > 4. 5 mg/dL**	***Hypophosphatemia* < 2.0 mg/dL**
See Hypocalcemia	Anorexia, weakness, osteomalacia, muscle weakness, tremors, seizures, coma, anemia, bleeding disorders, leukocytic alterations
Magnesium	
***Hypermagnesemia* > 3.0 mEq/L**	***Hypomagnesemia* < 1.5 mEq/L**
Skeletal muscle depression, muscle weakness, hypotension, bradycardia, respiratory depression	Hypocalcemia and hypokalemia, neuromuscular irritability, tetany, convulsions, tachycardia, hypertension

Note: Treatment of hypernatremia is to give water slowly and stop fluid loss. When intravenous replacement is required, 5% dextrose in water should be given because pure water lyses red blood cells. In hyponatremia, water is restricted and hypertonic saline solution is used cautiously with severe symptoms, such as seizures.

4. Differentiate between metabolic/respiratory acidosis and metabolic/respiratory alkalosis.
Study pages 109-114; refer to Figures 4-10 through 4-14 and Table 4-10. Important values include the following:

$pH = 7.35\text{-}7.45$
$K^+ = 5\,mEq/L$
$Na^+ = 142\,mEq/L$
$Cl^- = 104\,mEq/L$
$HCO_3^- = 24\,mEq/L$
$PaCO_2 = 35\text{-}45\,mm\,Hg$
$CO_2 = 28\,mEq/L$

Essentially, *acidosis causes nervous system depression, and alkalosis causes nervous system irritability.* The manifestations vary with the degree of alteration. (See the table "Comparison of Common Acid-Base Disturbances" on page 20.)

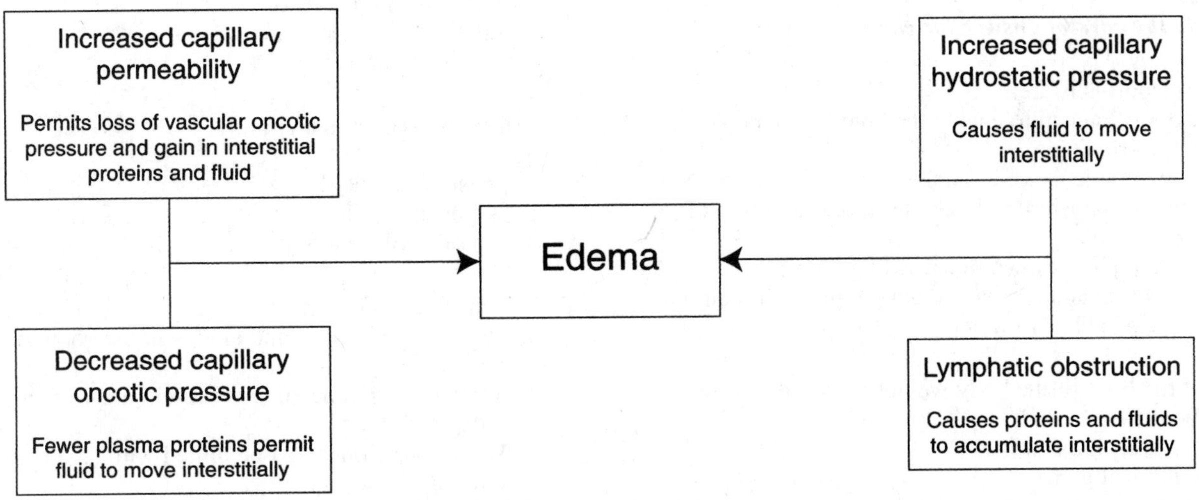

Mechanisms of Edema Formation

Comparison of Common Acid-Base Disturbances

Disturbance	Primary Disturbance	Correction/Compensation	Usual Causes
Metabolic acidosis $HCO_3^- < 24\,mEq/L$)	Excess endogenous acid depletes bicarbonate or bicarbonate is lost by kidneys	Hyperventilation (respiratory compensation) lowers $Paco_2$; kidneys (renal correction) excrete more hydrogen ions and retain more bicarbonate	Renal failure, ketosis, aspirin poisoning, overproduction of lactic acid
Respiratory acidosis ($Paco_2 > 45\,mm\,Hg$)	Hypoventilation increases $Paco_2$	Additional bicarbonate retention and H^+ excretion by kidneys (renal compensation)	Chronic pulmonary disease, drug depression of respiratory center
Metabolic alkalosis ($HCO_3^- > 26\,mEq/L$)	Excess plasma bicarbonate	Hypoventilation (respiratory compensation) raises $Paco_2$ to acidify blood; kidneys (renal correction) increase H^+ retention and excrete HCO_3^-	Loss of gastric juice, chloride depletion, excess corticosteroid hormones, ingestion of excessive bicarbonate or other antacids
Respiratory alkalosis ($Paco_2 < 35\,mm\,Hg$)	Hyperventilation lowers $Paco_2$	Increased excretion of bicarbonate and retention of H^+ by kidneys (renal compensation)	Severe anxiety with hyperventilation, central nervous system disease, hypoxia, pulmonary imbalances

PRACTICE EXAMINATION

Multiple Choice

Circle the correct answer for each question:

1. Aquaporins is/are:
   a. a mechanism to enable the body to adapt to hyperkalemia.
   b. restrictive to water intake.
   c. a mechanism that facilitates renal excretion of potassium.
   d. antibodies known to cause hypokalemia.
   e. water channel proteins that provide cell membrane permeability to water.

2. Of the 60% of the body weight made up of water, about two thirds is:
   a. extracellular water.
   b. intracellular water.
   c. intravascular water.
   d. interstitial water.
   e. None of the above is correct.

3. Sodium is responsible for:
   a. ICF osmotic balance.
   b. ECF osmotic balance.
   c. TBW osmolality.
   d. osmotic equilibrium.

4. A milliequivalent is a unit of:
   a. mass.
   b. physical activity.
   c. chemical activity.
   d. osmotic concentration.

5. Which statement is true?
   a. The number of ions and anions in the body must be equal.
   b. Intravascular molecules of protein are without charge.
   c. The sodium ions must be united with chloride ions.
   d. The positive and negative charges in blood plasma must be equal to each other.

6. Aldosterone controls ECF volume by:
   a. carbohydrate, fat, and protein catabolism.
   b. sodium reabsorption.
   c. potassium reabsorption.
   d. water reabsorption.
   e. Both b and d are correct.

7. The release of ADH is *not* stimulated by:
   a. stress.
   b. hyponatremia.
   c. hypernatremia.
   d. an increase in plasma osmolality.
   e. a decrease in plasma volume.

8. Laboratory studies of an adult reveal the following:
   Plasma sodium = 110 mEq/L
   Plasma chloride = 85 mEq/L
   Plasma potassium = 4.8 mEq/L
   Plasma calcium = 5.2 mEq/L
   Plasma bicarbonate = 26 mEq/L

   The most likely alteration is:
   a. base bicarbonate deficit (metabolic acidosis).
   b. hypokalemia.
   c. hyponatremia.
   d. base bicarbonate excess (metabolic alkalosis).
   e. calcium deficit.

9. An individual suffers from weakness, dizziness, irritability, and intestinal cramps. Laboratory studies reveal the following:
   Plasma sodium = 138 mEq/L
   Plasma potassium = 6.8 mEq/L
   Blood pH = 7.38
   Plasma bicarbonate = 25 mEq/L
   An EKG with tall, peaked T wave, but otherwise normal

   The individual is suffering from:
   a. hypernatremia.
   b. hyponatremia.
   c. hypercalcemia.
   d. hyperkalemia.
   e. hypokalemia.

10. An acid is:
    a. an anion.
    b. a cation.
    c. a substance/chemical that combines with a hydrogen ion to lower pH.
    d. a substance/chemical that donates a hydrogen ion or a proton to the solution.

11. Strong acids (more than one answer may be correct):
    a. include phosphoric acid.
    b. contribute many H^+ to the solution.
    c. have a pH of 7.
    d. have a pH of 14.
    e. are eliminated by the renal tubules.
    f. are good buffers.

12. The blood pH is maintained near 7.4 by buffering systems. The sequence from the fastest-acting to the slowest-acting system is:
    a. lungs, kidneys, blood buffers.
    b. blood buffers, lungs, kidneys.
    c. blood buffers, kidneys, lungs.
    d. lungs, blood buffers, kidneys.

13. The pH of saliva is about 7 and the pH of gastric juice is about 2. How many times more concentrated is the hydrogen ion in gastric juice than in saliva?
    a. 5
    b. 50
    c. 100
    d. 10,000
    e. 100,000

14. Which would *not* shift the blood pH toward alkalosis?
    a. hydrogen ion secretion into urine
    b. exhalation of carbon dioxide
    c. bicarbonate ion secretion into urine
    d. All of the above would shift the blood pH toward alkalosis.
    e. None of the above would do so.

15. A young female became agitated and apprehensive, and she eventually lost consciousness. At the hospital emergency room, the following laboratory values were obtained:
    Plasma sodium = 137 mEq/L
    Plasma potassium = 5.0 mEq/L
    Blood pH = 7.53
    Serum CO_2 = 22 mm Hg
    Plasma bicarbonate = 24 mEq/L

    Her immediate diagnosis was:
    a. hypokalemia.
    b. metabolic acidosis.
    c. metabolic alkalosis.
    d. respiratory acidosis.
    e. respiratory alkalosis.

16. As HCO_3^- shifts from the red blood cell to the blood plasma, it is expected that the plasma:
    a. Na^+ increases.
    b. Cl^- shifts into the red blood cell.
    c. K^+ increases.
    d. pH decreases.

17. An elevated anion gap is associated with an accumulation of:
    a. chloride anions.
    b. lactate anion.
    c. Both a and b are correct.
    d. Neither a nor b is correct.

Matching

Match the term with its definition:

_______ 18. Hydrostatic pressure

_______ 19. Oncotic pressure

a. water-pulling effect of plasma proteins
b. pressure of blood within the capillaries
c. mechanism to move fluid to lymph glands
d. movement of fluid through semipermeable membranes

Match the acid-base imbalance with the probable cause:

_______ 20. Respiratory acidosis

_______ 21. Respiratory alkalosis

_______ 22. Metabolic alkalosis

a. severe anxiety
b. diabetes
c. chronic diarrhea
d. emphysema
e. excessive ingestion of baking soda

Match the acid-base imbalance with the compensatory mechanism:

_______ 23. Respiratory acidosis

_______ 24. Respiratory alkalosis

_______ 25. Metabolic acidosis

a. kidneys retain H^+ and excrete HCO_3^-
b. kidneys excrete H^+ and retain HCO_3^-
c. respirations increase; more CO_2 is eliminated
d. respirations decrease; more CO_2 is retained

Fill in the Blank

Complete the following table comparing rapid with slow compensation for acid-base disturbances:

Acid-Base Corrections

Buffer System	Mechanism	Rate
Short term: Lungs Ionic shifts	 Exchange of intracellular K^+ and Na^+ for hydrogen	 2-4 hours
Long term: Kidneys Bone		

CASE STUDY

A 70-year-old woman was brought to an urgent care facility complaining, "I am weak and have been running off my bowels for 3 weeks." The onsite clinical laboratory provided the following electrolyte values:

Sodium = 142 mEq/L
Potassium = 2.1 mEq/L
Chloride = 94 mEq/L
Carbon dioxide = 30 mEq/L

What electrolyte levels are abnormal? Is there a medical emergency? If so, what is it, and what should be done?

5 Innate Immunity: Inflammation and Wound Healing

FOUNDATIONAL OBJECTIVES

After reviewing this chapter, the learner will be able to do the following:

a. Characterize the three human defensive lines.
Review pages 118-121; refer to Table 5-1.

Innate immunity, also known as *nonspecific* immunity, includes natural barriers (physical, mechanical, and biochemical) and inflammation. Innate barriers form the *first line* of defense at the body's surfaces and are present at birth to prevent damage by substances in the environment and to thwart infection by pathogenic microorganisms. Surface barrier may harbor a group of microorganisms known as the *"normal flora,"* which can protect against pathogens. If the surface barriers are breached, the *second line* of defense, the **inflammatory response**, is activated to protect the body from further injury, prevent infection of the injured tissue, and promote healing. The inflammatory response is a rapid activation of biochemical and cellular mechanisms that are relatively nonspecific. Similar responses are initiated against a wide variety of causes of tissue damage. The *third line* of defense, **adaptive immunity,** which is also known as *acquired or specific immunity,* is induced in a relatively slower and more specific process and targets particular invading microorganisms for the purpose of eradicating them. Adaptive immunity also involves *"memory,"* which results in a more rapid response during future exposure to the same microorganism.

b. Describe the first line of defense.
Review pages 119-121 and Figure 5-1.

The physical barriers are composed of tightly associated *epithelial cells* of the skin and of the linings of the gastrointestinal, genitourinary, and respiratory tracts. When pathogens attempt to penetrate this physical barrier, they may be removed by mechanical means. They are sloughed off with dead skin cells as the cells are routinely replaced, expelled by coughing or sneezing, vomited from the stomach, or sloughed from the urinary tract by urine.

Epithelial cells secrete several *biochemical substances* that protect against infection, including mucus, perspiration, saliva, tears, and earwax. These contain substances that kill microorganisms. Perspiration, tears, and saliva contain an enzyme, **lysozyme,** that attacks the cell walls of gram-positive bacteria. Sebaceous glands in the skin also secrete fatty acids and lactic acid that kill bacteria and fungi. These glandular secretions create an *acidic* and *inhospitable* environment for most bacteria.

Antimicrobial peptides kill or inhibit the growth of certain disease-causing bacteria, fungi, and viruses. The best-studied antimicrobial peptides are **cathelicidins** and **defensins.**

Bacteria have cholesterol-free membranes into which cathelicidins can insert to disrupt the membranes and kill the bacteria. Cathelicidin is stored in neutrophils, mast cells, and monocytes and can be released during inflammation. The alpha-defensins often require activation by proteolytic enzymes, whereas the beta-defensins are synthesized in active forms. Defensins may kill bacteria in the same way as cathelicidin.

The lungs produce and secrete a family of glycoprotiens, **collectins,** which react with carbohydrates on the surfaces of a wide array of pathogenic microorganisms and help macrophages to recognize and kill the microorganism. **Mannose-binding lectin (MBL)** is a powerful activator of complements, which lead to damage to bacteria or increased recognition by macrophages.

A spectrum of nonpathogenic microorganisms, collectively called the *normal flora,* resides on the body's surfaces. Each surface is colonized by a combination of mostly bacteria and occasionally fungi that is unique to the particular location. The relationship between humans and flora is *mutualistic* (to the benefit of both organisms). As an example, the environment of the intestine provides the needed temperature and nutrients for the growth of many bacterial species. To the benefit of humans, many of these microorganisms help digest fatty acids, large polysaccharides, and other dietary substances; produce biotin and vitamin K; and assist in the absorption of various ions, such as calcium, iron, and magnesium. These bacteria compete with pathogens for nutrients and block attachment to the epithelium. Members of the normal flora also produce chemicals and toxic proteins (*bacteriocins*) that *inhibit colonization* by pathogenic microorganisms. Prolonged treatment with broad-spectrum antibiotics can alter the normal intestinal flora, decreasing its protective activity, and lead to an overgrowth of pathogenic microorganisms, such as the yeast *Candida albicans* and the bacteria *Clostridium difficile*, which can cause pseudomembranous colitis and infection of the colon. Additionally, the normal flora of the gut help train the adaptive immune system by inducing growth of gut-associated lymphoid tissue, in which cells of the adaptive immune system reside, and the development of both local and systemic adaptive immune systems.

Also, *Lactobacillus* in women produces chemicals that help prevent infections of the vagina and urinary tract by other bacteria and yeast. Diminished colonization with lactobacilli as a result of *prolonged antibiotic treatment* increases the risk for urologic or vaginal infections.

Opportunistic microorganisms can cause disease if the individual's defenses are compromised. Severe burns compromise the integrity of the skin and may lead to life-threatening systemic pseudomonal infections.

c. Describe the second line of human defenses; diagram the sequence and consequences of the acute inflammatory process.

Review pages 121 and 122; refer to Figures 5-2 and 5-3.

Inflammation is the second line of defense and responds to injury to the body, whether the injured tissue is septic or sterile. This response rapidly initiates an interactive system of *humoral* and *cellular* systems. Inflammation is the *first immune response* to injury. This response: (1) occurs in tissues with a blood supply; (2) is activated within seconds after injury occurs; (3) involves the activity of both cellular and chemical components; and (4) is nonspecific, meaning that it takes place in approximately the same way regardless of the type of stimulus or whether exposure to the same stimulus has occurred in the past. Fluid and debris that accumulate at an inflamed site are drained by lymphatic vessels. This process facilitates the development of *adaptive immunity,* because microbial antigens in lymphatic fluid pass through the lymph nodes, where they encounter lymphocytes.

The acute inflammatory process continues only until the host's *threat* is eliminated, usually 8 to 10 days from onset to healing. The systemic effects of acute inflammation are *fever,* induced by interleukin-1 (IL-1) and increases in levels of circulating leukocytes (*leukocytosis*), and plasma proteins (*acute phase reactants*), which are either *proinflammatory* or *antiinflammatory* in nature.

d. Relate complement, clotting, and kinin systems to inflammation.

Review pages 122-124; refer to Figure 5-4.

The key **plasma protein systems** are essential to an effective inflammatory response. These are the complement system, the clotting system, and the kinin system. Each system consists of multiple proteins in the blood. They are normally in inactive forms; several are enzymes that circulate in inactive forms as proenzymes. Each system contains a few proteins that can be activated during inflammation. Activation of these first components results in sequential activation of other components of the system, leading to a biologic function that helps protect the individual. This sequential activation is referred to as a *cascade*.

The most important function of the **complement** cascade is activation of complement components C3 and C5, which results in a variety of molecules that are: (1) opsonins, (2) chemotactic factors, or (3) anaphylatoxins. **Opsonins** coat the surfaces of bacteria and increase their susceptibility to being phagocytized and killed by neutrophils and macrophages. **Chemotactic factors** diffuse from a site of inflammation and attract phagocytic cells to the site. **Anaphylatoxins** induce rapid degranulation of mast cells to release histamine, which causes vasodilation and increased capillary permeability. The most potent complement products are C3b (opsonins), C3a (anaphylatoxins), and C5a (anaphylatoxins, chemotactic factor). Activation of complement components C5b through C9 results in a complex that creates pores in the outer membranes of cells or bacteria. The pores disrupt the cell's membrane and permit water to enter, causing the cell to burst and die or at least preventing its reproduction.

Three major pathways control the activation of complement. The **classical pathway** is activated primarily by antibodies. Antibodies must first bind to their targets, called antigens. Antibodies activate the first component of complement, C1, which causes activation of other complement components, leading to activation of C3 and C5. Thus, antibodies of the acquired immune response can use the complement system to cell bacteria and activate inflammation. The **alternative pathway** is activated by several substances found on the surfaces of bacterial organisms *(endotoxin)* or yeast cell wall carbohydrates *(zymosan)*. This pathway uses unique proteins to form a complex that activates C3. C3 activation leads to C5 activation and convergence with the classical pathway. Thus, the complement system can be directly activated by certain infectious organisms without the presence of antibody. The **lectin pathway** is similar to the classical pathway but is independent of antibody. It is activated by several plasma proteins, particularly *MBL*. MBL is similar to C1 and binds to bacterial polysaccharides (endotoxins) containing the carbohydrate mannose. Thus, infectious agents that do not activate the alternative pathway may be susceptible to complement through the lectin pathway.

The **clotting (coagulation) system** is a group of plasma proteins that, when activated sequentially, form a blood clot. The clot is a network of *fibrin strands* that stabilizes the platelet plug and traps cells, such as erythrocytes, phagocytes, and microorganisms. Clots plug damaged vessels and stop bleeding, trap microorganisms and prevent their spread to adjacent tissues, and provide a framework for future repair and healing.

The clotting system can be activated by many substances that are released during tissue injury and infection, including collagen, proteinases, kallikrein, and plasmin, as well as by bacterial products, such as endotoxin. Like the complement cascade, the coagulation cascade can be activated through different pathways that converge and result in the formation of a clot. *Tissue factor (TF)* is released by damaged endothelial cells in blood vessels and reacts with factor VII (VIIa) to activate the *extrinsic pathway*. The *intrinsic pathway* is activated when *Hageman factor (factor XII)* in plasma contact substances exposed by vascular injury. Both pathways lead to a common pathway and activation of factor X. Activation of factor X begins a common pathway leading to activation of fibrin that polymerizes to form a fibrin clot.

As with the complement cascade, activation of the clotting cascade produces fragments known as *fibrinopeptides (FPs) A and B* that enhance the inflammatory response. FPs are released from fibrinogen when fibrin is produced. Both FPs are chemotactic for neutrophils and increase vascular permeability by enhancing the effects of bradykinin, which is formed from the kinin system.

The third plasma protein system, the **kinin system,** interacts closely with the coagulation system. Both the clotting and kinin systems can be initiated through activation of *Hageman factor (factor XII)* to factor XIIa. The final product of the kinin system is a low-molecular-weight molecule, **bradykinin,** which is produced from a larger precursor molecule, kininogen. Bradykinin causes dilation of blood vessels, acts with prostaglandins to induce pain, causes smooth muscle cell contraction, and increases vascular permeability.

e. Identify the source and function of some major cytokines involved in innate immunity.
Review pages 125-127; refer to Figures 5-5 through 5-7.

Cytokines

Types	Sources	Function
Interleukins (ILs)		
IL-1	Macrophages/lymphocytes	Increases inflammatory and immune responses
IL-6	Macrophages, lymphocytes, fibroblasts	Induces hepatocytes to produce proteins needed in inflammation; stimulates growth of blood cells and fibroblasts
Interferons (IFNs)	B and T cells, macrophages, fibroblasts, epithelial cells	Antiviral protection; decrease neoplastic growth; regulate interleukins
Tumor necrosis factors (TNFs)	T cells, macrophages	Tumor cytotoxicity; increase inflammatory and immune responses
Colony-stimulating factors (CSFs)	Various cells	Myelocytic stem cell growth factors; macrophage growth factors
Transforming growth factor (TGF)	Lymphocytes, macrophages, platelets, bone	Macrophage chemotaxis; stimulates fibroblasts

f. Describe mast cell degranulation products and the effects of its mediators.
Review page 127; refer to Figures 5-8 and 5-9.

Mast Cell Degranulation

Mediators from Granules	Action
Histamine	Dilation of postcapillary venules resulting in increased microcirculation blood flow; increases vascular permeability
Neutrophil chemotactic factor	Attracts neutrophils
Eosinophil chemotactic factor of anaphylaxis	Attracts eosinophils
Synthesized Mediators	
Leukotrienes	Stimulate slower and longer responses than histamine
Prostaglandins	Increase vascular permeability, neutrophil chemotaxis, and pain by direct effects on nerves
Platelet-activating factor (PAF)	Similar to that of leukotrienes

g. Describe phagocytosis and identify the phagocytic cells involved.
Review pages 129, 131, and 132; refer to Figures 5-10 and 5-11.

Phagocytosis is a multistep cellular process for the elimination of pathogens and foreign debris. The steps are recognition and attachment, engulfment, formation of a phagosome and phagolysosome, and destruction of pathogens or foreign debris. Phagocytic cells engulf microorganisms and enclose them in phagocytic vacuoles, *phagolysosomes*, wherein toxic products, especially *metabolites of oxygen*, and *degradative lysosomal enzymes* kill and digest the microorganisms. Opsonins, such as antibody and complement component C3b, coat microorganisms and make them more susceptible to phagocytosis by binding them more tightly to the phagocyte.

The **polymorphonuclear neutrophil (PMN),** the predominant phagocytic cell in the early inflammatory response, exits the circulation by diapedesis through the retracted endothelial cell junctions and moves to the inflammatory site by chemotaxis.

Eosinophils release products that control the inflammatory response and are the principal cell that kills parasitic organisms.

The **macrophage**, the predominant phagocytic cell in the late inflammatory response, is highly phagocytic, responsive to cytokines, and promotes wound healing.

Dendritic cells connect the innate and acquired immune systems by collecting antigens at the site of inflammation and transporting them to sites, such as the lymph nodes, where immunocompetent B and T cells reside.

h. Diagram the consequences of the acute inflammatory process.
Review pages 132 and 133.

i. Diagram the consequences of the chronic inflammatory process.
Review pages 133 and 134; refer to Figures 5-12 and 5-13.

Chronic inflammation can be a continuation of acute inflammation that lasts 2 weeks or longer, regardless of cause. It can be a distinct process without much preceding acute inflammation. Chronic inflammation is characterized by a dense infiltration of lymphocytes, monocytes, and macrophages. The body may wall off and isolate the infection to protect against tissue damage by formation of a *granuloma*.

j. Distinguish between regeneration (resolution) and repair.
Review pages 134-138; refer to Figures 5-14 and 5-15.

When little tissue has been lost or injured, it is capable of regeneration. This process is healing by *primary intention*. Tissues that have sustained extensive damage or those incapable of regeneration heal by the process of repair, resulting in the formation of a scar. This process is healing by *secondary intention*.

Resolution and repair occur in two separate phases, the *reconstructive phase* in which the wound begins to heal, and the *maturation phase,* in which the healed wound is remodeled.

Dysfunctional wound healing can occur as a result of abnormalities in either the inflammatory response or the reconstructive phase of resolution and repair.

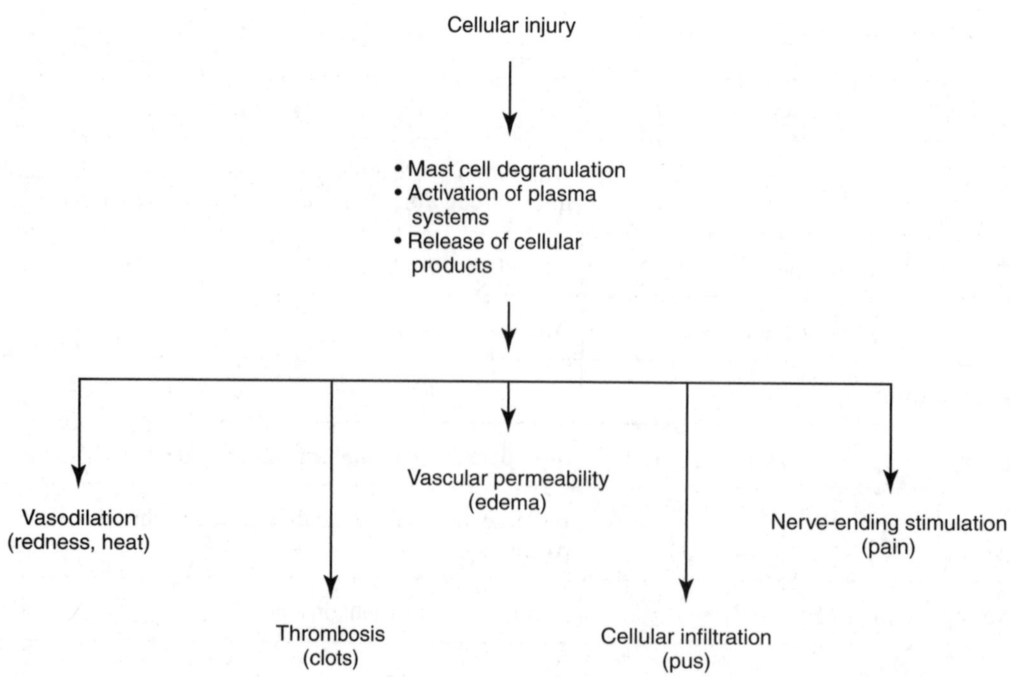

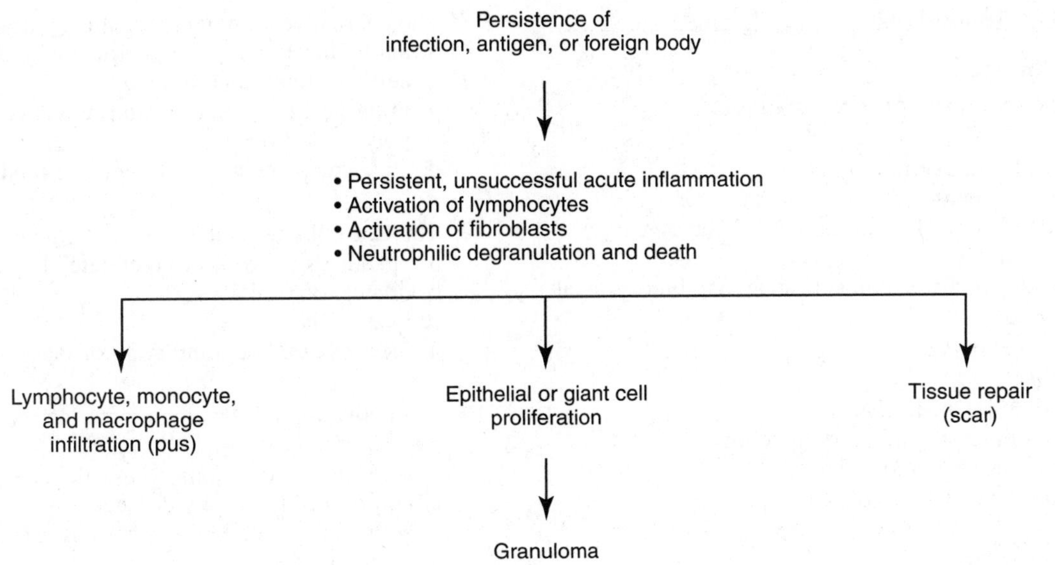

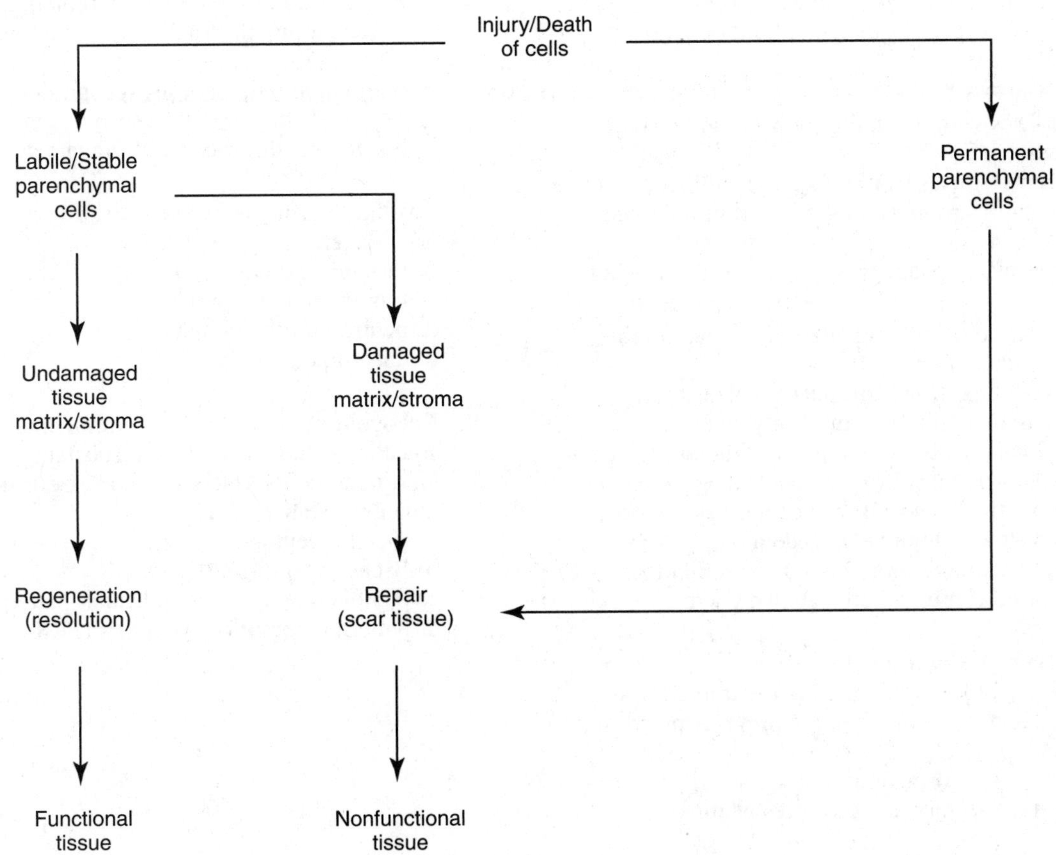

NOTE: If cells are to generate, they must:(1) possess a mitotic apparatus and (2) interact with growth/regulatory factors in the matrix.

PRACTICE EXAMINATION

Multiple Choice

Circle the best answer for each question:

1. Innate resistance or immunity:
   a. involves "memory."
   b. is a development of an individual's later years.
   c. is a relatively slow and specific process.
   d. depends on physical, mechanical, and biochemical barriers.

2. Collectins:
   a. are triple-stranded sheets.
   b. protect against respiratory infections.
   c. are produced by monocytes.
   d. are produced by neutrophils.

3. Complement is:
   a. a series of proteins in the blood.
   b. an antibody.
   c. a hormone.
   d. a lymphokine.

4. Diapedesis is a process in which:
   a. neutrophils migrate from the bloodstream to an injured tissue site.
   b. phagocytes stick to capillary and venule walls.
   c. bacteria are "coated" with an opsonin.
   d. there is oxygen-dependent killing of cells.

5. Interferon:
   a. interferes with the ability of bacteria to cause disease.
   b. prevents viruses from infecting healthy host cells.
   c. inhibits macrophage migration from inflamed sites.
   d. increases the phagocytic activity of macrophages.

6. The sequence of inflammatory events within the vasculature is:
   a. slower blood flow, arteriolar vasoconstriction, increased capillary permeability, edema.
   b. arteriolar vasoconstriction, vasodilation, increased capillary permeability, plasma leakage, edema.
   c. vasodilation, vasoconstriction, decreased local blood flow to injured site, edema.
   d. blood becoming more viscous, vasodilation, increased capillary permeability, edema.

7. The inflammatory response:
   a. prevents blood from entering the injured tissue.
   b. elevates body temperature to prevent spread of infection.
   c. prevents the formation of abscesses.
   d. minimizes injury and promotes healing.

8. The alternative complement pathway is activated by:
   a. antibodies binding to specific antigens.
   b. certain bacterial carbohydrates.
   c. gram-negative bacterial and fungal cell wall polysaccharides.
   d. a plasma protein called mannose-binding lectin.

9. The C3b subcomponent of complement:
   a. opsonizes microbes to facilitate phagocytosis.
   b. dilates arterioles.
   c. lyses cells.
   d. induces rapid degranulation of mast cells.

10. The activation of Hageman factor affects all three plasma protein systems through:
    a. activation of the clotting cascade through factor X.
    b. control of clotting by degradation of plasmin.
    c. activation of the kinin system by a fragment of Hageman factor.
    d. activation of C5 in the complement cascade.

11. The sequence for phagocytosis is:
    a. margination or pavementing, recognition of the target, adherence or binding, fusion with lysosomes inside the phagocyte.
    b. diapedesis, margination or pavementing, phagosome formation, recognition of the target, fusion with lysosomes inside the phagocyte.
    c. recognition of the target, margination or pavementing, destruction of the target by lysosomal enzymes.
    d. margination, diapedesis, recognition, adherence, ingestion, fusion with lysosomes inside the phagocyte, destruction of the target.

12. Swelling during acute inflammation is caused by:
    a. collagenase.
    b. the fluid exudate.
    c. lymphocytic margination.
    d. neutrophilic margination.
    e. anaerobic glycolysis.

13. Recognition of abnormal environmental components so cells can respond to these substances is by binding to cell surface receptors. Cells involved in innate resistance have:
    a. T-cell receptors (TCRs).
    b. B-cell receptors (BCRs).
    c. pathogen-associated molecular patterns (PAMPs).
    d. pattern recognition receptors (PRRs).

14. Mast cell degranulation releases:
    a. histamine, neutrophil chemotactic factor, and leukotrienes.
    b. histamine, IL-4, and eosinophil chemotactic factor of anaphylaxis.
    c. histamine and prostaglandins.
    d. histamine and platelet-activating factor.

15. Interleukin 6:
    a. is a myelocytic stem cell growth factor.
    b. increases the number of circulating neutrophils.
    c. stimulates growth of blood cells and fibroblasts.
    d. increases antiviral protection.

16. Tumor necrosis factor:
    a. is secreted by eosinophils.
    b. causes tumor cytotoxicity.
    c. induces fever by acting as an exogenous pyrogen.
    d. enhances expression of endothelial cell adhesion molecules.

17. Characteristic systemic manifestations of acute inflammation include:
    a. leukopenia.
    b. a "right shift" in the ratio of immature to mature neutrophils.
    c. reduced host susceptibility to the effects of endotoxins.
    d. fever caused by the release of IL-1 by neutrophils and macrophages.

18. Chronic inflammation is characterized by:
    a. hypertrophy.
    b. metaplasia.
    c. neutrophilic infiltration.
    d. lymphocytic and macrophagic infiltration.

19. Scar tissue is:
    a. nonfunctional collagenous and fibrotic tissue.
    b. functional tissue that occurs after wound healing.
    c. regenerated tissue formed in the area of injury.
    d. fibrinogen that has entrapped phagocytes and neurons.

Fill in the Blank

Supply the correct response for each statement:

20. ______________________ are the predominant phagocytes arriving early at inflammatory and infection sites.

21. ______________________, in comparison with neutrophils and basophils, function for a longer time and later in the inflammatory response and are involved in the activation of the adaptive immune system.

22. ______________________ serve as primary defenders against parasites and help regulate vascular mediators released from mast cells by preventing more inflammatory activity than is needed.

23. ______________________ recognize and eliminate virus-infected cells and cancerous cells.

24. ______________________ returns injured tissues to an approximation of their original structure and physiologic function.

25. ______________________ is filled with new capillaries and is surrounded by fibroblasts and macrophages.

Complete the following table distinguishing among the three lines of human defenses:

Human Defenses

Characteristics	Barriers	Innate Immunity	Adaptive Immunity
Defensive level	First defensive line against infection and tissue injury	Second defensive line responding to infection or tissue injury	Third defensive line initiated when innate immune system signals the cells of adaptive immunity
Defensive timing			Delay between first exposure to antigen and maximum response, immediate to second and subsequent antigenic exposure
Specificity	Broad, nonspecific		Specific response to antigen
Cells			T and B lymphocytes, macrophages, dendritic cells
Memory			Specific memory of T and B lymphocytes
Active molecules	Defensins, cathelicidins, lactoferrin, bacterial toxins		Antibodies, complement, cytokines
Protection	Skin and mucous membranes, lysosomes, low pH of stomach and urine, ciliary activity		Activated T and B lymphocytes, antibodies, cytokines

6 Third Line of Defense: Adaptive Immunity

FOUNDATIONAL OBJECTIVES

After reviewing this chapter, the learner will be able to do the following:

a. Characterize the third line of defense in the human body.
Review pages 142 and 143.

The third line of defense in the human body is **adaptive (acquired) immunity.** Once external barriers have been compromised and *innate immunity/inflammation* has been activated, the adaptive immune response occurs. It develops more slowly than the inflammatory and is *specific*—unlike inflammation, which is non-specific—and has *memory*. Adaptive immunity destroys infectious agents that are resistant to inflammation and provides long-term protection against *future exposure* to the same agents.

b. Compare innate (nonspecific) immunity with adaptive (specific) immunity (see p. 34).
Review Table 5-1.

c. Describe the sites of development, the antigenic challenge, macrophage processing, clonal selection, and the antigens neutralized and destroyed for specific adaptive immunity. (See p. 35.)
Refer to Tables 6-2 and 6-3 and Figures 6-19 through 6-21.

Antigen and *immunogen* are synonyms, but there are differences between the two. An antigen is a molecule that can bind with *antibodies or antigen receptors* on B and T cells. An immunogen is a molecule that induces an immune response. An immunogen must be foreign to the host, of adequate size, and present in sufficient quantity. *Supraantigens* activate a large population of T helper cells regardless of antigen specificity. An example is that they can cause food poisoning. *Self-antigens* are antigens on an individual's own cells. The individual's own immune system does not normally recognize self-antigens as immunogenic; this is a condition known as *tolerance*. *Human leukocyte antigen (HLA)* is a system used to assess *tissue compatibility*. White blood cells are used for testing, not red blood cells.

An *immunoglobulin (Ig)* or *antibody* consists of four polypeptide chains: two identical light (L) chains and two identical heavy (H) chains. An individual plasma cell produces only one type of L and H chain at a time. *Monoclonal antibody* is produced in the laboratory from one B cell that has been cloned; thus, it has antigenic specificity.

The response to antigen occurs in two phases: the primary and secondary immune responses. The *primary response* of humoral immunity is usually dominated by IgM with less IgG. The *secondary response* (anamnestic) has a more rapid production of antibody, mostly IgG. *Memory cells* facilitate this rapid response. IgE defends against *parasitic infections* and is the primary cause of *allergies*. Antibodies of the *systemic immune system* function internally, in the bloodstream and tissues. Antibodies of the *secretory immune system,* primarily IgA, function in the secretions of mucous membranes.

Induction of an immune response, or *clonal selection,* begins when the antigen enters the individual's body. Most antigens must first react with *antigen-presenting cells (APCs)* or macrophages. Antigen is processed in the macrophages and presented on cell surfaces by molecules of the *major histocompatibility complex (MHC)*. The particular MHC molecule, *class I or II*, presenting the antigen determines which cell will respond to that antigen. T helper cells require a complex with MHC class II molecules. T cytotoxic cells require class I molecules. The *natural killer (NK) cell* has some characteristics of the T cytotoxic cell and is important for killing target cells in which viral infection or malignancy has resulted in the loss of MHC molecules. The T cell sees the presented antigen through the *T-cell receptor (TCR)* and *accessory molecule*s of *CD4 or CD8,* which differentiate. CD4 is found on T helper cells and reacts specifically with MHC class II. CD8 is found on T cytotoxic cells and reacts specifically with MHC class I.

Compare innate to adaptive immunity.

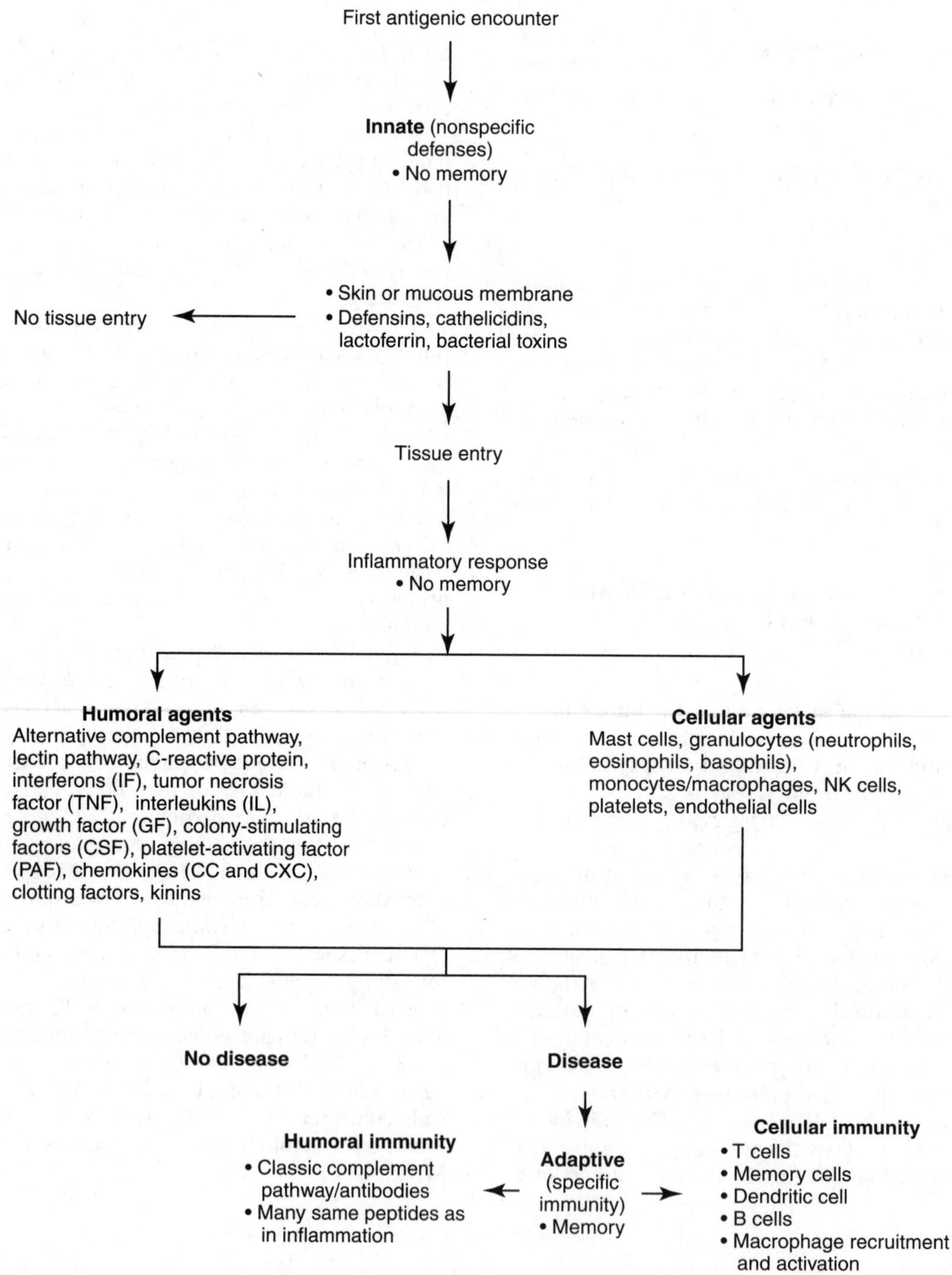

NOTE: Many of the same peptides, cytokines, and chemokines function on both innate and adaptive immunity.

Development and activities of cellular and normal immunity.

Refer to Tables 6.2 and 6.3 and Figures 6.19 through 6.21.

Bone marrow
↓
Lymphocyte stem cell

Cellular (left branch)		Humoral (right branch)
Thymus		Bone marrow
↓		↓
Immunocompetent T-cell receptors*		Immunocompetent B-cell receptors*
↓		↓
Secondary lymphoid tissue	← Antigenic challenge Macrophage processing selects and expands clones of T and B cells against specific antigens →	Secondary lymphoid tissue
↓		↓

Specific cellular immunity
Clonal selection

- Memory T cells
- Regulatory T cells
- Cytotoxic T cells
- Helper T cells
- T lymphokine producers
- Helper T cells

Specific humoral immunity
Clonal selection

- Memory T cells
- IgG producers
- IgM producers
- IgA producers
- IgE producers
- IgD producers
- IgE producers

Activities

Antigens neutralized

Cellular:

- Fungi
- Parasites
- Intracellular viruses
- Neoplastic cells
- Transplanted cells

Humoral:

- Bacteria
- Bacteria toxins
- Viruses

Antigenic destruction/removal

Cellular:

- Cell membrane perforation
- Recruitment and activation of macrophage mechanisms

Humoral:

- Phagocytosis

*Generation of clonal diversity produces receptors that can engage and react against all possible antigens but have not yet seen antigens.
NOTE: For lymphocyte activation, an antigen must be presented by an antigen-presenting cell (APC). Presenting and recognition structures include both classes of MHC, CD, HLA, BCR, and TCR molecules. Also, various cytokines stimulate binding of multiple cell-surface receptors.

d. Diagram the interrelationship between humoral and cell-mediated immunity.
Refer to Figure 6-17.

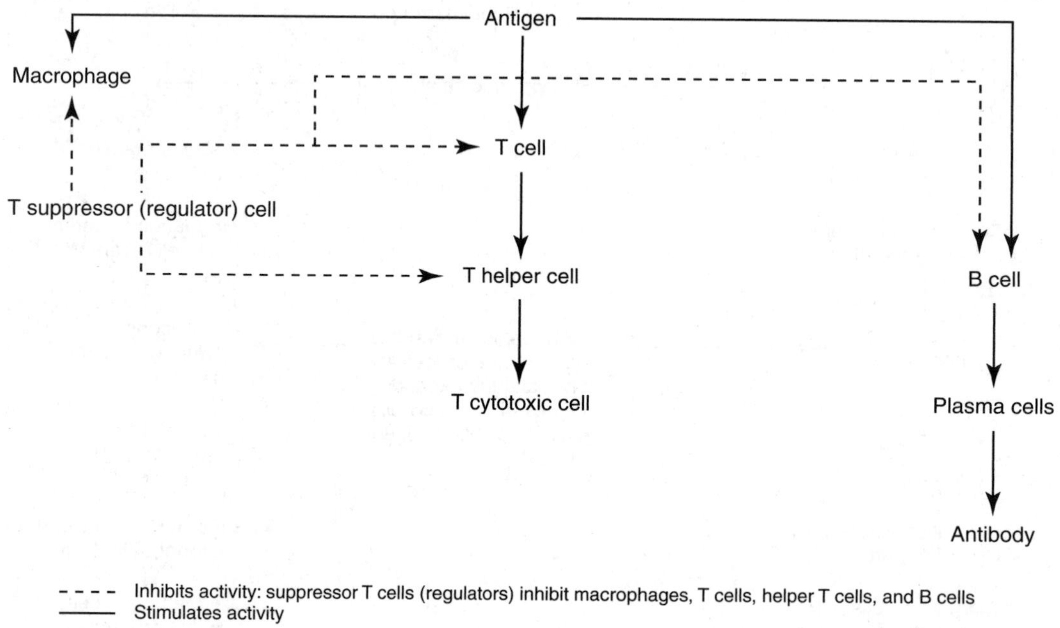

e. Diagram the interaction between lymphocytes and phagocytes.

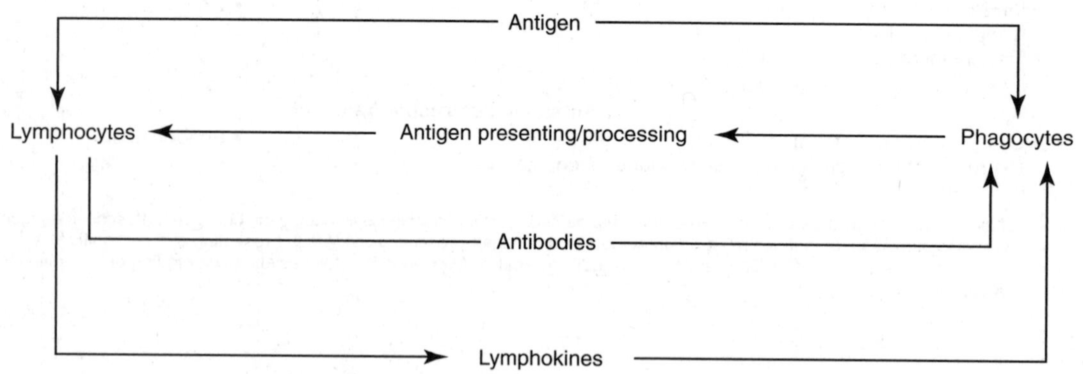

Note: There is interaction between specific and nonspecific areas of the immune system, The phagocytes cannot specifically recognize antigens but process and present them to the lymphocytes. Lymphocytes specifically recognize and produce antibodies or lymphokines, which help the phagocytes combat the antigen.

f. Compare adaptive immunity in pediatric individuals to that in elderly individuals.
Review page 162.

Pediatric Individuals	Elderly Individuals
Neonates often are transiently deficient in neutrophil chemotaxis and alternative complement pathway activity; T cell–independent immunity is adequate in the fetus and neonate, but the T cell–dependent immunity develops slowly during the first 6 months of life; maternal IgG antibodies cross the placenta into fetal blood to protect the neonate for 6 months, after which the child's own antibodies develop.	Chronic illnesses increase the risk for impaired wound healing; there is some deficiency in T cell function and antibody production, as well as a tendency for increased levels of autoantibodies or antibodies against self-antigens.

PRACTICE EXAMINATION

Multiple Choice

Circle the correct answer for each question:

1. Immunogenicity depends on:
   a. host foreignness.
   b. tolerance.
   c. chemical simplicity.
   d. low-molecular-weight molecules.

2. Which of the following are capable of forming clones?
   a. helper T cells
   b. cytotoxic T cells
   c. B cells
   d. both T and B cells

3. Which cells are stimulated by IL-2?
   a. B cells
   b. T cells and NK cells
   c. mast cells
   d. thymic epithelial cells

4. Which cells bind with MHC class I molecules?
   a. helper T cells
   b. cytotoxic T cells
   c. B cells
   d. both B and T cells

5. HLAs:
   a. have specific loci on chromosome 4.
   b. are not found on the surfaces of erythrocytes.
   c. are found on the surfaces of very few human cells.
   d. are not MHC molecules.

6. CD4 markers are associated with:
   a. cytotoxic T cells.
   b. suppressor T cells.
   c. helper T cells.
   d. APCs.

7. Antibodies are produced by:
   a. B cells.
   b. T cells.
   c. helper cells.
   d. plasma cells.
   e. memory cells.

8. An immunoglobulin contains:
   a. two heavy and two light polypeptide chains.
   b. four heavy and four light polypeptide chains.
   c. two heavy and four light polypeptide chains.
   d. four heavy and two light polypeptide chains.

9. The antibody class that has the highest concentration in the blood is:
   a. IgA.
   b. IgD.
   c. IgE.
   d. IgG.
   e. IgM.

10. Which of the following antibodies is matched with its appropriate role?
    a. IgA/allergic reactions
    b. IgD/found in respiratory secretions
    c. IgE/found in gastric secretions
    d. IgG/first to challenge the antigen
    e. IgM/first to challenge the antigen

11. The primary immune response involves:
    a. a rapid plasma cell response with peak antibody levels by 3 days.
    b. macrophage production of antibodies.
    c. T cell production of antibodies.
    d. a latent period followed by peak antibody production.

12. The B cell receptor (BCR) complex consists of:
    a. IgG or IgD antibody.
    b. IgE or IgD antibody.
    c. antibody-like transmembrane protein.
    d. antigen-recognition molecules.

13. Cytokines and their receptors function:
    a. as intracellular chemical signals.
    b. as chemical signals between cells.
    c. as negative regulators of acquired immune responses.
    d. to decrease the production of proteins.

14. Clonal selection:
    a. occurs primarily in the fetus.
    b. induces central tolerance.
    c. occurs primarily after birth and throughout life.
    d. occurs in central lymphoid organs.

15. Immunologic tolerance develops because:
    a. self-reactive lymphocytes are eliminated in the primary lymphoid organs.
    b. self-reactive lymphocytes are inactivated in the secondary lymphoid organs.
    c. lymphocytes remember their first exposure to the antigen.
    d. T cells may reprogram themselves by receptor editing.

16. Antigenic destruction/removal by humoral immunity requires:
    a. cell membrane lysis.
    b. histamine.
    c. phagocytosis.
    d. bradykinin.

17. Cytotoxic T cells:
    a. inhibit extracellular viruses.
    b. inhibit virus-infected cells.
    c. inhibit viral protein synthesis.
    d. decrease expression of MHC molecules.

18. Antibody is effective against:
    a. extracellular viruses.
    b. virus-infected cells.
    c. viral protein synthesis.
    d. expression of MHC molecules.

19. Adhesion molecule pairings involve:
    a. cytotoxic T cell CD4 ↔ MHC class II on APC.
    b. cytotoxic T cell CD8 ↔ MHC class I on APC.
    c. helper T cell CD2 ↔ CD58 on APC.
    d. helper T cell CD4OL ↔ MHC class II on APC.

20. Transforming growth factor (TGF) functions to:
    a. increase phagocytosis.
    b. increase expression of MHC class II.
    c. be chemotactic for neutrophils and T cells.
    d. stimulate wound healing.

Fill in the Blanks

Supply the correct response for each statement:

21. ______________________ are necessary to induce both humoral and cellular immune responses.

22. A second challenge by the same, earlier antigen results in an ______________________ immune response characterized by more antibody production in a shorter time than the initial or first challenge.

23. ______________________ function to avoid attacking self-antigens or to avoid overactivation of immune responses.

24. ______________________ cause activation of large populations of T lymphocytes irrespective of antigen specificity.

25. The ______________________ consists of antibodies in bodily secretions that protect the body against antigens yet to penetrate the skin or mucous membranes.

Complete the following table identifying characteristics of clonal selection:

Generation of Clonal Selection

Generation of Clonal Selection	
Characteristic	**Clonal Selection**
Purpose	Select, expand, and differentiate clones of T and B cells against a specific antigen
Time of occurrence	
Site of occurrence	
Foreign antigen involvement	
Cytokines involved	
Final products	Plasma cells to produce antibodies; effector T cells that help kill targets or regulate immune responses; memory B and T cells

7 Infection and Defects in Mechanisms of Defense

FOUNDATIONAL OBJECTIVES

a. **Completely review all foundational objectives in Chapters 5 and 6.**

LEARNING OBJECTIVES

1. **Describe the relationships between humans and microorganisms.**
   Study pages 165-166; refer to Table 7-1.

True pathogens have devised means to avoid controls by the host's defensive barriers, the inflammatory response, and immune system. Several factors influence the ability of pathogens to cause disease:

Communicability is the capacity to spread from one individual and cause disease in others.

Immunogenicity is the ability of pathogens to induce an immune response.

Infectivity enables pathogens to invade and multiply in a susceptible host.

Action mechanism is how the microbe damages tissue.

Pathogenicity is the production of a disease.

Portal of entry is the route by which the pathogen enters and infects the host. It may by direct contact, inhalation, ingestion, or by animal or insect bites.

Toxigenicity is the ability to produce soluble toxins or endotoxins.

Virulence is the pathogen's capacity to cause disease; measles virus has low virulence, while rabies virus is highly virulent.

2. **Describe the mechanisms of infection and cellular injury by bacteria, viruses, fungi, and parasites. Identify counter measures against pathogens.**
   Study pages 166-168, and 171-178; refer to Figures 7-1 through 7-3 and Tables 7-2 to 7-10.

Bacteria are prokaryotes lacking discrete nuclei; they are relatively small. Their survival and growth depend on the effectiveness of the *host's defense mechanisms* and on *the bacterium's ability to resist these defenses.* Some bacteria have *coatings* that protect them from phagocytosis. These coatings include polysaccharide coverings for the *Pneumococcus,* the waxy capsule surrounding the tubercle bacillus, and the M protein cell wall of the *Streptococcus.*

Other bacteria survive and proliferate in the body by producing *hemolysins, leukocidins, coagulases, exotoxins,* and *endotoxins* that injure cells and tissues. **Exotoxins** are metabolic proteins released into the environment primarily from gram-positive bacteria during bacterial growth. These proteins have highly specific effects on host cells. **Endotoxins** are lipopolysaccharides contained in the cell walls of gram-negative bacteria that are released from cell walls during lysis or destruction of the bacteria. Their effects are generalized. Endotoxins can be released from the bacterial membrane during treatment with antibiotics. Therefore, antibiotics cannot prevent the toxic effects of endotoxins. Once in the host's blood, endotoxins cause the release of vasoactive peptides that produce *vasodilation.* This, in turn, reduces blood pressure, decreases oxygen delivery, and can result in cardiovascular shock. **Endotoxic shock** is a complication of sepsis and can be fatal. Tumor necrosis factor-α (TNF-α) is involved in its pathogenesis.

Viruses are *intracellular parasites* that take over the genetic and metabolic machinery of host cells and use them for their own survival and replication. Viruses contain genetic information in either DNA or RNA. This genetic material is protected by a protein coat that must be removed in the cytoplasm of the host cell if the virus is to replicate. Viruses are *incapable of independent reproduction*; replication depends totally on their ability to infect a **permissive** host cell—a cell unable to resist viral invasion and replication. Infection with a virus requires its binding to a **specific receptor** on the plasma membrane of the host cell. Viral replication depends on absorption, penetration, uncoating, replication, assembly, and release of new virions.

Once inside the host cell, virions have many harmful effects, including the following: (1) cell protein synthesis cessation, (2) disruption of lysosomal membranes resulting in release of enzymes that can kill the host cell, (3) fusion of host cells, (4) alteration of antigenic properties causing the immune system to attack the host cell as if it were foreign, (5) transformation of host cells into cancerous cells, and (6) promotion of secondary bacterial infections that result from tissue damage by the viral infection.

Fungi are relatively large organisms with thick walls that grow as either single-celled yeasts or multicelled molds. *Molds are aerobic,* and *yeasts are facultative anaerobes.* Pathogenic *fungi release mycotoxins* and *enzymes* that damage connective tissues.

Diseases caused by fungi are called *mycoses.* Most fungi grow as *parasites* on or near skin or mucous membranes and usually produce mild and superficial disease. Injury to tissue can lead to secondary bacterial infection.

Fungi causing deep infection enter the body through inhalation or through open wounds. Deep infections are most common in association with other diseases or as opportunistic infections in immunosuppressed individuals. Some *fungi are part of the normal body flora and become pathogenic when antibiotics kill bacteria* that normally compete for nutrients and preclude fungal growth. For example, yeasts in the vagina may undergo rapid proliferation when antibiotics kill vaginal bacteria.

Parasites range from unicellular protozoa, which *are eukaryotic*, to large worms. Parasitic worms include *Helminthes,* roundworms, and tapeworms. Tissue damage may result from *infestation* in the tissue or may be *secondary to the individual's immune and inflammatory responses.* Parasitic and protozoal infections are rarely transmitted from human to human. Infection spreads mainly through vectors or through contaminated water or food.

Chemicals or antimicrobials prevent growth or destroy pathogens by: (1) inhibiting synthesis of cell walls, (2) damaging cytoplasmic membranes, (3) altering metabolism of nucleic acids, (4) inhibiting protein synthesis, and (5) altering energy metabolism. *Vaccines* are biologic preparations of weakened or dead pathogens that, when administered, stimulate production of antibodies or cellular immunity against the pathogen without causing disease. The purpose of *vaccination* is to induce long-lasting protective immune responses. The primary immune response from vaccination is generally short-lived; therefore, booster injections are used to aid the immune response through multiple secondary responses. This process results in large numbers of memory cells and sustained protective levels of antibody or T cells, or both.

3. Characterize immune deficiencies; describe examples of congenital or primary diseases.

Study pages 178-181; refer to Figure 7-4 and Table 7-11.

Immune deficiencies occur because of *impaired function* of one or more components of the *inflammatory or immune response*. B cells, T cells, phagocytic cells, or complement may be involved. The clinical manifestation of immune deficiency is a tendency to develop *unusual or recurrent severe infections*. Deficiencies in T cell immune responses are suspected when certain viruses, fungi, and yeasts or certain atypical organisms cause recurrent infections. B cell deficiencies are suspected if the individual has recurrent infections with encapsulated bacteria or viruses against which humoral immunity is normally effective.

Primary or congenital immune deficiency occurs if lymphocyte development is disturbed in the fetus or embryo or if there is a genetic anomaly. Most primary deficiencies *involve a single gene*. Some diseases are primarily caused by a defect in one or the other of the cell lines, although both T and B cell lines may be partially deficient.

A common defect in which a particular class of antibody is affected is selective immunoglobulin A **(IgA) deficiency**. Individuals with selective IgA deficiency are able to produce other classes of immunoglobulin but fail to produce IgA. Individuals with IgA deficiency often present with chronic intestinal candidiasis. IgA may normally prevent the uptake of allergens from the environment. Therefore, IgA deficiency may lead to *increased allergen uptake* and a more intense challenge to the immune system because of prolonged exposure to environmental antigens.

Bruton agammaglobulinemia is caused by failure of B cell precursors to become mature B cells because of the lack of normal bursal-equivalent tissue. There are few or no circulating B cells, though T cell number and function are normal.

DiGeorge syndrome is the complete lack of or, more commonly, partial lack of the thymus. This thymus deficiency causes lymphopenia and greatly decreased T cell numbers and function.

Severe combined immune deficiency (SCID) occurs when few lymphocytes exist in the circulation or in secondary lymphoid tissue. Individuals with the disorder are deficient in lymphocyte development rather than in all white blood cells. T and B lymphocytes are few or totally absent in the circulation, the spleen, and the lymph nodes. The thymus is usually underdeveloped. IgM and IgA levels are absent or greatly reduced. Other forms of SCID are caused by autosomal recessive enzymatic defects. These altered enzyme levels enable the accumulation of metabolites that are toxic to rapidly dividing lymphocytes.

Some immune deficiencies involve a defect that results in depressed development of a small portion of the immune system. An example is **Wiskott-Aldrich syndrome**, an X-linked recessive disorder, in which IgM antibody production is greatly depressed, and therefore, antibody responses against polysaccharide antigens from bacterial cell walls are deficient.

Complement deficiencies are possible. When a **C3 deficiency** exists, individuals are at risk for recurrent life-threatening infections with encapsulated bacteria, such as streptococcal pneumonia. **Phagocytic deficiencies** also permit recurrent infections to develop in association with antibody and complement deficiencies.

4. Cite causes of secondary or acquired immune deficiencies.

Study page 181; refer to Box 7-2.

Secondary or acquired and inflammatory deficiencies develop after *birth and are not related to genetic defects*. They are *more common than primary deficiencies*. Acquired immune deficiencies *are caused by superimposed conditions*, such as physiologic and psychologic stressors (pregnancy and aging), medical therapies (cancer therapy and immunosuppression), dietary insufficiencies (malnutrition), malignancies (lymphoid tissues, sarcomas, and carcinomas), and physical trauma (burns).

Although secondary immune deficiencies are common, many are not clinically relevant. In many cases, the immune deficiency is relatively minor and without any apparent increased susceptibility to infection. Some secondary immune deficiencies; however, are extremely severe and may cause life-threatening recurrent infections.

5. Describe acquired immune deficiency syndrome (AIDS).

Study pages 183-184 and 186-187; refer to Figures 7-5 through 7-8.

AIDS is caused by a virus currently named human immunodeficiency virus, or HIV. HIV is *retrovirus* carrying genetic information in RNA rather than DNA. A viral enzyme, *reverse transcriptase*, converts the viral

RNA to DNA and another enzyme, *integrase*, inserts that DNA into the infected cell's genetic material. Viral proliferation may occur, resulting in the lysis and death of the infected cell. If, however, the cell remains relatively dormant rather than active, the viral genetic material integrated into the infected cell's DNA may *remain latent for years*, if not for the life of the individual. HIV infects and *destroys the helper T cell*, which is necessary for the development of both plasma cells and cytotoxic T cells.

HIV is a blood-borne pathogen with the typical routes of transmission through blood or blood products, intravenous drug abuse, both heterosexual and homosexual activity, and from mother to child before or during birth.

CD4 is an antigen on the surface of cells that acts as a receptor for the HIV. The virus primarily *infects CD4-positive T helper lymphocytes*, but it may also infect and lyse various other cells that express the CD4 antigen. The major immunologic finding in AIDS is the striking *decrease in T helper cells or CD4-positive cells*.

At the time of diagnosis, the individual may manifest one of several different conditions: serologically negative (no detectable antibody), serologically positive but asymptomatic, early stages of HIV disease, and AIDS. The most common laboratory test is for antibodies against HIV. Antibody appears soon after infection through blood products, usually within 4 to 7 weeks. After sexual exposure, the individual *can be infected yet seronegative* for 6 to 14 months, in one case for years. The period between infection and the appearance of antibody is referred to as the window period. Although the patient may not have antibody, he or she may be *viremic and infectious to others*, implying that seronegativity can be meaningless. The average time from infection to development of full-blown AIDS has been estimated at just over 10 years.

The current regimen for treatment of HIV infection is a combination of drugs, termed **highly active antiretroviral therapy (HAART).** The combination involves inhibitors of reverse transcriptase (**reverse transcriptase inhibitors**) and of viral protease (**protease inhibitors**). Inhibitors of the initial viral entrance into the target cell (**entrance inhibitors**) and inhibitors of the viral integrase (**integrase inhibitors**) have undergone clinical trials and are being added to the combination.

Drug therapy for AIDS is difficult because *the AIDS retrovirus incorporates into the genetic material of the host and may never be removed by antiviral therapy*. Therefore, drug administration may have to continue for the lifetime of the individual. Thus, the need for a vaccine is significant.

The development of an effective AIDS vaccine has been slowed by several major difficulties. *The AIDS virus is genetically and antigenically variable*. Therefore, a vaccine created against one variant may not protect against another variant. This is a real problem, because as many as 30 to 40 different genetic variants have been isolated from the same individual during the progression of the disease. Many of these variants may coexist in the individual. Although individuals with AIDS have high levels of circulating antibodies against the virus, these antibodies do not appear to be protective. The AIDS virus is transmitted from cell to cell and may initially enter the body in an infected cell that is not susceptible to circulating antibody. Also, HIV-infected cells tend to fuse with other cells, so infection can spread to uninfected cells without production of viral particles.

6. Indicate some replacement therapies and laboratory tests for immune deficiencies.
Study page 182; refer to Table 7-12.

Immunodeficiency syndromes usually are treated using replacement therapy. Deficient antibody production is treated by replacement of missing immunoglobulins with commercial gamma (γ) globulin preparations. Lymphocyte deficiencies are treated with the replacement of host lymphocytes by means of transplantation of bone marrow, fetal liver, or fetal thymus from a donor.

7. Compare the four hypersensitivities.
Study pages 189, 190, 191, 193, and 195-197; refer to Figures 7-9 through 7-14 and Tables 7-13 through 7-16.

Hypersensitivity is an excessive immunologic reaction to an antigen that results in a pathologic response after *reexposure* to the same antigen. *Allergy, autoimmunity, and alloimmunity are all hypersensitivity responses*. The difference is the source of the antigen to which the hypersensitivity is directed.

Comparison of Hypersensitivity Disorders

Hypersensitivity	Immunity/ Response Time	Effectors	Examples
Type I: IgE-mediated Anaphylactic	Humoral/immediate	*Antigen* reacts with IgE bound to mast cells; *histamine* release, histamine effects	Allergy: Allergic rhinitis, asthma, urticaria, food allergies, anaphylactic shock
Type II: Cytotoxic Tissue-specific	Humoral/immediate	*IgG or IgM* reacts with *antigen* on cell's membrane; *complement* is activated; lysis or phagocytosis of cells, cell-mediated cytolysis, antibody binding to receptors	Allergy: Immediate drug reaction

Continued

Comparison of Hypersensitivity Disorders—Cont'd

Hypersensitivity	Immunity/ Response Time	Effectors	Examples
			Autoimmunity: Hemolytic anemia, Graves disease Alloimmunity: Transfused blood cells, hemolytic disease of the newborn
Type III: Immune complex	Humoral/immediate	*IgG or IgM* unites with *antigen* to form a complex that is deposited in vessel walls or tissues, neutrophil attraction; *complement activation; lysosomal enzymes* injure tissue	Allergy: Arthus reaction, allergic alveolitis Autoimmunity: Serum sickness, celiac disease glomerulonephritis, systemic lupus erythematosus
Type IV Cell-mediated	Cellular/delayed	Reaction of sensitized *T lymphocytes* with *antigen* leads to *lymphokine* release, recruitment of macrophages, and subsequent lysosomal release	Allergy: Contact dermatitis Autoimmunity: Hashimoto thyroiditis, rheumatoid arthritis Alloimmunity: Graft rejection, tuberculin reaction

8. Describe the likely causes of autoimmune and alloimmune diseases; cite examples.
Study pages 197-200; refer to Figures 7-15 through 7-17.

Self-antigens are usually tolerated by the host's own immune system. This *immunologic tolerance* develops in humans during the embryonic period. Autoreactive lymphocytes are either eliminated or suppressed. **Autoimmunity** is a breakdown of tolerance in which the body's immune system begins to recognize *self-antigens as foreign.* The mechanisms of tolerance breakdown are varied and often unknown. Mechanisms implicated in the development of autoimmunity include *alterations of self-antigenic markers* by infectious diseases and *genetic factors associated with the products of the histocompatibility leukocyte antigen (HLA) locus* or the histocompatibility complex–linked immune response genes.

Alloimmunity occurs when an individual's immune system *reacts against antigens* of the tissues of other members of *the same species.* Two examples of this reactivity are transient neonatal diseases and transplant rejection and transfusion reactions. Because a fetus has mother and father antigens, fetal paternal antigens that are different from maternal antigens can cross the placenta and elicit an immune response in the mother. Maternally produced antibody may be transported into the fetal circulation to produce alloimmune disease in the fetus. Examples of diseases that can affect the fetus, neonate, or child include Graves disease, myasthenia gravis, systemic lupus erythematosus, immune thrombocytopenic purpura, and erythroblastosis fetalis.

Transplantation of organs is commonly complicated by an immune response against donor antigens. The primary mechanism of *the rejection of transplanted organs is a type IV, cell-mediated reaction.* HLA antigens are the principal targets of the rejection reaction.

Transplant rejection is classified as hyperacute, acute, or chronic depending on the amount of time that elapses between transplantation and rejection. *Hyperacute rejection* usually occurs in recipients who have preexisting IgG or IgM antibody to antigens in the graft. As circulation to the graft is reestablished, antibody binds to the grafted tissue and activates the inflammatory response. This response initiates the coagulation or blood-clotting cascade, which results in cessation of blood flow into the graft.

Acute rejection is a cell-mediated immune response that occurs within days to a month after transplantation. The recipient develops an immune response to unmatched HLA antigens and shows an infiltration of lymphocytes and macrophages that are characteristic of type IV hypersensitivity reaction. The Th1 cells release cytokines that activate the infiltrating macrophages, and the Tc cells directly attack the endothelial cells in the transplanted tissue.

Chronic rejection may occur after months or years of normal function. It is characterized by slow, progressive organ failure. Chronic rejection may be caused by inflammatory damage to endothelial cells that line the blood vessels; it is likely a result of a weak immunologic reaction against minor histocompatibility antigens on the grafted tissue.

PRACTICE EXAMINATION

Multiple Choice

Circle the correct answer for each question:

1. Immunologic responses recognized as disease are:
   a. immediate hypersensitivities.
   b. delayed hypersensitivities.
   c. Both a and b are correct.
   d. Neither a nor b is correct.

2. Which is *not* characteristic of hypersensitivity?
   a. specificity
   b. immunologic mechanisms
   c. inappropriate or injurious response
   d. prior contact unnecessary to elicit a response

3. When the body produces antibodies against its own tissue, the condition is called:
   a. a hypersensitivity.
   b. an antibody reaction.
   c. a cell-mediated immunity.
   d. an autoimmune disease.
   e. an opsonization.

4. Which hypersensitivity is caused by poison ivy?
   a. type I
   b. type II
   c. type III
   d. type IV

5. The mechanism of hypersensitivity for drugs is:
   a. type I.
   b. type II.
   c. type III.
   d. type IV.
   e. a, b, and c are correct.

6. Which is *not* an autoimmune disease?
   a. multiple sclerosis
   b. pernicious anemia
   c. transfusion reaction
   d. ulcerative colitis
   e. Goodpasture disease

7. Damage in systemic lupus erythematosus (SLE) results from the formation of antigen/antibody complexes mediated by:
   a. IgE.
   b. mast cells.
   c. the cell-mediated immune system.
   d. the humoral immune system and complement.
   e. lymphokines.

8. The classical complement cascade begins with:
   a. antigen/antibody complexes binding to a component of the complement system.
   b. opsonization.
   c. chemotaxis.
   d. cytolysis.

9. Which of the following is/are an alloimmune disorder(s)?
   a. erythroblastosis fetalis
   b. insulin-dependent diabetes
   c. myxedema
   d. All of the above are correct.
   e. None of the above is correct.

10. Immunodeficiencies occur because of impaired function of:
    a. B and T cells.
    b. phagocytic cells.
    c. complement.
    d. All of the above are correct.
    e. Both a and c are correct.

11. An X-linked recessive disorder of immune deficiency involves a deficit of:
    a. IgA.
    b. IgD.
    c. IgE.
    d. IgG.
    e. IgM.

12. Deficiencies in B cell immune responses are suspected when unusual or recurrent severe infections are caused by:
    a. fungi.
    b. yeasts.
    c. encapsulated bacteria.
    d. Both a and b are correct.
    e. a, b, and c are correct.

13. DiGeorge syndrome is a primary immune deficiency caused by:
    a. failure of B cells to mature.
    b. congenital lack of thymic tissue.
    c. failure of the formed elements of blood to develop.
    d. selective deficiency of IgG.
    e. selective deficiency of IgA.

14. Secondary or acquired immunodeficiencies:
    a. develop after birth.
    b. may be caused by viral infections.
    c. may develop following immunosuppressive therapy.
    d. Both a and c are correct.
    e. a, b, and c are correct.

15. Rejection of a kidney transplant occurred after 2 weeks. The reaction occurred because of:
    a. immune response against recipient HLA antigens.
    b. immune response against donor HLA antigens.
    c. a type IV hypersensitivity.
    d. Both a and b are correct.
    e. Both b and c are correct.

16. SCID exhibits:
    a. B cell deficits.
    b. T cell deficits.
    c. complement deficits.
    d. B and T cell deficits.

17. A positive HIV antibody test signifies that the:
    a. individual is infected with HIV and likely so for life.
    b. asymptomatic individual will absolutely progress to AIDS.
    c. individual is not viremic.
    d. sexually active individual was infected the previous weekend.

18. Which is *incorrect* regarding AIDS?
    a. Antibody usually appears within 4 to 7 weeks after infection.
    b. The patient will be anti-HIV.
    c. The patient will likely experience opportunistic infections and cancer.
    d. The patient will have increased numbers of CD4+ cells or helper T cells.

Matching

Match the condition with the immunologic mechanism:

________ 19. Graves disease

________ 20. Serum sickness

________ 21. Allergic rhinitis

________ 22. Systemic lupus erythematosus

________ 23. Contact dermatitis

________ 24. Hemolytic anemia

________ 25. Tuberculin reaction

a. IgE-mediated
b. cytotoxic/tissue-specific reaction
c. immune complex reaction
d. cell-mediated reaction

Complete the following table comparing primary and secondary immunodeficiencies:

Primary and Secondary Immunodeficiencies

Primary Deficiencies		Secondary Deficiencies	
Cause	Example	Cause	Example
Lack of B cells			
No IgA production			
Lack of T cells			
Lack of B cells, T cells, phagocytes	SCID	Physical trauma	Burns
Decreased IgM			

Complete the following table comparing defense mechanism of bacteria to viruses that resist immune responses:

Pathogen's Resistance to Immune Responses

	Mechanisms	Effect on Immunity
Bacteria		
Viruses		

CASE STUDY 1

A 23-year-old male financial adviser sought relief from itchy eyes, repetitive sneezing, and nasal congestion that worsen at night. He said, "If I could only sleep at night, I could handle this." His history revealed that these symptoms occur every spring/summer and last for 6 to 8 weeks. As a teenager, he worked in his father's hay fields. His mother had asthma as a child. The physical examination showed his internal nares swollen and moist, with a clear discharge without purulence. There was no wheezing, and the lungs were clear to auscultation and percussion.

What is your diagnosis? What do you recommend?

CASE STUDY 2

C.E., a 27-year-old white man, was admitted to the emergency department with shortness of breath and a productive cough. He said, "I have no appetite and have lost 10 pounds over the past 2 weeks. Also, I have had pneumonia several times in the past 2 years." C.E. volunteered information about his homosexual practices. Physical examination revealed perianal vesicular lesions of herpes simplex infection, as well as fine crackles on the lower half of the lung fields with inspiratory and expiratory rhonchi.

Considering the circumstances, what laboratory tests are appropriate? What test results would you expect?

8 Stress and Disease

FOUNDATIONAL OBJECTIVE

After reviewing the primary text where referenced, the learner will be able to do the following:

a. Identify the function of some important biochemicals that regulate the stress response.

Refer to Figures 8-2 through 8-6 and Tables 8-2 through 8-4.

MEMORY CHECK!

There is a relationship between the nervous, endocrine, and immune systems that involves the common usage of molecules and receptors in each system. Central nervous system and autonomic nervous system neuropeptides affect immune cells. Endocrine products influence immune and neuroimmune cell function. The immune cell cytokines affect both nervous and endocrine cell function.

These intersystem effectors and their actions include the following:

- Corticotropin-releasing hormone (CRH) is a hypothalamic hormone that regulates many stress-induced alterations. It activates the pituitary gland and the sympathetic nervous system. Also, direct suppressive effects of CRF occur on two immune cell types possessing CRH receptor: the monocyte-macrophage and the helper T lymphocyte.
- ACTH controls the production and secretion of glucocorticoids by the cortex of the adrenal glands. ACTH is produced by the anterior pituitary and in small amounts by lymphocytes.
- Cortisol is secreted by the adrenal cortex, and it then circulates in the blood plasma. It elevates blood glucose and is anabolic for liver RNA and protein but catabolic for muscle and lymphoid tissue. When excessive, it stimulates gastric secretion. Cortisol is immunosuppressive for immunoglobulins and reduces eosinophils, macrophages, and lymphocytes; it is generally anti-inflammatory.
- Growth hormone (GH) is secreted by the anterior pituitary; it elevates blood glucose and promotes protein anabolism, tissue repair, and antibody production by plasma cells. Prolonged stress suppresses GH.
- Interleukin-1 (IL-1) and interleukin-6 (IL-6) are substances produced by macrophages that stimulate the release of ACTH through CRF. These factors affect B cell and T cell proliferation and body temperature.
- Interleukin-2 (IL-2) is produced by T cells and potentiates B cells and T cells, monocyte, and natural killer cell activity and increases pituitary ACTH levels. Prolactin acts as a second messenger for IL-2 and has a positive influence on B cell activation and differentiation.
- Interferons (IFN) are produced by lymphocytes, macrophages, and fibroblasts. These proteins are antiviral; they enhance phagocytic activity, suppress neoplastic growth, and stimulate the hypothalamus, pituitary, and adrenal pathway.
- Tumor necrosis factor (TNF) is produced mostly by macrophages. It stimulates inflammatory and immune mediators.
- Substance P is found in sensory nerves, spinal cord pathways, and parts of the brain; it stimulates the perception of pain.
- Endorphins are concentrated in the pituitary gland and inhibit pain by blocking the release of substance P; they may inhibit CRF secretion and inhibit or delay blood pressure increases.
- Epinephrine and norepinephrine levels are controlled by sympathetic preganglionic neurons that stimulate their secretion by the adrenal medulla. Both increase heart rate, blood pressure, and blood glucose concentration. Epinephrine dilates skeletal muscle blood vessels. Lymphoid tissue is innervated and, therefore, is influenced by these substances.
- Neuropeptide Y (NPY) is a neurotransmitter and neurohormone released from the sympathetic nerves and the adrenal medulla. NPY increases both vasoconstriction and the action of catecholamines.
- Histamine and serotonin are both vasoactive amines that participate in inflammation. Serotonin is found in the brain stem and in blood platelets. Histamine is found in basophils, mast cells, and platelets.
- Testosterone is immunosuppressive, whereas estrogen enhances resistance to infection but increases risk for autoimmune disease.
- Oxytocin likely is associated with reduced hypothalamic-pituitary-adrenal (HPA) axis activation and diminished anxiety, so it has antistress properties.
- Estrogen works in concert with oxytocin, exerting a calming effect during stress.
- Melatonin reverses lymphocyte suppression.

LEARNING OBJECTIVES

After studying this chapter, the learner will be able to do the following:

1. Define stress, identify stressors, and state the effects of stress.
Study text pages 204, 205, and 207; refer to Figure 8-1.

Stress involves daily hassles, such as fast-paced scheduling; pressure to remain in constant contact through social media, cell phones, or both; family member loss; loss of employment; and mental and physical abuse or trauma.

Stress arises when a person *interacts* or *transacts* with situations in certain ways. People are not disturbed by situations as they exist, but by the ways they individually appraise and react to situations. Stress is a condition in which a demand *exceeds* a *person's coping abilities*. Stress reactions may include disturbance of cognition, emotion, and behavior that can adversely affect an individual's well-being.

2. Describe Selye's original general adaptation syndrome; cite its stages.
Study text pages 204 and 205; refer to Figures 8-2 and 8-3.

While attempting to discover a new sex hormone, Selye injected crude ovarian extracts into rats. Repeatedly, he found the following *triad* of structural changes: (1) enlargement of the cortex of the adrenal gland, (2) atrophy of the thymus gland and other lymphoid structures, and (3) development of bleeding ulcers of the stomach and duodenal lining. Selye discovered that this triad of manifestations was not specific for his ovarian extracts, but also occurred after he exposed the rats to other noxious stimuli, such as cold, surgical injury, and restraint. Selye concluded that this triad or syndrome of manifestations represented *a nonspecific response to noxious stimuli.* Because many diverse agents caused the same syndrome, Selye suggested that it be called the **general adaptation syndrome (GAS).**

Selye later defined three successive stages in the development of the GAS: (1) the *alarm stage*, (2) the *stage of resistance* or adaptation, and (3) the *stage of exhaustion.* The nonspecific physiologic response identified by Selye consists of interaction among the sympathetic branch of the autonomic nervous system and two glands, the pituitary gland and the adrenal gland; hence, the interaction was known as the **hypothalamic-pituitary-adrenal (HPA) axis** system.

The alarm phase of the GAS begins when a stressor triggers the actions of the *pituitary gland and the sympathetic nervous system.* The resistance or adaptation phase begins with the actions of *cortisol, norepinephrine, and epinephrine.* Exhaustion occurs if stress continues and *adaptation is not successful; it marks the onset of disease.* The ultimate signs of exhaustion are impairment of the immune response, heart failure, and kidney failure, leading to death. Selye identified three components of the physiologic stress: (1) the exogenous or endogenous stressor initiating the disturbance, (2) the chemical or physical disturbance produced by the stressor, and (3) the body's counteracting (adaptational) response to the disturbance.

3. Identify current concepts that modify Selye's work.
Study text pages 205 and 207.

Selye believed that stressors cause a general or nonspecific, but purely physiologic, response. However, research has shown the remarkable *sensitivity of the central nervous system and endocrine system to psychological and social influences.* As with a physically mediated stress response, psychological stressors can elicit a reactive stress response. The *reactive response* is a physiologic response derived from psychological stressors. For example, the stress of an examination may produce an increased heart rate and dry mouth in the unprepared student. Although there is no physical stressor, the psychological stress of an examination elicits a reactive physiologic response.

Another type of psychologically-mediated stress response is the *anticipatory response.* Rather than reacting to an obvious stressor, the body mounts a physiologic stress response in anticipation of disruption of the optimal steady state, also known as *homeostasis.* These anticipatory responses can be generated either by species-specific innate programs, such as predators and unfamiliar situations, or by experience-dependent memory programs created by *conditioning.* Under some circumstances these memory programs may become so strong that psychological disorders, such as phobias, develop. Some individuals demonstrate *posttraumatic stress disorders* in response to the memory of traumatic events. These disorders are characterized by flashback memories, sleep disturbances, depression, and other symptoms that render the victim incapable of being employed or maintaining personal relationships.

Stressors also cause *psychoneuroimmunology responses.* Psychoneuroimmunology assumes that all immune-related disease is multifactorial, or the result of interrelationships among psychosocial, emotional, genetic, neurologic, endocrine, and immune systems and behavioral factors.

Specifically, CRH is released from the hypothalamus, the sympathetic nervous system, the pituitary gland, and the adrenal gland. CRH is also released peripherally at inflammatory sites called peripheral or immune CRH. Sufficient data now exist to conclude that immune modulation by psychosocial stressors or interventions leads directly to health outcomes, with the strongest data in studies of infectious disease and wound healing.

4. Summarize the major interactions of the nervous, endocrine, and immune systems in the stress response and develop an abbreviated flow chart showing these relationships.

Study the stress response in the summary review on page 219; refer to Figure 8-7.

CRH is the primary mediator of many stress-induced alterations to immune functions because of its role as an initiator of biologic brain responses to stress. It activates the *HPA axis,* which regulates many stress-induced responses by the *anterior pituitary,* the locus coeruleus–norepinephrine (*LC-NE) system and the adrenal medulla, and the posterior pituitary*. However, direct suppressive effects of CRH have also been reported on two immune cell types that process CRH receptors: the *monocyte-macrophage and the CD4 (helper T) lymphocyte*. The production of CRH is initiated by a high level of IL-1. Production of *IL-1* by activated macrophages and monocytes is inhibited by circulating *glucocorticoids*. The stimulation of CRH production in the hypothalamus by IL-1 demonstrates immune-induced regulation of the CNS and the cytokines (TNF and IFN). The T cell growth factor IL-2 can increase pituitary ACTH as well. It is likely that chronic inflammation can cause dysfunctional HPA stimulation. The parasympathetic nervous system also plays a role opposing the catecholamine responses and has anti-inflammatory effects. Sleep deprivation can elevate evening cortisol, insulin and blood glucose, blood pressure, proinflammatory cytokines, and appetite, while reducing parasympathetic activity. These alterations can increase caloric intake, depress mood, and cause cognitive disorders and a host of other problems from insomnia.

Communication among these three systems involves the common use of signal molecules and their similarly designed receptors. These signal/receptor interactions then regulate cellular behavior in each system, thereby linking each to the other(s).

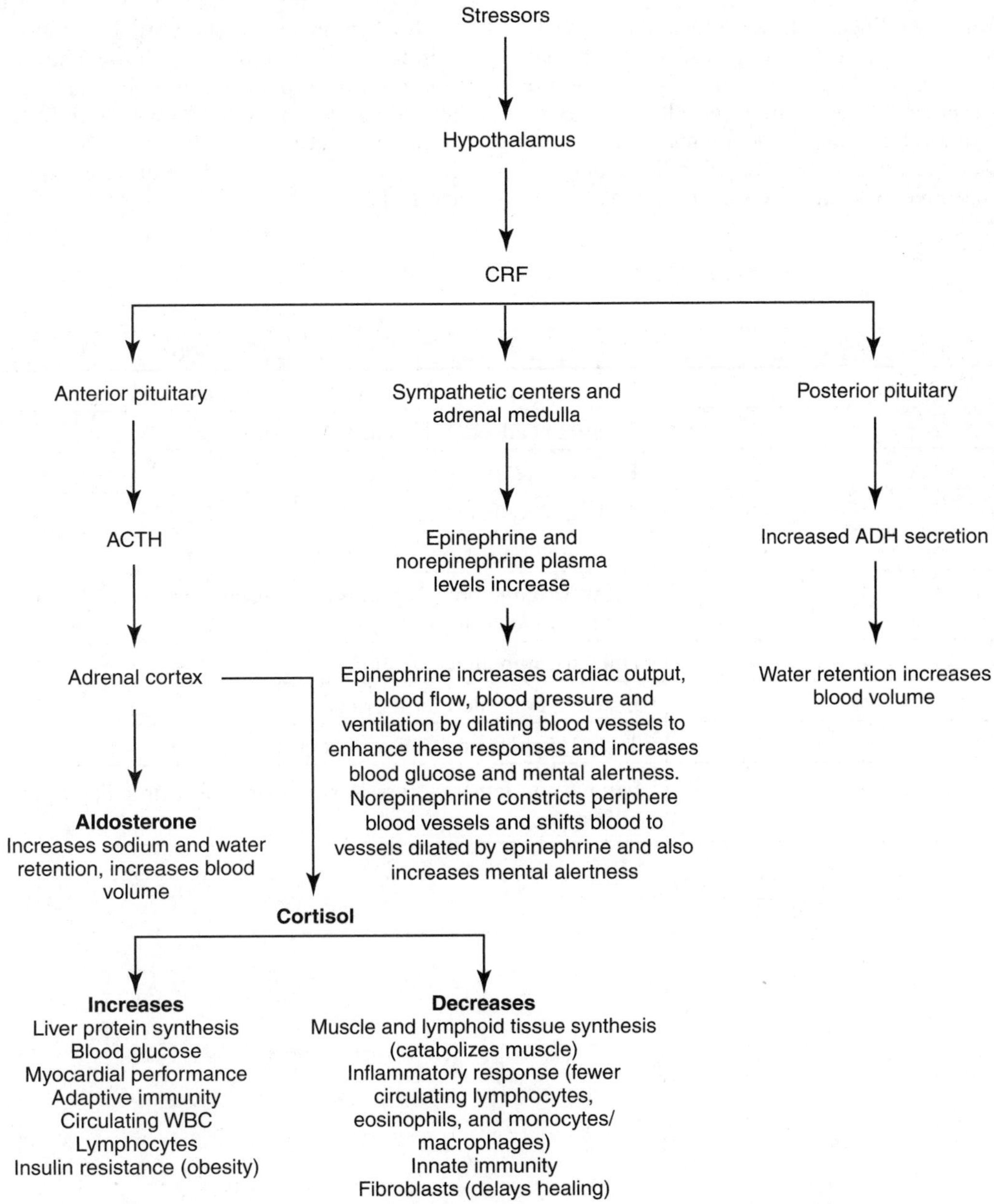

5. Distinguish between ineffective and effective methods of coping with stress.
Study pages 216-218; refer to Figure 8-8.

Stress is not an independent entity, but rather a system of *interdependent processes* that are moderated by the nature, intensity, and duration of the stressor. The perception, appraisal, and coping efficacy of the affected individual mediate the psychological and physiologic responses to stress. *Coping is managing the stressful demands that exceed the individual's resources.*

Coping responses may be adaptive or maladaptive. *Maladaptive coping* can result in a behavior change contributing to potentially adverse health effects such as smoking and eating and sleeping disturbances. *Adverse life events* that have the most *negative effect on immunity* have been characterized as those events that are uncontrollable and undesirable and that overtax the individual's ability to cope. Those individuals unable to cope may develop immune dysfunction.

Factors that may influence stress susceptibility or resilience include age, socioeconomic status, gender, social support status, personality, self-esteem, genetics, life events, past experiences, and current health status. With aging, a set of neurohormonal and immune alterations, including tissue and cellular changes, occur. Some of these changes are adaptive, whereas others are damaging.

Problem-focused and social support coping processes have a beneficial influence during stressful experiences. An individual who is experiencing distress may draw upon internal and external resources to meet the demands. Social support groups can improve psychological coping and immune function by increasing natural killer cell activity.

6. Cite examples of stress-related diseases.
Refer to Table 8-1. See the table below.

The table below includes an abbreviated grouping of stress-related disease. However, there is also convincing evidence linking cancer with psychological distress with three possible mechanisms involved. First, natural killer cell activity is inhibited in stressed or depressed people. Second, stress and depression are also associated with poorer repair of damaged DNA, and third, alterations occur in the rates of apoptosis of immune and cancer cells.

New evidence is showing a relationship among immune stimulation, infections, and heart disease. The relationship between stress and cardiovascular health may be mediated by stress-induced changes in immune function, which may potentiate proinflammatory processes and permit infections that lead to heart disease.

Stress-Related Diseases

Organ or System	Disease or Condition
Cardiovascular	Coronary artery disease, hypertension, stroke, arrhythmia
Muscles	Tension headaches, backache
Connective tissues	Rheumatoid arthritis
Pulmonary	Asthma, hay fever
Immune	Immunosuppression, deficiency, autoimmunity
Gastrointestinal	Ulcer, irritable bowel syndrome, diarrhea, nausea and vomiting, ulcerative colitis
Genitourinary	Diuresis, impotence, frigidity
Integumentary	Eczema, neurodermatitis, acne
Endocrine	Type 2 diabetes mellitus, amenorrhea
Central nervous	Fatigue and lethargy, type A behavior, overeating, depression, insomnia

PRACTICE EXAMINATION

Multiple Choice

Circle the correct answer for each question:

1. Which of the following is a characteristic of Selye's stress syndrome?
   a. adrenocortical enlargement
   b. thymus enlargement
   c. It is a specific response to stress.
   d. lymphatic organ enlargement

2. Which of the following characterizes the alarm stage?
   a. increased lymphocytes
   b. increased sympathetic activity
   c. increased parasympathetic activity
   d. increased eosinophils

3. In stressed or depressed individuals:
   a. natural killer cells are stimulated.
   b. damaged DNA is repaired properly.
   c. apoptosis of immune and cancer cells is altered.
   d. cellular immunity is increased and humoral immunity is decreased.

4. Which is the correct sequence of Selye's hypothesis for stress?
   a. increased ACTH secretion, alarm
   b. increased ACTH in the blood, hypertrophy of the adrenal cortex
   c. stimulation of the sympathetic centers, alarm
   d. increased secretion of epinephrine, increased ACTH in the blood

5. Corticotropin-releasing hormone (CRH) is released by the:
   a. adrenal medulla.
   b. adrenal cortex.
   c. anterior pituitary.
   d. hypothalamus.

6. Stress may be defined as any factor that stimulates the:
   a. posterior pituitary.
   b. anterior pituitary.
   c. hypothalamus to release CRH.
   d. hypothalamus to release ADH.

7. Which of the following is true?
   a. Stressors initially stimulate the adrenal cortex.
   b. Stressors stimulate immunity.
   c. The emotions fear, anxiety, and grief can act as stressors.
   d. Stressors are the same for all individuals.

8. Glucocorticoids are highest during the stage of:
   a. exhaustion.
   b. alarm.
   c. resistance.

9. The physiologic response to the stress of a student's final exam may be:
   a. reactive.
   b. a conditioned behavior.
   c. anticipatory.
   d. caused by a physical stressor.

10. The production of cortisol in response to stress can be initiated by:
    a. the hypothalamus, anterior pituitary, and adrenal cortex.
    b. the hypothalamus, posterior pituitary, and adrenal cortex.
    c. the hypothalamus, sympathetic nerve fibers, and adrenal cortex.
    d. the hypothalamus, sympathetic nerve fibers, and adrenal medulla.

11. Cortisol:
    a. affects protein catabolism.
    b. decreases blood sugar.
    c. increases immune response.
    d. increases allergic reactions.

12. Which of the following would occur in response to stress?
    a. increased systolic blood pressure
    b. decreased epinephrine
    c. constriction of the pupils
    d. decreased adrenocorticoids

13. Which of the following would be least useful in the assessment of stress?
    a. total blood cholesterol
    b. eosinophil count
    c. lymphocyte count
    d. adrenocorticoid levels

14. In response to stress, the adrenal cortex secretes:
    a. norepinephrine.
    b. norepinephrine and cortisol.
    c. cortisol and aldosterone.
    d. norepinephrine and aldosterone.

15. Coping:
    a. slows natural killer cell activity.
    b. best involves solving the stress circumstance by oneself.
    c. effectively leads to immune dysfunction.
    d. manages stressful demands exceeding an individual's resources.

Fill in the Blanks

***Supply the correct response for each statement*:**

16. Biochemicals secreted by the adrenal cortex in response to stress are ________________________.

17. ________________________ cause disturbances in cognition, emotion, and behavior.

18. The bodily changes initiated by noxious stimuli cause the ________________________.

19. The stage of GAS wherein the immunity of an individual is most impaired is the ________________________.

20. The stage of GAS that triggers the sympathetic nervous system is the ________________________.

21. The cytokine produced by macrophages stimulating release of CRH is ________________________.

22. An interleukin that increases ACTH levels is ________________________.

23. A neurotransmitter augmenting the action of catecholamines is ________________________.

24. A substance produced by lymphocytes, macrophages, and fibroblasts that enhances phagocytic activity is ________________________.

25. ________________________ inhibit pain, CRH secretion, and blood pressure increases.

Complete the following table comparing the effects of epinephrine/norepinephrine to the actions of cortisol:

Epinephrine/Norepinephrine vs. Cortisol Actions

Effects	
Catecholamines (Epinephrine and Norepinephrine)	Cortisol

9 Biology, Clinical Manifestations, and Treatment of Cancer

FOUNDATIONAL OBJECTIVES

a. Describe the phases of cellular mitosis and cytokinesis and cell differentiation.
Review pages 22-24; refer to Figure 1-26.

MEMORY CHECK!

- The reproduction or division of somatic cells involves two sequential phases: *mitosis*, or nuclear division, and *cytokinesis*, or cytoplasmic division. These phases occur in close succession, with cytokinesis beginning toward the end of mitosis. Before a cell can divide, it must double its mass and duplicate all of its contents. Most of the preparation for division occurs during the growth phase or interphase. The alternation between mitosis and interphase in all tissues that have cellular turnover is known as the cell cycle.
- There are four designated phases of the cell cycle. They are: (1) the S phase (synthesis), in which DNA is synthesized in the cell nucleus; (2) the G2 phase, in which RNA and protein synthesis occurs; (3) the M phase (mitosis), which includes both nuclear and cytoplasmic division; and (4) the G1 phase, which is the period between the M phase and the start of DNA synthesis. Interphase, consisting of the G1, S, and G2 phases, is the longest period of the cell cycle.
- The M phase of the cell cycle, mitosis and cytokinesis, begins with *prophase* or the first appearance of chromosomes. Each chromosome has two identical halves called chromatids that lie side by side and are attached together at a site called a centromere. The nuclear membrane disappears in this phase. Spindle fibers are microtubules formed in the cytoplasm that radiate from two centrioles located at opposite poles of the cell.
- During *metaphase*, the next phase of mitosis and cytokinesis, the spindle fibers pull the centromeres until they are aligned in the middle of the spindle or at the equatorial plate.
- *Anaphase* begins when the centromeres separate and the genetically identical chromatids are pulled apart. The chromatids are pulled, centromeres first, toward opposite sides of the cell. When the identical chromatids are separated, each is considered to be a chromosome. Thus, the cell has 92 chromosomes during this stage. By the end of anaphase, there are 46 chromosomes at each side of the identical cell. Each of the two groups of 46 chromosomes should be identical to the original 46 chromosomes present at the start of the cell cycle.
- During *telophase*, a new nuclear membrane is formed around each group of 46 chromosomes, the spindle fibers disappear, and the chromosomes begin to uncoil. Cytokinesis causes the cytoplasm to divide into roughly equal parts during this phase. At the end of telophase, two identical diploid cells, called daughter cells, have formed from the original cell.
- The difference between slowly and rapidly dividing cells is the length of time spent in the *G1 phase* of the cell cycle. Some cells that divide slowly can remain in the G1 phase for years. Once the S phase begins, progression through mitosis requires a relatively constant amount of time. Once a cell has progressed out of the G1 phase, it must complete the S, G2, and M phases.

b. Identify mechanisms that control cell division.
Review pages 23-27; refer to Figure 1-27 and Table 1-5.

MEMORY CHECK!

- Protein *growth factors* govern the proliferation of different cell types in *conjunction with genes* involved in the social control or relationship of cells within tissues. It is likely that some genes code for growth factors, some for growth factor receptors, some for intracellular regulatory proteins involved in cell adhesion, and some for proteins that help relay signals for cell division to the cell nucleus.
- Cells require highly specific proteins to stimulate cell division. These growth factors are present in the serum in very low concentrations. For example, *platelet-derived growth factor* stimulates the production of *connective tissue* cells. Another important growth factor is *interleukin*, which stimulates proliferation of *T cells*. Cells responding to a particular growth factor have specific receptors for the specific growth factor in their plasma membrane. Some growth factors also are regulators of cellular differentiation.

c. Describe mechanisms that confine cells and tissues to a specific anatomic site.
Review page 24.

MEMORY CHECK!

- All cells are within a network of extracellular macromolecules known as the *extracellular matrix*. The extracellular matrix holds cells and tissues together and provides an organized framework in which cells can interact with one another.
- To confine themselves and form tissues, cells must have *intercellular recognition, adhesion, and memory*. Communication ensures that new cells are produced only when and where they are required. Different cell types have different adhesion molecules in their plasma membranes, sticking selectively to other cells of the same type. They can also adhere to extracellular matrix components. Cells have memory because of specialized pattern of gene expression evoked by signals that acted during embryonic development. Memory allows cells to autonomously preserve their distinctive character and pass it on to the progeny.

LEARNING OBJECTIVES

After studying this chapter, the learner will be able to do the following:

1. Define tumor, neoplasia, and cancer.
Study page 222.

The term **tumor** originally referred to any swelling due to inflammation, but is now generally reserved for a *new growth, or* ***neoplasm***. Not all tumors or neoplasms, however, are cancer. The term **cancer** refers to a malignant tumor and is not used to refer to *benign* growths such as lipomas and hypertrophy of an organ.

2. Name and classify tumors; distinguish between benign and malignant tumors.
Study page 223; refer to Figures 9-1 and 9-2 and Table 9-1.

Cancers are named according to the cell types from which they *originate*. Those arising from epithelial tissue are named **carcinomas;** if from ductal or glandular structures, they are **adenocarcinomas.** Cancers arising from mesenchymal tissue are **sarcomas.** Cancers from lymphatic tissue are **lymphomas**, whereas cancers of blood-forming tissues are **leukemias.**

Early stage growths that relocalized to the epithelium but have not invaded the local basement membrane

Properties of Benign/Malignant Tumors

Characteristic	Benign	Malignant
Differentiation	Yes, resembles tissue of origin	No, little resemblance to tissue of origin
Mitotic figures	Normal	Abnormal
Growth rate	Slow	Rapid
Growth mode	Expansive	Infiltrative
Capsulation	Yes	No
Cellular cohesiveness	Yes	No
Metastasis	No	Yes

or the surrounding stroma have a specific classification. These growths are not malignant and are called **carcinoma in situ (CIS).** CIS lesions can have three fates: (1) they can remain stable for long periods, (2) they can progress to invasive and malignant cancers, or (3) they can regress and disappear.

Now, diagnosis and treatment is commonly accompanied by immunohistochemical analysis of protein expression. Frequently, this analysis is supplemented by molecular analysis of the tumor.

3. Describe tumor cell markers; cite marker examples that suggest the existence of cancer.
Study pages 225-227; refer to Table 9-2.

Tumor cell markers are substances that are produced by cancer cells and found on tumor plasma membranes or in the blood, spinal fluid, or urine. They include hormones, enzymes, genes, antigens, and antibodies.

Tumor cell markers can be used in three ways: (1) to identify individuals at high risk for cancer, (2) to help diagnose the specific type of tumor in an individual with clinical manifestations of cancer, and (3) to observe the clinical course of cancer. The presence of a tumor marker may *increase the probability of cancer*, but it is not used alone as a diagnostic test. If the tumor marker itself has biologic activity, it can cause symptoms. This is known as a paraneoplastic syndrome.

Examples of Tumor Markers

Marker	Name	Type of Cancer Suggested
AFP	α-fetoprotein	Hepatic, germ cell
CEA	Carcinoembryonic antigen	GI, pancreas, lung, breast
b-hCG	Beta subunit of human chorionic gonadotropin	Germ cell
PSA	Prostate-specific antigen	Prostate
Catecholamines (epinephrine and metabolites)		Pheochromocytoma (adrenal medulla, neuroblastoma)
Urinary Bence-Jones protein		Multiple myeloma
ACTH	Adrenocorticotropic hormone	Pituitary adenomas

4. **Identify some changes that occur in cancerous cells and their functional significance.**
Study page 227; refer to Figure 9-4.

Cancerous Cell Changes and Their Significance

Change	Significance
Transformation (autonomy)	Decreased need for external growth factors, lack contact inhibition
Anchorage-independent (fewer anchoring junctions)	Cells continue to grow and divide when not attached to firm surface; favors growth in new area
Immortal	Unlimited life span, continue to divide
Anaplasia	Loss of differentiation or specialization; loss of ability to function and control its growth and division
Pleomorphism	Variable size and shape

Note: The most malignant tumors have the most anaplasia.

5. **Postulate a model for the causes and sequence of carcinogenesis.**
Study pages 227-229, 231, and 233-241; refer to Figures 9-5 through 9-18 and Tables 9.3 through 9-5.

Oncogenes are genes that can transform a normal cell into a cancerous cell when inherited or activated by oncogenic viruses. Oncogenes can develop from normal genes **(proto-oncogenes)** that regulate growth and development by encoding for growth factors and growth factor receptors. These genes may undergo some change that either causes them to produce an abnormal product or disrupts their control so that they are expressed inappropriately and accelerate proliferation.

Some cancers are not caused by oncogenes but rather by genes called **tumor suppressor genes** that have mutated. These genes produce proteins that normally oppose the action of an oncogene or inhibit cell division. Carcinogenesis inactivates tumor suppressor genes by loss of **heterozygosity** (loss of one gene copy), which unmasks mutations in recessive genes, or by **epigenetic silencing** (in which methylation of DNA shuts off genes without mutation without change in he DNA sequence), activates oncogenes, and turns off tumor suppressor genes. Changes in gene regulation can affect not only single genes but entire networks of signaling. Gene expression networks can be regulated by changes in microRNAs and other non-coding RNAs.

Cells have a self-destruct mechanism, known as **apoptosis,** which is triggered by normal development and excessive growth. The most common mutations causing resistance to apoptosis occur in the *p53* gene.

Other than germ cells, cells in the body can divide only a limited number of times. **Telomeres** are at the ends of each chromosome and block unlimited cell division.

Causes and Sequence of Carcinogenesis

Several mutagenic "hits" to DNA

↓

Alteration or mutation of genetic molecules
Proto-oncogenes
Oncogenes
Tumor suppressor genes
Telomeres/reactivation of telomerase
Apoptosis prevention gene
Caretaker genes
Micro RNAs, oncomirs and non-coding RNAs

↓

Activate growth-promoting pathways
Block antigrowth signals
Prevent apoptosis
Activate angiogenesis

↓

Cancerous cell changes
Limitless replication/immortal cells
Loss of differentiation

↓

Clonal proliferation, expansion and selection of fast growing subclones

↓

Benign tumor/carcinoma in situ

↓

Sequential mutagenic changes

↓

Advanced tumor/malignant neoplasia

Note: Genetic mutations can occur in response to exposure to a large number of environmental agents. See Chapter 12 for agent exposures related to cancer. Epigenetic changes in genes by DNA methylation and covalent histone modification can mimic mutation by heritably turning off tumor suppressor genes.

Telomerase maintains telomeres. Cancer cells activate telomerase to restore and maintain telomeres so cells can divide over and over again.

Whenever normal DNA integrity is disrupted during mitosis or by external mutagens, multiple mechanisms have evolved to protect and repair the genome. These repair mechanisms are directed by **caretaker genes.** These genes encode proteins that repair damaged DNA, and loss of caretaker genes leads to increased mutation rates.

The successful cancer cell divides rapidly and has a consequent need for building blocks for new cancerous cells. Also, cancer genes promote aerobic glycolysis and high glucose utilization within the cell.

6. Identify the genetic events occurring within cancer-prone families.

Study page 234; refer to Figure 9-11 and Table 9-4.

Most of the genetic and epigenetic alterations causing cancer occur during the lifetime of the individual within the *somatic tissues*. Because they occur in the somatic cells rather than germline cells, they are *not transmitted to future generations*; they are not inherited. It is possible, however, for cancer-producing mutations to occur in germline cells. When mutations are present in *germline cells*, transmission of cancer-causing genes occurs from *one generation to the next generation,* producing families with a high incidence of specific cancers. These inherited mutations are almost invariably *in tumor suppressor genes*. Individuals who inherit the germline mutant allele will suffer loss of the normal allele by loss of heterozygosity or genetic silencing in some cells, and the tumor develops.

7. Describe the mechanisms involved in metastasis.

Study pages 241-243; refer to Figure 9-19.

Most cancer cells are unable to cause metastases. The reason lies both in the "seed" and the "soil." Cancer cells (*the seeds*) must overcome multiple physical and physiologic barriers to spread, survive, and proliferate in distant locations (*the soil*), which must be receptive to the cancer cells. As cancers grow, they develop increasing **heterogeneity.** As this diversity increases, the number of cells in the cancer mass rises with new abilities that facilitate metastasis.

For cells to move from their normal, original niche, they must *detach* from the stroma and migrate. To spread, many tumors and their associated inflammatory cells secrete proteases and protease activators. *Proteases* digest the extracellular matrix and basement membranes and thus *create pathways* through which cancer cells move. Another mediator of cell detachment is the decrease in the cancer cell of specific adhesion molecules, such as *E-cadherin and integrins*. When E-cadherin is lost, cells are able to *detach* from their extracellular attachments, become more slippery, and migrate more readily. To *transition* from local to distant metastasis, the cancer cell must be able *to invade local blood vessels and lymphatic vessels*. This task is facilitated by stimulation of *neoangiogenesis and lymphangiogenesis* by factors such as VEGF.

Once in the circulation, metastatic cells must withstand the *stresses of travel* in the blood and lymphatic vessels, as well as exposure to immune cells. Metastatic cells must move to a distant site through veins and lymphatics and then *escape* from the *circulation*. Cancer cells arrive at a new location and attach therein to *develop a new microenvironment*. It is possible that successful metastatic tumor cells secrete factors that recruit circulating mesenchymal stem cells to the metastatic site. These newly recruited stem cells then differentiate into tumor-supporting stroma and new blood vessels.

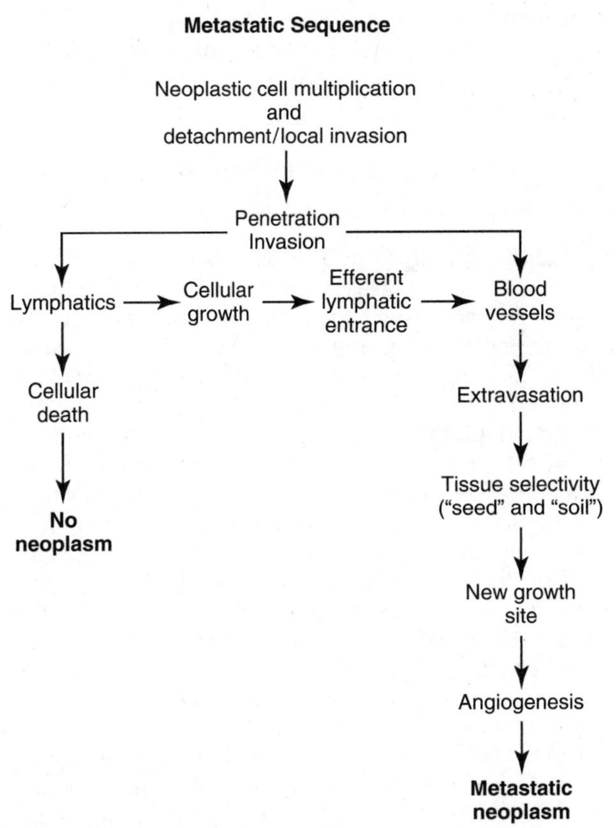

Note: Mobile tumor cells enter the circulation because of chemoattractive mediators released from neovascularization. Specific interactions between the cancer cells and receptors on small blood vessels create the microenvironment ("soil").

8. Describe the diagnosis and staging of cancer.
Study pages 243 and 244; refer to Figure 9-20 and Table 9-6.

The diagnostic symptoms a cancer produces are as diverse as the types of cancer. The location of the cancer can *determine symptoms by physical pressure, obstruction, and loss of normal function.* Cancer can cause problems far away from its source by pressing on nerves or secreting bioactive compounds. Once the diagnosis of cancer is suspected or identified, tumor tissue must be obtained to establish a *definitive diagnosis* and correctly classify the disease. The classification of cancer can be further facilitated by other available tests, including immunohistochemical stains, flow cytometry, electron microscopy, chromosome analysis, and nucleic acid-based molecular studies.

If cancer exists, it is critical to know the extent of its spread, or its **stage**. Staging the tumor is an important component of cancer diagnosis. In general, a four-stage system is used, with carcinoma in situ regarded as a special case. Cancer *confined to the site of origin is stage 1*, cancer that *is locally invasive is stage 2*, cancer that has *spread to regional* structures such as *lymph nodes is stage 3*, and cancer that has spread to *distant sites is stage 4.* In general, the lower the stage, the more amenable the cancer is to treatment. Also, staging alters the choice of therapy; more aggressive therapy is delivered to more invasive disease.

9. Describe the clinical manifestations of cancer.
Study pages 243-248; refer to Figure 9-21 and Table 9-8.

Usually little or no **pain** is associated with the early stages of malignant disease, but pain will affect individuals who are terminally ill with cancer. Cancer-associated pain arises from multiple sources. Direct pressure, obstruction, invasion of sensitive structures, stretching of visceral surfaces, tissue destruction, infection, and inflammation all can cause pain. Pain can occur at the site of the primary tumor or from a metastatic lesion. Furthermore, it can be referred from any involved site.

Fatigue is the most frequently reported symptom of cancer and cancer treatment. Likely causes of fatigue include sleep disturbance, biochemical changes, psychological factors, altered nutritional status, and level of activity. Decreased muscle contractibility and function are observed in individuals with cancer. Muscle loss may result from cancer treatment or from circulating tumor necrosis factor (TNF) and IL-1.

Cachexia is a wasting, emaciation manifesting symptoms of anorexia; early satiety; anemia; marked weakness; taste alteration; and altered protein, lipid, and carbohydrate metabolism, which is a loss of appetite. Individuals show hyperinsulinemia, insulin resistance, hyperglycemia, and abnormal blood glucose tests. In cancer, protein is used to meet energy needs rather than spared to protect vital tissues. Cytokines including IL-6, TNF, and an interferon appear to cause the metabolic alterations associated with tissue loss in cancer wasting.

Anemia is also commonly associated with malignancy. The majority of individuals with cancer have a mild anemia, although 20% may have hemoglobin concentrations below 9 g/dL. Chronic bleeding, severe malnutrition, medical therapies, or malignancy in blood-forming organs may cause anemia by depleting erythrocyte building blocks or destroying the site for synthesis of erythrocytes.

Direct tumor invasion into the bone marrow causes **leukopenia** and **thrombocytopenia.** Many chemotherapeutic drugs are toxic to the bone marrow and cause **granulocytopenia** as well as thrombocytopenia. Radiation therapy that involves the bone marrow also may cause granulocytopenia.

Infection is the most significant cause of complications and death in individuals with malignant disease. Individuals with cancer are very susceptible to infection because of reductions in immunologic functions, debility from advanced disease, and immunosuppression from radiotherapy and chemotherapy. Surgery can create favorable sites for infection. The incidence of hospital-related or nosocomial infections is increased in patients with cancer because of indwelling medical devices, compromised wound care, and the introduction of microorganisms from visitors and other patients.

10. Compare the modalities for the treatment of neoplasms.
Study pages 248 and 249; refer to Table 9-9.

Cancer is treated with chemotherapy, radiotherapy, surgery, immunotherapy, and combinations of these modalities. The goal of **chemotherapy** is to kill cells that are undergoing mitosis and cytokinesis and those in interphase. *Combination chemotherapy* is the synergistic use of several agents, each with an effect against a certain cancer, used to avoid single-agent resistance and acquired drug resistance. Also, lower doses of each agent may be used, causing fewer side effects and less toxicity. Faster-growing neoplasms are generally more sensitive to chemotherapy. *Induction chemotherapy* seeks to cause shrinkage or disappearance of tumor; it may or may not cure the recipient. *Adjuvant chemotherapy* is given *after* surgical excision of a cancerous lesion with the goal of eliminating micrometastases. *Neoadjuvant chemotherapy* is given prior to localized surgery or radiation.

To eradicate neoplastic cells without producing excessive toxicity and to avoid damage to normal structures are the challenges of **radiation therapy**. Ionizing radiation damages important macromolecules, especially DNA. *Rapidly renewing and dividing cells* are generally more *radiosensitive* than other cells. Because radiation produces irreversible changes in normal tissue, there is a *maximum lifetime* dose that tissue can tolerate. Radiation therapy is well suited to treat localized disease in areas that are difficult to reach surgically. A common radiation delivery system is a targeted external beam. Radioactive iodine capsules can be placed temporarily into body cavities for treatment of cervical, prostate, and head and neck cancers; this delivery method is termed **brachytherapy**.

Surgical therapy is useful and definitive if the neoplasm is accessible and has *not yet spread beyond the limits of surgical excision.* Lymph node removal during surgery will provide valuable staging information necessitating further treatment. Debulking surgery, in which the majority of a tumor is removed, can allow greater success with adjuvant chemotherapy or irradiation. Palliative surgery (alleviation without cure) may be used to relieve or avoid symptoms of malignancy. The key principle that applies to cancer surgery involves obtaining *adequate surgical margins* during resection to prevent local recurrences and scrupulously avoiding the spread of cancer cells during the surgical procedures.

PRACTICE EXAMINATION

Multiple Choice

Circle the correct answer for each question:

1. Which characterize(s) cancer cells?
   a. poorly differentiated
   b. metastasis
   c. infiltrative growth mode
   d. poor cellular cohesiveness
   e. All of the above are correct.

2. Tumor cell markers:
   a. are proteases.
   b. are absolutely diagnostic for cancer.
   c. can monitor the course of cancer.
   d. indicate metastasis.

3. Telomeres:
   a. block unlimited cell division.
   b. activate oncogenes.
   c. encode repair proteins for damaged DNA.
   d. lead to increased mutation rates.

4. Metastasis is:
   a. an alteration in normal cellular growth.
   b. growth of benign or malignant neoplastic cells.
   c. mutational.
   d. the ability to establish a secondary neoplasm at a new site.

5. Carcinoma in situ is:
   a. preinvasive.
   b. a glandular or epithelial lesion.
   c. a teratoma.
   d. a carcinoma that has broken through the basement membrane.
   e. Both a and b are correct.

6. Known routes of metastasis include:
   a. continuous extension.
   b. lymphatic spread.
   c. bloodstream dissemination.
   d. Both b and c are correct.
   e. a, b, and c are correct.

7. Tumor suppressor genes are:
   a. genes that have the ability to transform a normal cell into a cancerous cell.
   b. normal genes that regulate growth and development.
   c. genes that produce proteins that inhibit cellular division.
   d. Both b and c are correct.

8. In the current theory of carcinogenesis:
   a. the sequence is initiation-promotion-progression.
   b. several mutagenic "hits" are required.
   c. mutations in somatic cells are transmitted to future generations.
   d. sequential genetic changes occur.
   e. Both b and d are correct.

9. Which is *not* involved in metastasis?
   a. initial establishment
   b. interference
   c. invasion
   d. dissemination
   e. proliferation

10. Loss of E-cadherin:
    a. stimulates protease production.
    b. digests extracellular matrix.
    c. increases cellular receptiveness to cancer cells.
    d. transforms a normal cell to a cancerous cell.
    e. causes cells to detach from their extracellular attachments.

11. The *p53* gene:
    a. enables cells to cope with DNA damage.
    b. blocks the proliferation of cells that have suffered carcinogenic mutations.
    c. mutations are the most common genetic lesion in human cancer.
    d. mutations disable an emergency brake on cell proliferation.
    e. All of the above are correct.

12. Local invasive factors include all *except:*
    a. increased cellular adhesion.
    b. lytic enzymes.
    c. mechanical pressure.
    d. cellular multiplication.

13. The sequence of carcinogenesis is:
    a. exposure to carcinogens, selection of subclones, and mutation of genetic molecules.
    b. ionizing radiation, caretaker gene activity, and point mutations.
    c. several mutagenic "hits" to DNA, reactivation of telomerase, and development of immortal cells.
    d. carcinoma in situ, altered genetic molecules, and sequential mutagenic changes.

14. Adjuvant chemotherapy:
    a. produces irreversible tissue alteration.
    b. is well suited to treat localized disease.
    c. seeks to shrink tumors.
    d. is used prior to localized surgery.
    e. follows surgery to eliminate micrometastases.

Matching

Match the term with its definition:

_______ 15. Neoplasia

_______ 16. Anaplasia

_______ 17. Autonomy

a. variation in size, shape, and arrangement of cells
b. differentiation of dividing cells into cellular types not ordinarily found in a given area
c. abnormal, proliferating cells possessing a higher degree of autonomy than normal cells
d. increase in absolute number of cells
e. lack of cellular differentiation or specialization, primitive cells
f. cancer cells' independence from normal cellular controls

Match the term with its definition/characteristic:

_______ 18. Stage 3

_______ 19. Tumor markers

_______ 20. Loss of heterozygosity

_______ 21. Silencing

a. increased metabolite transport
b. cancer has spread to regional structures
c. unmasks mutations in recessive genes
d. methylation of DNA shuts off genes
e. "rounded-up" cells
f. substances produced by cancer cells
g. increased extracellular proteolysis

Match the tumor markers with their expressing neoplastic cells:

_______ 22. AFP

_______ 23. CEA

_______ 24. Urinary Bence-Jones protein

_______ 25. PSA

a. multiple myeloma
b. retinoblastomas
c. hepatic, germ cells
d. GI, pancreas
e. Wilms tumor
f. prostate gland

Complete the following table by relating benign and malignant tumors to their sites of origin:

Common Benign and Malignant Tumor Origin Sites

Tissue	Benign Tumor	Malignant Tumor
Connective/mesenchymal Tissue	Fibroma Chondroma Osteoma Lipoma Leiomyoma Rhabdomyoma Hemangioma	
Hematopoietic	Infectious mononucleosis	
Nerve Tissue	Neuroma Neurilemmoma	
Epithelial Tissue	Papilloma Adenoma	

10 Cancer Epidemiology

LEARNING OBJECTIVES

After studying this chapter, the learner will be able to do the following:

1. Generalize gene-environment-lifestyle interactions.
Study pages 253 and 257; refer to Table 10-1.

Cancer arises from a complicated and an interacting web of multiple causes. At the cellular level, cancer is genetic. Preventing exposures to *individual carcinogens*, or cancer-causing substances, can prevent many cancers. Widespread general exposures to pollutants from water, air, and the work environment; personal lifestyle choices, such as smoking, excessive alcohol, and poor diet; and involuntary or unknowing exposures in air, water, and occupational environments are major contributors to cancer.

It appears that the majority of excess cancer in populations exposed to carcinogens is from the exposure itself and not from rare genetic predispositions. For example, in women who have mutated cancer susceptibility genes *BRCA1* or *BRCA2,* the risk of having breast cancer at age 50 years is 24% for those born before 1940 but 67% for those born later. The implication is related to lifestyle factors that have changed since 1940, including, most notably, hormone therapy, later age of first pregnancy, and increased nulliparity.

Studies comparing different populations around the world illustrate the large role of **environment-lifestyle** contributions to cancer. Breast cancer, for example, is prevalent among northern Europeans and Americans but is relatively rare among women in developing countries. If ethnicity played a major role, then immigrants should retain the cancer incidence rates of their country of origin. Instead, immigrants acquire the cancer rates of the environment they move to within one to two generations.

Elevated cancer rates are more common in cities, in farming locations, near hazardous waste sites, downwind of industrial and radiation activities, and near contaminated water wells. In addition, cancers are associated with areas of high pesticide use, toxic work exposures, waste incinerators, and other sources of pollution.

Susceptibility to disease is set *in utero* or *neonatally* as the result of nutrition and exposures to environmental toxins or stressors, or both. Children also may be affected by prenatal exposures, parental exposures prior to conception, and breast milk. Epidemiologic studies have linked higher risks of childhood leukemia and brain and CNS cancers with parental and childhood exposure to particular solvents, pesticides, petrochemicals, dioxins, and polycyclic aromatic hydrocarbons.

2. Describe the relationship between epigenetics and genetics.
Study pages 257 and 260; refer to Figure 10-1 and Tables 10-3 and 10-4.

It is clear that inherited variation in DNA sequence influences individual risk of cancer; however, it constitutes a small percentage of the population. An explosion of data now indicates the importance of epigenetic processes, especially those with resultant gene silencing of *key* regulatory genes. Epigenetic changes collaborate with genetic changes with environmental-lifestyle factors to cause the development of cancer. These changes are mitotically and meiotically heritable.

The three major areas of **epigenetics** are: (1) **methylation** (the addition of a methyl group [CH_3] to a cytosine ring), an aberrant methylation that can lead to silencing of tumor-suppressor genes; (2) **histone modifications** (histone acetylation, alterations in chromatin); and (3) **microRNAs** (miRNAs), small RNA molecules that can target gene expression post-transcriptionally. The expression of miRNAs has recently been linked to carcinogenesis because they can act as either oncogenes or tumor-suppressor genes.

An important feature of epigenetic mechanisms and their role in development and disease is that epigenetic processes can be modified by lifestyle, particularly diet and the environment, pharmacologic interventions, or both. **Environmental-lifestyle** factors act on individuals throughout life, changing **gene expression** through epigenetic mechanisms with subsequent implications for health or disease.

Biologically active food components modify DNA methylation directly. Nutrition influences metabolic effects associated with energy balance. Because adipose tissue is endocrine tissue, obese individuals accumulate macrophages that secrete various proinflammatory signaling molecules and cytokines. *Inflammation is strongly associated with cancer development,* and inflammatory bowel disease is related to methylation in the colon.

3. Indicate the role of in utero and early life conditions in cancer development.
Study pages 260 and 261; refer to Figure 10-2 and Tables 10-3 and 10-4.

It is widely accepted that a *long latency period* precedes the onset of adult cancers. Early life events influence later susceptibility to certain chronic diseases.

Developmental plasticity is the ability to develop in particular ways depending on the environment or setting. It requires stable gene expression, which appears to be modulated by epigenetic processes, such as DNA methylation and histone modification. Sensitivity to environmental-lifestyle factors influences the mature phenotype and depends on the interactions of the genome and epigenome.

Perhaps one of the best examples of early life events and future cancer was the chemical exposure to *diethylstilbestrol (DES),* a synthetic estrogen. Studies have revealed that daughters of women who took DES during pregnancy may have a slightly increased risk of breast cancer before age 40 years. Epigenetic mechanisms are responsible for tissue-specific gene expression during cellular differentiation, and these mechanisms modulate developmental phenotypic changes. The phenotypic effects of epigenetic modifications during development may need long latency periods, such as in cancer, thus manifesting later in life.

4. Describe tobacco use as a carcinogenic agent.
Study page 261.

Cigarette smoking is carcinogenic and remains the most important cause of cancer. The risk is greatest in those who begin to smoke when young and continue throughout life. Cigarette smoking accounts for one of every five deaths each year in the United States. Tobacco use is also associated with squamous and small cell adenocarcinomas. In addition, smoking causes even more deaths from vascular, respiratory, and other diseases than from cancer. Smoking tobacco is linked to cancers of the lower urinary tract, upper digestive tract, paranasal sinuses, liver, kidney, pancreas, cervix, uterus, and myeloid leukemia.

Secondhand smoke, also called *environmental tobacco smoke (ETS)*, is the combination of sidestream smoke (burning end of a cigarette, cigar, or pipe) and mainstream smoke (exhaled by the smoker). More than 4000 chemicals have been identified in mainstream tobacco smoke (250 chemicals as toxic), of which 60 are considered carcinogenic. Nonsmokers who live with smokers are at greatest risk for lung cancer as well as numerous noncancerous conditions.

5. Relate diet and obesity to carcinogenesis.
Review pages 261, 262 and 264-266; refer to Figures 10-3 through 10-6 and Table 10-6.

People are constantly exposed to a variety of compounds termed *xenobiotics* that include toxic, mutagenic, and carcinogenic chemicals. Many of these chemicals are found in the human **diet.** These chemicals can react with cellular macromolecules, such as proteins and DNA, or can react directly with cell structures to cause cell damage. The body has two defense systems for counteracting these effects: (1) detoxification enzymes and (2) antioxidant systems. Enzymes that activate xenobiotics are called *phase I activation enzymes* and are represented by the multigene cytochrome P450 family, aldehyde oxidase, xanthine oxidases, and peroxidases. *Phase II detoxification enzymes* then protect further against a large array of reactive intermediates and nonactivated xenobiotics. These enzymes are located predominantly in the liver and provide clearance of compounds through the portal circulation, thereby preventing the potentially carcinogenic agent(s) from entering the body through the gastrointestinal tract and portal circulation.

The most relevant carcinogens produced by cooking are the polycyclic aromatic hydrocarbons and heterocyclic aromatic amines generated by meat protein. The greatest levels are found in well-done, charbroiled beef. People also ingest xenobiotics that are found in environmental or industrial contaminants such as the particulate matter of diesel exhaust, contaminating pesticides in food and water supplies, and in certain prescribed and over-the-counter medicines.

Specific nutrients may directly affect the *phenotype* or expression of key genes, for example, epigenetically through abnormalities of methylation of the promoter regions of genes or histones. DNA also can be hypomethylated. *Hypomethylation* can cause overexpression of the transcription of proto-oncogenes, increased recombination and mutation, and loss of imprinting. These alterations can all promote cancer. Aberrant DNA methylation patterns occur in colon, lung, prostate, and breast cancers. Dietary factors may be related to DNA methylation in four ways: (1) they may influence the supply of methyl groups; (2) they may modify the use of methyl groups; (3) they may reduce methyl groups called demethylation; and (4) DNA methylation patterns may influence the response to a dietary factor.

Because **obesity** is associated with other chronic diseases, such as cardiovascular disease and diabetes, it can increase overall mortality; however, it may not be the causal factor involved in cancer mortality. Yet, obesity is related to increased incidence of several cancer types. Compared with men whose *body mass index (BMI)* was in the normal range (18.5 to 24.9), men with substantial obesity (BMI > 40.0) were found to have significant increases in cancer mortality. In men with higher BMI, there were higher rates of death from esophageal, stomach, colorectal, liver, gallbladder, pancreatic, prostate, and kidney cancers as well as non-Hodgkin lymphoma, multiple myeloma, and leukemia. Among women, high BMI was correlated with greater morbidity from colorectal, liver, gallbladder, pancreatic, breast, uterine, cervical, ovarian, and kidney cancers, non-Hodgkin lymphoma, and multiple myeloma.

Abdominal obesity, as defined by waist circumference or waist/hip ratio, has been shown to be more strongly related to some tumor types than obesity as defined by BMI. Possible associated mechanisms include insulin resistance and resultant chronic hyperinsulinemia as well as increased insulin-like growth factors (IGFs), steroid hormones, tissue-derived hormones, and cytokines (adipokines) or inflammatory mediators.

Adiposity influences the synthesis and bioavailability of *endogenous sex steroids*, the estrogens, progesterone, and androgens. Three mechanisms are involved: (First, adipose tissue expresses various sex-steroid metabolizing enzymes that promote the formation of estrogens from androgenic precursors secreted by the gonads and adrenal glands. Second, *adipose* cells increase the circulating levels of insulin and increase IGF biologic activity. Third, *high insulin levels* can increase ovarian and, possibly, adrenal androgen synthesis and, in some genetically susceptible premenopausal women, cause the development of polycystic ovary syndrome. Adiposity-induced alterations in blood levels of sex steroids explain the correlation noted between indices of excess weight and risks of postmenopausal breast cancer and endometrium cancer.

For breast and endometrial cancers, a central role of estrogens and progesterone is established from a large body of experimental and clinical evidence. These sex steroids are important regulators of cellular proliferation, differentiation, and apoptosis. Among men, prostate carcinogenesis is thought to be related to endogenous hormone metabolism.

Chronically increased insulin levels have been correlated with the pathogenesis of colon, breast, pancreatic, and endometrial cancers. These cancer-causing effects of insulin might be mediated by insulin receptors in the preneoplastic or neoplastic target cells or could be due to alterations in endogenous hormone metabolism secondary to hyperinsulinemia. Excess body weight and a high plasma level of C-peptide both predispose men to prostate cancer and to a greater likelihood of dying from their disease.

6. Relate alcohol consumption to carcinogenesis.
Review pages 266 and 267.

Chronic **alcohol consumption** is a strong risk factor for cancer of the oral cavity, pharynx, hypopharynx, larynx, esophagus, and liver. Breast carcinogenesis can be enhanced with relatively low daily amounts of alcohol. Alcohol interacts with smoke, raising the risk of malignant tumors, possibly by acting as a solvent for the carcinogenic chemicals in smoke products. Carcinogenic promotion may occur because of the generation of reactive oxygen species (ROS), increased procarcinogenic activation (nitrosamines), and nutritional deficiencies that alter mucosal integrity, metabolic function, and structure.

7. Identify the carcinogenic risks to individuals of ionizing, ultraviolet, and electromagnetic radiation exposure.
Review pages 267, 268, and 270-277; refer to Figures 10-7 through 10-13 and Table 10-7.

Ionizing radiation (IR) is a mutagen and carcinogen; it can penetrate cells and tissues and deposit energy in tissues at random in the form of ionization, which excites or removes an electron from the target atom. These ionizations can lead to irreversible damage or indirect damage from formation and attack by water-based free radicals. IR affects many cell processes, including gene expression, disruption of mitochondrial function, cell cycle arrest, and cell death. IR is a potent DNA damaging agent that causes cross-linking, nucleotide base damage, and single- and double-strand breaks. Damage to DNA and disrupted cellular regulation processes can lead to carcinogenesis. The double-strand break (DSB) is considered the characteristic lesion observed for the effects of IR. DSBs are mostly repaired by the nonhomologous end joining (NHEJ) pathway. This pathway is efficient for joining the DNA broken ends; however, errors can occur. Irradiated human cells unable to execute the NHEJ are supersensitive to the introduction of large-scale mutations and chromosomal aberrations.

It is known that radiation may induce a type of *genomic instability* in the progeny of the directly irradiated cells over many generations of cell irradiation. The instability leads to an increased rate of mutations/chromosomal aberrations in these distant progeny. This process is called *transgeneration effects.* In addition, the directly irradiated cells can lead to genetic effects in *bystander cells* or innocent cells, even though these latter cells received no direct radiation exposure. The bystander and genomic instability effects also have been termed "*nontargeted*" *effects.* Although bystander and transgeneration IR effects are associated with induced genomic instability leading to chromosome aberrations, gene mutations, late cell death, and aneuploidy, all of these effects may be epigenetically mediated. The epigenetic changes include DNA methylation, histone modification, and RNA-associated silencing. Bystander effects are considered manifestations of a radiation-induced genomic instability. These effects could lead to a "hypelinearity" response—that is, a higher level of risk per unit dose. Oxidizing mediators increase the expression of proteins involved in *gap junction intercellular communication (GJIC).* Some data support a role for *oxidative* stress and GJIC in radiation-induced bystander effects.

Ultraviolet radiation (UVR) can emanate from both natural and artificial sources; however, the principal source of exposure for most people is sunlight. UVR is now known to cause specific gene mutations; for example, squamous cell carcinoma involves mutation in the *p53* gene, basal cell carcinoma in the *patched* gene, and melanoma in the *p16* gene. The development of melanoma is associated with the loss of E-cadherin and the appearance of N-cadherin adhesion molecules. UV light induces the release of tumor necrosis factor (TNF) in the epidermis, which may reduce immune surveillance against skin cancer. Skin exposure to UVR and IR, as well as xenobiotic agents or drugs, produces *ROS* in large quantities that can overwhelm tissue antioxidants and other oxygen-degrading pathways.

Antioxidants decrease ROS and oxidative stress and other protective mechanisms, including DNA repair and apoptosis. UVR activates free radicals important in regulating genes that induce inflammation; inflammation is critical for tumor progression. A point mutation in the *B-raf* (BRAF) proto-oncogene increases BRAF kinase, which activates the mitogen-activated protein kinase pathway.

Health risks associated with **electromagnetic radiation** (EMR) are controversial. Exposure to electric and magnetic fields is widespread. EMRs are a type of nonionizing, low-frequency radiation without enough energy to break off electrons from their orbits around atoms and ionize the atoms. Microwaves, radar, and power frequency radiation associated with electricity and radio waves, fluorescent lights, computers, and other electric equipment all create EMRs of varying strength. A meta-analysis found a consistent pattern of an increased risk for acoustic neuroma and glioma in individuals using cell phones for more than 10 years.

Increasing evidence has indicated that the mechanism of harm from EMR involves induction of cell stress and damage to intracellular components, free radical formation, and altered protein conformation. Adverse EMR has been reported to affect DNA synthesis and alter cell division, electrical charge of ions, and molecules within cells.

8. Identify behaviors and environment agent exposures associated with carcinogenesis.
Study pages 277, 278, and 281; refer to Boxes 10-4 through 10-6.

Sexually transmitted infection with carcinogenic types of human papilloma virus (HPV), referred to as *high-risk types of HPV,* causes most cervical cancers. In addition, HPV is an identified causal factor for oral pharyngeal cancers. HPV infections, however, are very common in sexually active women, and the majority of these infections resolve or cause only transient, minor problems. One hundred HPV types have been sequenced, 30 of which infect both the female and male genital tracts; two thirds of these 30 are classified as high-risk types. **HPV-16,** in most countries, accounts for 50% to 60% of cervical cancer cases, followed by HPV-18 (10%-12%). HPV types correlated with genital warts, HPV-6 and HPV-11, are called low risk because they are rarely associated with cancer.

For colon cancer, **physical activity** increases gut motility, which reduces the length of time (transit time) that the bowel lining is exposed to potential mutagens. For breast cancer, vigorous physical activity may decrease exposure of breast tissue to ovarian hormones, insulin, and *insulin-like factor.* A randomized trial found that after 12 months of moderate-intensity exercise, postmenopausal women had significantly decreased serum estrogens. Physical activity also helps prevent type 2 diabetes, which has been associated with risk of cancer of the colon and pancreas.

One notable **occupational factor** is *asbestos*, which increases the risk of mesothelioma and lung cancer. Carcinoma of the bladder has been linked with the manufacture of dyes, rubber, paint, and aromatic amines. *Benzol inhalation* is linked to leukemia in shoemakers and in workers in the rubber cement, explosives, and dyeing industries. Other notable occupational hazards include high-nickel alloy, chromium VI compounds, inorganic arsenic, silica, polycyclic aromatic hydrocarbons, sulfuric acid, and chloromethyl ether. Studies of occupational exposure to **diesel exhaust** indicate an increased risk of lung cancer.

Air pollution can be carcinogenic. A person inhales about 20,000 L of air in 1 day; thus, even modest contamination of the atmosphere can result in inhalation of appreciable doses of pollutants. Contaminants include outdoor and indoor air pollutants. Concerns include *industrial emissions*, including arsenicals, benzene, chloroform, formaldehyde, sulfuric acid, mustard gas, vinyl chloride, and acrylonitrile. Living close to certain industries is a recognized cancer risk factor. Indoor pollution generally is considered worse than outdoor pollution, partly because of cigarette smoke. *Environmental tobacco smoke (ETS)* can cause the formation of reactive oxygen free radicals and, thus, DNA damage. *Radon* is a natural radioactive gas derived from the radioactive decay of uranium that is ubiquitous in rock and soil; it can become trapped in houses and gives rise to radioactive decay products known to be carcinogenic to humans. The most hazardous houses can be identified by testing and then modified to prevent further radon contamination. Exposure levels are greater from underground mines than from houses. Most of the lung cancers associated with radon are bronchogenic; however, small cell carcinoma does occur with greater frequency in underground miners. Strong evidence indicates a higher risk of bladder, skin, and lung cancers after consumption of water with high levels of *arsenic*.

PRACTICE EXAMINATION

Fill in the Blank

1. Preventing exposure to ____________________ can prevent many cancers.

2. The expression of ____________________ is linked to carcinogenesis because they can act as either oncogenes or tumor-suppressor genes.

3. ____________________ is the ability to develop in a particular way depending on the environment.

4. ____________________ is a combination of sidestream and mainstream smoke.

5. ____________________ include toxic, mutagenic, and carcinogenic chemicals.

6. The most relevant carcinogens produced by cooking

   are generated by ____________________ proteins.

7. ____________________ can cause loss of imprinting.

8. ____________________ increase the circulating levels of insulin.

9. Exposure to asbestos increases the risk for

______________________.

10. Prolonged exposure to UVR increases the risk for

______________________.

11. An inhaled chemical within the dyeing industry linked to leukemia is ______________________.

12. At the cellular level, cancer is

______________________.

13. IR causes mutation to clonal progeny and to

______________________.

14. UVR induces the release of

______________________, which may reduce immune surveillance.

15. Enzymes that activate xenobiotics are known as

______________________.

16. Among men, prostate carcinogenesis is related to production of ______________________.

17. Higher ______________________ is associated with gastrointestinal, reproductive, renal, and lymphoid cancers.

18. ______________________ changes are mitotically and meiotically heritable.

19. Estrogen and progesterone play a central role in ______________________ and ______________________ cancers.

20. The double-strand break is considered the characteristic affected by

______________________.

21. ROS in large quantities can overwhelm ______________________ and ______________________ pathways.

22. ______________________ can silence tumor-suppressor genes.

23. The phenotypic effects of epigenetic modification during development require ______________________ before manifesting in later life.

24. ______________________ accounts for 50% to 60% of cervical cancer.

25. ______________________ is derived from radioactive decay of uranium, can be trapped in homes, and is carcinogenic to humans.

Complete the following table comparing foods that may increase or decrease the risk of cancer development:

Possible Carcinogenic/Noncarcinogenic Foods

Increase Risk of Cancer	Decrease Risk of Cancer

11 Cancer in Children

FOUNDATIONAL OBJECTIVES

a. Describe mechanisms that regulate cellular reproduction and differentiation and determine their specific anatomical site selection.
Review Foundational Objectives in Chapter 9.

LEARNING OBJECTIVES

After studying this chapter, the learner will be able to do the following:

1. Describe the incidence and types of childhood cancers.
Study pages 288 and 289; refer to Tables 11-1 and 11-2.

An analysis of cancer incidence rates for children 0 to 19 years of age by primary site for all types of childhood cancers was completed for the period 1999 through 2006. The statistics showed rates per 100,000 individuals. For Caucasian children, the incidence was 18.7, for African-American children, it was12.9, and for Hispanic children, it was 18.0.

Most childhood cancers originate from the *mesodermal germ layer* that gives rise to connective tissue, bone, cartilage, muscle, blood and blood vessels, gonads, kidney, and the lymphatic system. Thus, the more common childhood cancers are leukemias, sarcomas, and embryonic tumors. *Embryonic tumors* originate during intrauterine life and contain immature tissue unable to mature or differentiate into functional cells. Embryonic tumors are diagnosed early, usually by 5 years of age.

Carcinomas rarely occur in children because these cancers usually result from environmental carcinogens and *require a long time from exposure to the appearance* of the lesion. However, epithelial tumors begin to increase between the ages 15 and 19 years and become the most common cancer type after adolescence.

The most common malignancy in children is leukemia, accounting for more than one third of childhood cancers. The second most common group is cancers of the nervous system, primarily brain lesions. All other pediatric malignancies occur much less often. *Neuroblastoma* is a tumor of the sympathetic nervous system. *Wilms tumor* is a malignancy of the kidney; its histologic name is nephroblastoma. *Rhabdomyosarcoma* is a soft tissue sarcoma of striated muscle. Two major bone tumors, *osteosarcoma* and *Ewing sarcoma*, occur in children.

Childhood cancers usually are diagnosed during peak times of growth and maturation. In general, they are extremely *fast-growing cancers*. Many childhood cancers have a peak incidence before the child is 5 years of age. Among these are the leukemias, neuroblastoma, Wilms tumor, and retinoblastoma. Central nervous system tumors are more common in children younger than 15 years. Bone tumors, soft tissue sarcomas, and lymphomas are more likely to occur in children between 15 and 19 years of age.

2. Describe the genetic etiologic factors for childhood cancers.
Study pages 289 and 290; refer to Tables 11-3 and 11-4.

Some environmental and host factors predispose a child to cancer, but causal factors have not been established for most childhood cancers. Many host factors are genetic risk factors or congenital conditions. Childhood cancer most likely can be attributed to the complex interaction of *both genetic and environmental factors*.

Genetic factors may involve chromosome aberrations, single-gene defects, or chromosome abnormalities, including aneuploidy, deletions, translocations, and fragility. Some congenital malformations and syndromes herald the onset of pediatric malignancies. One of the more recognized syndromes is the association of *Down syndrome with an increased susceptibility to acute leukemia*. For children with this syndrome, the risk for development of leukemia is 10 to 20 times greater during the first 10 years of life than the risk is in healthy children.

Wilms tumor is particularly recognized for its association with a number of genitourinary malformations, congenital absence of the iris of the eye, and muscular overgrowth of half of the body or face. Approximately 10% of children diagnosed with Wilms tumor demonstrate one of these abnormalities. Wilms tumor *genes—WT1, WT2, and WTC*—have been found. *Retinoblastoma,* a malignant embryonic tumor of the eye, occurs as an inherited defect or as an acquired mutation of the retinoblastoma gene, the *RBI* gene. Single-gene defects have been associated with the subsequent development of childhood tumors. Two autosomal recessive diseases involving increased chromosomal fragility, *Fanconi anemia* and *Bloom syndrome*, are risk factors predisposing to acute lymphocytic leukemia.

The relative *ineffectiveness of the immune surveillance system during intrauterine life* may explain the occurrence of embryonic tumors. During rapid proliferation and differentiation of cells in the developing fetus, cell mutation could result in embryonic tumors.

A few malignancies seem to demonstrate a *familial tendency* because these specific cancers cluster in particular families. A child who has a sibling with leukemia has a risk for leukemia that is two to four times greater than that for a child with a normal sibling. The occurrence of leukemia in monozygous twins is estimated as being as high as 25%.

In families with *Li-Fraumeni syndrome (LFS),* an autosomal dominant disorder involving the *TP53* tumor suppressor gene, the risk for development of cancer in childhood or adulthood is significantly higher than that in the unaffected population. Individuals in these families are at risk for soft tissue sarcoma, breast cancer, leukemia, osteosarcoma, melanoma, and cancer of the colon, pancreas, adrenal cortex, and brain.

3. Describe environmental factors for childhood cancer.
Study page 291; refer to Table 11-5.

Prenatal exposures *to some drugs and to ionizing radiation* have been linked to subsequent cancers. Perhaps the best-known such drug is diethylstilbestrol (DES), a drug taken to avert early abortion. *DES is a transplacental chemical carcinogen.* Adenocarcinoma of the vagina has developed in a small percentage of the daughters of mothers who took DES while pregnant.

Childhood exposures to drugs, ionizing radiation, and viruses have been implicated as risk factors for specific cancers. Drugs implicated include: (1) anabolic androgenic steroids, which are used in the treatment of aplastic anemia or used illegally by teenaged athletes for body development and have been associated with subsequent hepatocellular carcinoma; (2) cytotoxic agents used in the treatment of pediatric cancers, which may predispose a child to leukemia in later years; and (3) immunosuppressive agents, particularly those used for transplantation, which have been shown to increase the risk for lymphoma. In children, the strongest viral carcinogenic relationship is between the Epstein-Barr virus and Burkitt lymphoma, nasopharyngeal carcinoma, and Hodgkin disease. Children with AIDS have an increased risk of non-Hodgkin lymphoma and Kaposi sarcoma.

4. Indicate the prognosis for childhood cancers.
Study pages 291 and 292.

More than 70% of children diagnosed with cancer can now be expected to survive for 5 years or more. Estimates indicate that these survivors are at *increased risk for a second cancer* because of their *previous exposure to cancer therapy* and, possibly, their genetic constitution. Overall, children have a more favorable prognosis than adults. Children appear to be *more responsive to available treatments* and are better able to tolerate the immediate side effects of therapies.

Some of the factors in the improvement in cure rates in pediatric oncology are the use of combination chemotherapy, multimodal treatment for childhood solid tumors, improvement in supportive care, and development of research centers for childhood treatment.

Even those cancers that cannot be cured can be treated, resulting in significant quality time. Cured children do face *residual and late effects* of treatment. These late effects are more significant in children than in adults because childhood treatment occurs in a physically immature, growing individual.

Indicate some differences between childhood and adult cancers.
Study all chapter pages and tables.

The incidence for adult cancers is much higher than that for childhood cancers. A much greater environmental and lifestyle causation relationship is found in adult than in childhood cancers. In childhood cancers, the origin is connective tissue; in adult cancers, it is epithelial tissue. Toxic side effects of treatment in children seem less than those in adults, but long-term consequences are more significant in children than adults. The prognosis is better for children than adults.

PRACTICE EXAMINATION

True/False:

1. Childhood cancers are more common than adult cancers.
2. Childhood cancers have a strong relationship to environmental agents.
3. There is an association between the gene *N-myc* and neuroblastoma.
4. Childhood cancers involve tissues more than organs.
5. Childhood cancers involve epithelial cells more often than connective tissue cells.
6. There is an association between the gene *WTC* and Wilms tumor.
7. There is an association between the gene *ATM* and leukemia.
8. Among childhood cancers in Caucasian children, lymphoma has the highest incidence.
9. Childhood cancers have more long-term consequences than adult cancers.
10. Childhood cancers have a better prognosis than adult cancers.

Matching

Match the syndrome/disorder with the risk factor:

_______ 11. Down syndrome

_______ 12. Wilms tumor

_______ 13. Retinoblastoma

_______ 14. Fanconi anemia

_______ 15. Vaginal adenocarcinoma

_______ 16. Li-Fraumeni syndrome

a. *Rb1* gene
b. DES
c. *TP53* gene
d. nonlymphocytic leukemia
e. acute leukemia
f. congenital absence of iris of the eye

True/False

17. Most childhood cancers originate from the mesoderm.

18. Embryonic tumors are diagnosed during teenage years.

19. Carcinomas are prevalent before adolescence.

20. Cancer is more common in Caucasian than in African-American children.

21. The overall incidences of cancer are nearly equal in Caucasian and Hispanic children.

22. Fewer than 50% of children diagnosed with cancer can expect to survive for 5 years.

23. Cured children face few residual and late effects from their therapy.

Fill in the Blank

Complete the following table identifying childhood cancer groupings and some possible associated gene groupings:

Childhood Cancers and Their Associated Genes

Cancer	Oncogenes	Tumor-Suppressor Genes

12 Structure and Function of the Neurologic System

FOUNDATIONAL OBJECTIVES

After reviewing this chapter, the learner will be able to do the following:

1. **Identify the structural and functional subdivisions of the nervous system.**
   Review page 293.

2. **Compare the functions of neurons with those of neuroglia; identify the parts of neurons.**
   Review pages 293-296; refer to Figures 12-1 through 12-3 and Table 12-1.

3. **Describe the circumstances under which nervous tissue can regenerate.**
   Review page 297; refer to Figure 12-4.

4. **Describe transmission of impulses by neurotransmitters.**
   Review page 297 and 298; refer to Figures 12-2 and Table 12-2.

5. **Identify the three main divisions of the brain; characterize their associated structures and functions.**
   Review pages 299, 301, 303, and 304; refer to Figures 12-5 through 12-9 and Table 12-3.

6. **Identify the significance of contralateral control of motor fibers.**
   Review page 301; refer to Figure 12-8.

7. **Describe the location and structure of the spinal cord; define reflex arc.**
   Review pages 304-307; refer to Figures 12-10 through 12-14.

8. **Identify the structures responsible for maintaining and protecting the central nervous system.**
   Review pages 307-309; refer to Figures 12-15 through 12-17 and Table 12-4.

9. **Identify the route of blood circulation within the central nervous system; note the significance of the circle of Willis.**
   Review pages 310, 311, and 313; refer to Figures 12-18 through 12-23 and Table 12-5.

10. **Describe the structure of cranial and spinal nerves; locate plexuses.**
    Review pages 311-313; refer to Figure 12-24.

11. **Name the cranial nerves and state functions of each.**
    Refer to Table 12-6.

12. **Identify the subdivisions of the autonomic nervous system, their origins, and their general functions.**
    Review pages 313 and 316; refer to Figures 12-25 through 12-27.

13. **Identify the type of neurotransmitter secreted by preganglionic and postganglionic fibers in the autonomic nervous system.**
    Review pages 317, 320, and 321; refer to Figures 12-28 and 12-29 and Table 12-7.

14. **Identify the structural, cellular, vascular, and functional changes that occur with aging.**
    Review page 302.

PRACTICE EXAMINATION

Multiple Choice

Circle the correct answer for each question:

1. One function of the somatic nervous system that is *not* performed by the autonomic nervous system is conduction of impulses:
   a. to involuntary muscles and glands.
   b. to the central nervous system.
   c. to skeletal muscles.
   d. between the brain and spinal cord.

2. A neuron with a single dendrite at one end of the cell body and a single axon at the other end of the cell body would be classified as:
   a. unipolar.
   b. multipolar.
   c. monopolar.
   d. bipolar.

3. Neurons that carry impulses away from the CNS are called:
   a. afferent neurons.
   b. sensory neurons.
   c. efferent neurons.
   d. association neurons.

4. Neurons are specialized for the conduction of impulses, whereas neuroglia:
   a. support nerve tissue.
   b. serve as motor end plates.
   c. synthesize acetylcholine and cholinesterase.
   d. All of the above are correct.

5. There is one-way conduction at a synapse because:
   a. only postsynaptic neurons contain synaptic vesicles.
   b. acetylcholine prevents nerve impulses from traveling in both directions.
   c. only the presynaptic neuron contains neurotransmitters.
   d. only dendrites release neurotransmitters.

6. Which contains the thalamus and hypothalamus?
   a. diencephalon
   b. cerebrum
   c. medulla oblongata
   d. brain stem

7. The reticular activating system:
   a. programs for fine repetitive motor movements.
   b. maintains wakefulness.
   c. maintains constant internal environments.
   d. affects the positioning of the head to improve hearing.

8. Which phrases best describe the spinal cord? (More than one answer may be correct.)
   a. descends inferior to the lumbar vertebrae
   b. conducts motor impulses from the brain
   c. descends to the fourth lumbar vertebra
   d. conducts sensory impulses to the brain

9. Which is *not* a protective covering of the CNS?
   a. cauda equine
   b. dura mater
   c. arachnoid
   d. cranial bone

10. The composition of cerebrospinal fluid is:
    a. the same as blood.
    b. distilled H_2O with dissolved salts.
    c. a plasma-like liquid with glucose, salts, and proteins.
    d. a heavy mucous solution with dissolved salts, glucose, and urea.

11. An autonomic ganglion can be described as:
    a. the site of synapses between visceral efferent neurons.
    b. a site where spinal reflexes occur.
    c. a point of synapse between parasympathetic and sympathetic neurons.
    d. the place where unconscious sensations occur.

12. The sympathetic division of the autonomic nervous system:
    a. mobilizes energy in times of need.
    b. is innervated by cell bodies from T1 through L2.
    c. is innervated by cell bodies located in the cranial nerve nuclei.
    d. Both a and b are correct.
    e. Both a and c are correct.

13. The parasympathetic division of the autonomic nervous system:
    a. conserves and stores energy.
    b. has relatively short postganglionic neurons.
    c. Both a and b are correct.
    d. has paravertebral ganglia.

Matching

Match the structure with its function or description:

_______ 14. Schwann cell

_______ 15. Dendrite

a. is the outer, nucleated layer of a certain cell type
b. produces a myelin sheath
c. carries impulses away from the perikaryon
d. covers neuron fibers
e. conducts impulses to cell body

Match the component of a reflex arc with its descriptor:

_______ 16. Sensory neuron

_______ 17. Effector

a. carries impulses to the CNS
b. carries impulses to a responding organ
c. responds to motor impulse
d. is stimulated by one neuron and passes impulse on to another neuron
e. responds directly to changes in environment

Match the function with the cranial nerve:

_______ 18. Tasting

_______ 19. Balance maintenance

a. facial
b. olfactory
c. vestibulocochlear
d. hypoglossal
e. optic

Match the characteristic with the related division of the autonomic nervous system:

_______ 20. More extensive use of norepinephrine as a transmitter substance

_______ 21. More widespread and generalized effects

_______ 22. Elicits rest-response

a. sympathetic
b. parasympathetic

Match the effect of sympathetic nerve stimulation with the structure:

_______ 23. Breathing passageways

_______ 24. Intestines

_______ 25. Liver

a. increases diameter
b. decreases diameter
c. increases activity
d. decreases activity

Complete the following table comparing adrenergic responses to cholinergic responses:

Responses of Selected Effector Organs to Automatic Nerve Impulses

Effector	Receptor	Adrenergic Response	Cholinergic Response
Eye			
Radial muscle, iris	δ		—
Sphincter muscle, iris	β_1	—	
Heart			
SA node	β_1	Increases heart rate	
Ventricles	β_1		—
Arterioles			
Pulmonary	δ, β_2		—
Skeletal muscle	δ, β_2		—
Cerebral	δ		—
Lung			
Bronchial muscle	β_2		
Adrenal medulla	—	—	

13 Pain, Temperature, Sleep, and Sensory Function

FOUNDATIONAL OBJECTIVES

a. Describe the neuroanatomy of pain and its neuromodulation.
Review pages 325-327; refer to Figures 13-1 through 13-3 and Table 13-1.

MEMORY CHECK!

- Pain receptors, also known as **nociceptors**, are small unmyelinated and lightly myelinated nerve endings of afferent neurons found in nearly every tissue in the body. These neurons respond to chemical, thermal, and mechanical stimuli. Sensory nerves transmit the stimuli from pain receptors into the dorsal horn of the spinal cord. The impulses ascend by either the neospinothalamic tract or the paleospinothalamic tract. The paleospinothalamic tract carries information to the midbrain and is responsible for reflex responses to pain, thus changing autonomic function. The neospinothalamic tract carries information to the lateral thalamus and then projects to the cortex, where precision and discrimination occur. Afferent stimulation of the ventromedial medulla and periaqueductal gray matter in the midbrain stimulates efferent pathways, which modify or inhibit afferent signals to the dorsal horn.
- According to the **gate control theory**, nociceptive impulses are transmitted from specialized skin receptors to the spinal cord through large A delta and small C fibers. These fibers terminate in the dorsal horn of the spinal cord. Cells in the substantia gelatinosa of the dorsal horn function as a gate and permit some impulses to reach the central nervous system for interpretation. Stimulation of larger, faster-transmitting fibers causes the cells in the substantia gelatinosa to "close the gate," which diminishes pain perception. Pain perception occurs primarily in the limbic systems and the cerebral cortex. Slower-transmitting small-fiber input inhibits cells in the substantia gelatinosa and "opens the gate," enhancing pain perception. In addition to gate control through stimulation of large and small fibers, the central nervous system, through its efferent pathways, may close, partially close, or open the gate. The **sensory-discriminative system** is mediated by the somatosensory cortex and identifies the presence, character, location, and intensity of the pain. The **affective-motivational system** determines conditioned avoidance behaviors and emotional response to pain. **Pain modulation** increases or decreases the transmission of pain throughout the nervous system. This gate control theory does not explain chronic pain problems such as phantom limb pain. The **neuromatrix theory of pain** proposes that in the absence of discernable causes for chronic pain, the brain produces nerve impulses triggered from the periphery or they originate independently within the brain.
- Tissue injury and chronic inflammation result in the release of prostaglandins and lymphokines, which trigger the release of neuromodulators that mediate information about painful stimuli. These neuromodulators include *substance P, calcitonin gene–related peptide, norepinephrine,* and *5-hydroxytryptamine (serotonin).*
- **Endorphins** (endogenous morphines) are neuropeptides that inhibit transmission of pain impulses in the spinal cord and brain. All endorphins attach to opiate receptors on the plasma membrane of the afferent neuron. The combination of the opiate receptor and endorphin inhibits the release of excitatory neurotransmitters, thereby blocking the transmission of the painful stimulus.

b. Describe thermoregulation.
Review pages 330 and 331; refer to Table 13-5.

- The control of body temperature is a function of centers located in the **hypothalamus. Thermoreceptors** provide the hypothalamus with information about peripheral and core temperatures. If the temperature is low, the body initiates heat conservation measures by a series of hormonal mechanisms. Heat production begins with the hypothalamic release of thyroid-stimulating hormone (TSH) from the anterior pituitary. The TSH causes the release of thyroxine from the thyroid gland. This hormone causes the release of epinephrine from the adrenal medulla. *Epinephrine* causes *vasoconstriction,* glycolysis, and increased metabolic rates, which increase heat production. Warmer peripheral and core temperatures reverse the process. Decreasing the sympathetic pathway produces *vasodilation,* decreased muscle tone, and increased perspiration.
- Because of their greater body surface/mass ratio and decreased subcutaneous fat, infants do not conserve heat well. Elderly individuals have poor responses to environmental temperature extremes as a result of slowed blood circulation, changes in the skin, and an overall decrease in heat-producing activities.

c. Identify the normal sleep stages; describe nervous system control of sleep.
Review pages 333 and 334.

- Several areas of the brain process are associated with sleep and sleep-awake cycles. A small group of hypothalamic nerve cells, the **suprachiasmatic nucleus (SCN),** controls the timing of the sleep-wake cycle and coordinates this cycle with the circadian rhythms (24 hours rhythm cycles) in other areas of the brain and other tissues. Normal sleep has two phases that can be documented by electroencephalography (EEG): *rapid eye movement (REM) sleep* and *non-REM (slow-wave) sleep.*
- REM and non-REM sleep succeed each other in 90- to 120-minute intervals. Four to six cycles occur during a normal sleep period based on changes in the EEG pattern. Non-REM sleep is initiated by the withdrawal of neurotransmitters from the reticular formation and by the inhibition of arousal mechanisms. The *restorative, reparative,* and *growth processes occur during slow-wave sleep.* Altering periods of REM and NREM occur through the night, with lengthening intervals of REM and fewer intervals of the deeper stages of non-REM toward the morning. Many neurotransmitters are associated with excitatory and inhibitory sleep patterns. Sleep promoting neurotransmitters include prostaglandin D, 1-tryptophan, serotonin, adenosine, melatonin, GABA, and growth hormones. Awake-promoting neurotransmitters include hypocretin, acetylcholine, and glutamate. The pontine reticular formation is primarily responsible for generating REM sleep. Projections from the reticular formation and other areas of the mesencephalon and brainstem produce non-REM sleep. The sleep patterns of the newborn and young child vary from those of the adult in total sleep time, cycle length, and percentage of time spent in each sleep cycle. Sleep for infants and children is important for growth and neurocognitive development. Elderly individuals experience a total decrease in time.

d. Describe the eye and its structure.
Review page 335; refer to Figures 13-6 through 13-8.

MEMORY CHECK!

- Three layers form the wall of the eye: the sclera, choroid, and retina. It becomes transparent at the cornea in the central anterior region, which allows light to enter the eye. The choroid is the pigmented middle layer that prevents light from scattering inside the eye. The iris, part of the choroid, has a round opening, the pupil, through which light passes.
- The innermost layer of the eye, the retina, contains the rods and cones. These photoreceptors convert light energy into nerve impulses.
- Nerve impulses pass through the optic nerves to the optic chiasm. Nerves from the nasal halves of the retinas cross and join fibers from the temporal halves of the retinas to form the optic tracts. The optic tracts connect to the primary visual cortex in the occipital lobe of the brain. Light entering the eye is focused on the retina by the lens, which is a flexible, biconvex, crystal-like structure. The lens separates the anterior cavity from the vitreous chamber. The aqueous humor of the anterior cavity helps maintain pressure inside the eye and provides nutrients to the lens and the cornea. The vitreous chamber is filled with a gel-like vitreous humor that prevents the eyeball from collapsing inward.
- Six extrinsic eye muscles allow gross eye movements and permit eyes to follow a moving object. The external structures protecting the eye include the eyelids, conjunctiva, and lacrimal apparatus.

e. Describe the parts of the ear.
Review pages 338-340; refer to Figures 13-11 and 13-12.

MEMORY CHECK!

- The ear is divided into three areas: the external ear, involved only with hearing; the middle ear, involved only with hearing; and the inner ear, involved with hearing and equilibrium.
- The external ear is composed of the pinna, which is visible, and the external auditory canal that leads to the middle ear. Sound waves entering the external auditory canal cause the tympanic membrane to vibrate. This membrane separates the external ear from the middle ear.
- The middle ear is composed of the tympanic cavity within the temporal bone. Three ossicles transmit the vibration of the tympanic membrane to the inner ear and set the fluids of the inner ear in motion.
- The inner ear is a system of osseous labyrinths filled with perilymph. The bony labyrinth is divided into the cochlea, the vestibule, and the semicircular canals.
- Sound waves that reach the cochlea through vibrations of the tympanic membrane, ossicles, and oval window set the cochlear fluids in motion. Receptor cells on the basilar membrane are stimulated and transmit impulses along the cochlear nerve, a division of the vestibulocochlear nerve, to the auditory cortex of the temporal lobe for sound interpretation.
- The semicircular canals and vestibule of the inner ear contain equilibrium receptors. In the semicircular canals, the dynamic equilibrium receptors respond to changes in direction of movement. The vestibule in the inner ear contains receptors essential to the body's sense of static equilibrium. Both of these impulses are transmitted through the vestibular nerve, a division of the vestibulocochlear nerve, to the cerebellum.

LEARNING OBJECTIVES

After studying this chapter, the learner will be able to do the following:

1. Describe clinical categories of pain; characterize pain threshold and pain tolerance.
Study pages 327-329; refer to Figure 13-4 and Tables 13-2 through 13-4.

Somatogenic pain is pain with an identifiable cause. **Psychogenic pain** is pain without a known physical cause. "Pain perception is real and is best acknowledged as what the affected individual says it is."

Acute pain may be somatic, visceral, or referred. **Somatic pain** comes from the skin or close to the surface of the body and is well localized. **Visceral pain** occurs in internal organs, the abdomen, or skeleton. It is poorly localized. It is associated with nausea and vomiting, hypotension, restlessness, and possible shock. Visceral pain often radiates or is referred. **Referred pain** is present in an area removed or distant from its point of origin. The area of referred pain is supplied by the same spinal segment as the actual site of injury. Impulses from many cutaneous and visceral neurons converge on the same ascending neuron, and the brain cannot distinguish between the origins of the two.

Chronic pain is prolonged; it may last longer than 3 to 6 months and may either persist or be intermittent. Causes of chronic pain include decreased levels of endorphins or a predominance of C neuron stimulation. Physiologic responses to chronic pain depend on the persistent or intermittent nature of the pain. **Intermittent pain** produces a physiologic response similar to acute pain, whereas **persistent pain** permits physiologic adaptation. Individuals with chronic pain often are depressed, have difficulty sleeping and eating, and may spend a large amount of time seeking relief.

Neuropathic pain results from abnormal processing of sensory information by the peripheral and central nervous systems. *Central pain* is caused by a lesion or dysfunction in the brain or spinal cord, such as phantom pain or reflex sympathetic dystrophy. *Peripheral pain* is the result of trauma or disease that affects peripheral nerves, such as nerve entrapment or diabetic neuropathy.

The **pain threshold** is the lowest intensity at which a stimulus is perceived as pain and may be influenced by genetics. Intense pain at one location may increase the threshold in another location. **Pain tolerance** is the amount of time or intensity of pain that an individual will endure before initiating overt pain responses. It generally decreases with repeated exposure to pain, fatigue, anger, boredom, apprehension, and sleep deprivation. Tolerance increases with alcohol consumption, medication, hypnosis, warmth, distracting activities, and strong beliefs of faith.

2. Describe the alterations occurring in fever, hyperthermia, and hypothermia.
Study pages 331-333; refer to Figure 13-5.

Fever is not the failure of the normal thermoregulatory mechanism. Instead, it is considered *a resetting of the hypothalamic thermostat to a higher level.* The normal thermoregulatory mechanisms are raised so that the thermoregulatory center adjusts heat production, conservation, and loss to maintain the core temperature at a new, higher set-point temperature.

The pathophysiology of fever begins with exogenous pyrogens or *endotoxins* stimulating the release of interleukin-1, tumor necrosis factor, interleukin-6, and interferon, which raise the set point. As the set point is raised, the hypothalamus signals an increase in heat production and conservation to raise body temperature to the new level.

As fever breaks, the set point is returned to normal. The hypothalamus signals a decrease in heat production and an increase in heat reduction.

Fever can be beneficial. Elevated body temperature kills many microorganisms and has adverse effects on the growth and replication of others. Increased temperature causes lysosomal breakdown with auto destruction of cells; this prevents viral replication in infected cells. Heat increases lymphocytic transformation and motility of polymorphonuclear neutrophils, which facilitate the immune response.

Hyperthermia can produce nerve damage, coagulation of cell proteins, and death. At 41° C (106° F), nerve damage produces seizures in the adult. At 43° C (109° F), death follows. In hyperthermia, there is no resetting of the hypothalamic set point. Forms of accidental hyperthermia are heat cramps, heat exhaustion, and heatstroke.

Heat cramps are severe, spasmodic cramps in the abdomen and extremities subsequent to prolonged sweating and associated sodium loss. Heat cramps usually appear in individuals who are unaccustomed to heat or who perform strenuous work in very warm climates. Fever, rapid pulse, and increased blood pressure often accompany the cramps.

Heat exhaustion or collapse results from prolonged high body core or environmental temperatures. These high temperatures cause profound vasodilation and profuse sweating. Over a prolonged period of elevated temperatures, the hypothalamic responses produce dehydration, decreased plasma volumes, hypotension, decreased cardiac output, and tachycardia.

Heatstroke is a potentially lethal consequence of a breakdown in control of an overstressed thermoregulatory center. In cases of very high core temperatures (>40° C or 104°F), the regulatory center may cease to function appropriately.

High core temperatures and vascular collapse produce cerebral edema, degeneration of the central nervous system, and renal tubular necrosis. Death results unless immediate, effective treatment is initiated.

Malignant hyperthermia is a potentially lethal complication of an inherited muscle disorder that may be triggered by inhaled anesthetic or depolarizing muscle reactants. Malignant hyperthermia causes intracellular calcium levels to rise, producing sustained, uncoordinated muscle contractions. As a result of these contractions, acidosis develops. Cardiac dysrhythmias, hypotension, decreased cardiac output, or cardiac arrest may follow.

Hypothermia (marked cooling of core temperature) produces depression of the central nervous and respiratory systems. In severe hypothermia, ice crystals form on the inside of the cell, causing cells to rupture and die. Tissue hypothermia slows cell metabolism, increases the blood viscosity, slows microcirculatory blood flow, facilitates blood coagulation, and stimulates profound vasoconstriction. Hypothermia may be accidental, traumatic, or therapeutic.

Fever of unknown origin (FUO) is a fever greater than 38.3°C or 101° F that remains undiagnosed after three days of hospital investigation or 2 or more outpatient visits. The clinical categories of FUO include infectious, rheumatic/inflammatory, neoplastic, and miscellaneous disorders.

3. Describe sleep disorders; cite examples.
Study pages 334 and 335.

Sleep disorders include dyssomnias-sleep initiating disorders (insomnia, disordered breathing, hypersomnia, or sleep-wake disorders)-and parasomnias-sleep walking or night terrors.

Insomnia, the inability to fall or stay asleep, is transient and related to travel across time zones, or it may result from acute stress. Long-term insomnia is associated with drug or alcohol abuse, chronic pain disorders, or chronic depression.

In **obstructive sleep apnea syndrome (OSAS)**, the periodic breathing and apneic periods are generally caused by obesity, decreased chemosensitivity to carbon dioxide and oxygen tensions, or upper airway obstruction occurring while sleeping. The periodic breathing eventually produces arousal and reduces total sleep time. The sleep apnea reduces oxygen saturation and eventually produces polycythemia, pulmonary hypertension, right-sided congestive heart failure, liver congestion, cyanosis, and peripheral edema.

Hypersomnia (excessive daytime sleepiness) is a disorder associated with OSAS. Individuals may fall asleep while driving a car, working, or even while conversing. Treatment is symptomatic with reinforcement of good sleeping habits and may be related to sleep-disordered breathing requiring continuous positive air pressure.

Common **disorders of the sleep-wake schedule** include rapid time-zone change or "jet-lag syndrome" (an altered sleep schedule with an advance or a delay of 3 hours or more in sleep time) or a change in total sleep time from day to day. Vigilance of psychomotor performance and arousal are markedly depressed after alterations in the sleep-wake schedule.

Parasomnias are unusual behaviors occurring during sleep and are common in children. **Somnambulism**, or sleepwalking, appears to resolve itself within several years after the onset of the sleepwalking episodes. During the sleepwalking episode, the child functions at a low level of arousal and has no memory of the event upon awakening.

Night terrors are characterized by sudden apparent arousals in which the child expresses intense fear or emotion. However, the child is not awake and is difficult to arouse. Once awakened, the child has no memory of the night terror event. Neither somnambulism nor night terrors are associated with dreams.

Restless leg syndrome (RLS) is a common sensorimotor disorder associated with prickling, tingling, crawling that occurs at rest and is worse at night. It is associated with a circadian fluctuation of dopamine in the substantia nigra. The disorder is more in women, the elderly, and iron deficit individuals; iron is a cofactor in dopamine production.

4. **Identify common diseases that are associated with the special senses and describe their etiologies and manifestations.**
Study pages 335 and 342; refer to Figures 13-9 and 13-10 and Tables 13-6 and 13-7.

Vision

Blepharitis is an inflammation of the eyelids caused by staphylococcal infections or seborrheic dermatitis.

Conjunctivitis is an inflammation of the conjunctiva, the mucous membrane covering the front part of the eyeball. It may be caused by bacteria, viruses, allergies, or chemical irritations.

Keratitis is an infection of the cornea usually caused by bacteria or viruses. Bacterial infections often cause corneal ulceration and require extensive antibiotic treatment. Type I herpes virus usually infects the cornea and conjunctiva.

Strabismus is the deviation of one eye from the other when the person is looking directly at an object. It is caused by a weak or hypertonic muscle in one of the eyes. The deviation may be upward, downward, inward, or outward. **Diplopia** (double vision) is a symptom of strabismus. **Nystagmus** is the involuntary lateral, rhythmic movement of the eyes.

Amblyopia is a vision reduction or dimness caused by cerebral blockage of visual stimuli. Amblyopia is associated with diabetes mellitus, renal failure, malaria, and toxic substances such as alcohol and tobacco.

A **scotoma** is a circumscribed defect of the central field of vision. It is most often a sequel to an inflammatory lesion of the optic nerve and is often associated with multiple sclerosis.

A **cataract** is a cloudy or opaque ocular lens. The most common form of cataract is degenerative.

Papilledema is edema and inflammation of the optic nerve at its point of entrance into the eyeball. Generally, papilledema is caused by obstruction to the venous return from the retina.

Dark adaptation affects visual acuity. Changes in rhodopsin, a substance found in the rods and responsible for low-light vision, are likely responsible for reduced dark adaptation in older adults. Vitamin A deficiencies can cause the same disorder in individuals of any age.

Glaucoma is characterized by intraocular pressures above the normal range of 12 to 20 mm Hg maintained by the aqueous fluid in homeostasis. Intraocular fluid accumulation blocks the flow of nutrients to optic nerve fibers, leading to their death.

Age-related macular degeneration (AMD) is a severe and irreversible loss of vision and a major cause of blindness in older individuals. Hypertension, cigarette smoking, and diabetes are risk factors. There are two forms: atrophic (dry) and neovascular (wet). The atrophic form may involve limited night vision and difficulty reading. The neovascular form consists of abnormal blood vessel growth, leakage of blood or serum, retinal detachment, fibrovascular scarring, and loss of photoreceptors.

Loss of accommodation associated with aging is termed **presbyopia**, a condition in which the ocular lens becomes larger, firmer, and less elastic. The major symptom is reduced near vision, causing reading material to be held at arm's length.

In **myopia**, or nearsightedness, light rays are focused in front of the retina when the person is looking at a distant object. In hyperopia, or farsightedness, light rays are focused behind the retina when the person is looking at a near object. Astigmatism is caused by an unequal curvature of the cornea; light rays are bent unevenly and do not come to a single focus on the retina.

Hearing

A conductive hearing loss occurs when a change in the outer or middle ear impairs sound conduction from the outer to the inner ear. Conditions that commonly cause a conductive hearing loss include impacted cerumen, foreign bodies lodged in the ear canal, neoplasms of the external auditory canal or middle ear, eustachian tube dysfunction, otitis media, cholesteatoma, and otosclerosis. Symptoms of conductive hearing loss are diminished hearing and soft speaking voice. The voice is soft because the individual may hear his or her voice conducted by bone ossicles.

A sensorineural hearing loss is caused by impairment of the organ of Corti and its hearing receptors or its central connections. Conditions that commonly cause sensorineural hearing loss include congenital and hereditary factors, noise exposure, aging, ototoxicity, and systemic diseases. Congenital and neonatal sensorineural hearing loss is caused by impairment of the organ of Corti on its control connections. **Presbycusis** is the most common form of sensorineural hearing loss in the elderly. Drugs and chemicals may cause **tinnitus** (ringing in the ear), followed by progressive high-tone sensorineural hearing loss that is permanent. **Ménière disease** is a disorder of the middle ear of unknown etiology; excessive endolymph and pressure in the membranous labyrinth disrupts both vestibular and hearing functions. Recurring symptoms include profound vertigo, nausea, and vomiting with deafness and tinnitus.

Otitis externa is a bacterial infection of the outer ear associated with prolonged exposure to moisture. Drainage accumulation causes pain. Topical antimicrobials are usually effective.

Otitis media is an infection of the middle ear common in children. Acute otitis media (AOM) is associated with an inflamed, bulging tympanic membrane and fluid in the middle ear. The presence of fluid behind the membrane without acute infection is ostitis media with effusion. Antimicrobial therapy and possible placement of tympanotomy tubes may be required for its treatment and prevention.

Olfaction

Hyposmia is an impaired sense of smell; **anosmia** is the complete loss of smell. **Olfactory hallucinations** arise from hyperactivity in cortical neurons and involve the smelling of odors that are not actually present. **Parosmia** is an abnormal or perverted sense of smell.

Taste

Hypogeusia is decreased taste sensation; **ageusia** is the absence of taste. **Dysgeusia** is a perversion of taste in which substances possess an unpleasant flavor, such as metallic. These disorders are the result of cranial nerve injuries and can be specific to the area of tongue innervated.

Parageusia is a perversion of taste in which substances that are usually palatable instead elicit an unpleasant flavor. It is common in individuals receiving chemotherapy for cancer. Parageusia often leads to anorexia.

Touch

Any impairment of reception, transmission, perception, or interpretation of touch alters tactile sensation. Trauma, tumor, infection, metabolic changes, vascular changes, and degenerative disease may cause tactile dysfunction.

Proprioception

Proprioception is the perception and awareness of the position of the body and its parts. It depends on impulses from the inner ear and from receptors in joints and ligaments.

Proprioceptive dysfunction may be caused by alterations at any level of the nervous system, similar to that observed in tactile dysfunction.

Vestibular nystagmus is the constant, involuntary movement of the eyeball caused when the semicircular canal system is overstimulated.

Vertigo is the sensation of spinning that occurs with inflammation of the semicircular canals in the ear.

Peripheral neuropathies are probably associated with renal disease and diabetes mellitus. The result is diminution or absence of the sense of body position or position of body parts. Gait changes often occur in affected persons.

PRACTICE EXAMINATION

Multiple Choice

Circle the correct answer for each question:

1. Endorphins:
   a. increase pain sensations.
   b. decrease pain sensations.
   c. may increase or decrease pain sensations.
   d. have no effect on pain sensations.

2. Referred pain from upper abdominal diseases involves:
   a. the sacral region.
   b. L2 to L4.
   c. T8, L1, and L2.
   d. the gluteal regions, posterior thighs, and calves.

3. In the gate control theory of pain:
   a. a "closed gate" increases pain perception.
   b. stimulation of large A fibers "closes the gate."
   c. Both a and b are correct.
   d. Neither a nor b is correct.

4. Which is *not* a neuromodulator of pain?
   a. prostaglandins
   b. 5-hydroxytryptamine
   c. norepinephrine
   d. lymphokines
   e. heparin

5. Interleukin-1:
   a. raises the hypothalamic set point.
   b. is an endogenous pyrogen.
   c. is stimulated by exogenous pyrogens.
   d. None of the above is correct.
   e. a, b, and c are correct.

6. Increased serum levels of epinephrine increase body temperature by:
   a. increasing shivering.
   b. increasing muscle tone.
   c. increasing heat production.
   d. decreasing basal metabolic rate.

7. In heatstroke:
   a. core temperature usually does *not* exceed 101° F.
   b. sodium loss follows sweating.
   c. core temperature increases as the regulatory center fails.
   d. Both b and c are correct.

8. Which is involved in fever?
   a. tumor necrosis factor
   b. endotoxins
   c. elevation of the set point in the hypothalamus
   d. Both a and b are correct.
   e. a, b, and c are correct.

9. In hypothermia:
   a. the viscosity of blood is decreased.
   b. acidosis can develop.
   c. the hypothalamic center prevents shivering.
   d. All of the above are correct.

10. Although non-REM sleep and REM sleep are defined by electrical recordings, they are characterized by physiologic events. Which does *not* occur?
   a. During non-REM sleep, muscle tone decreases.
   b. Non-REM sleep is initiated by withdrawal of neurotransmitters from the reticular formation.
   c. During non-REM sleep, cerebral blood flow to the cortex decreases.
   d. During non-REM sleep, levels of corticosteroids increase.

11. Ménière disease:
   a. affects the outer ear.
   b. disrupts both vestibular and hearing functions.
   c. is the common cause of sensorineural hearing loss.
   d. is caused by impacted cerumen.

12. Acute otitis media (AOM):
   a. has no genetic determinants.
   b. displays a tympanic membrane progressing from erythema to opaqueness with bulging.
   c. risk factors include breast-feeding.
   d. is commonly caused by *Staphylococcus aureus*.

13. Age-related macular degeneration (AMD):
   a. has a higher incidence in hypotensive individuals.
   b. occurs before age 60 years.
   c. exhibits retinal detachment and loss of photoreceptors.
   d. exhibits loss of accommodation.

14. Vestibular nystagmus:
   a. is the constant, involuntary movement of the eyeball caused by ear disturbances.
   b. is the sensation of spinning.
   c. may be caused by alterations in the nervous system from the receptor to the cerebral cortex.
   d. causes a diminished sense of the position of body parts.

15. Sleep apnea:
   a. is lack of breathing during sleep.
   b. can result from airway obstruction during sleep.
   c. is associated with jet-lag syndrome.
   d. All of the above are correct.
   e. Both a and b are correct.

16. Individuals affected by sleep apnea may experience:
   a. polycythemia.
   b. cyanosis.
   c. pulmonary hypertension.
   d. All of the above are correct.

Matching

Match the pain characteristic with the nervous system component:

17. Basic perception of pain
18. Initiation of pain stimulus
19. Discrimination and precision given to painful stimulus

a. nociceptive receptors
b. postcentral gyrus
c. brainstem
d. A fibers
e. cortex

Match the term with its defining characteristic:

_______ 20. Suprachiasmatic nucleus
_______ 21. Strabismus
_______ 22. Anosmia
_______ 23. Hypogeusia
_______ 24. Vertigo
_______ 25. Glaucoma

a. inflammation of mucous membrane covering the eyeball
b. infection of the cornea
c. weak muscle in one of the eyes
d. reduction or dimness of vision
e. coordinates sleep-awake cycle with circadian rhythm
f. decreased intraocular pressures
g. elevated intraocular pressure
h. inflammation of the semicircular canals
i. decreased taste sensation
j. complete loss of smell

Fill in the Blank

Complete the following table comparing acute to chronic pain:

Comparison of Acute and Chronic Pain

Characteristic	Acute Pain	Chronic Pain
Experience		
Onset		
Duration		
Identification	Generally well defined	
Pattern		
Course		
Prognosis		

CASE STUDY

Mrs. D. is a 45-year-old woman who sought care for chronic insomnia of 15 months' duration. She stated, "I wake up 15 to 20 times a night and rarely sleep more than 4 hours." Various hypnotics have been unsuccessful in relieving her symptoms.

Her history showed that about 18 months earlier, some important stressful life changes occurred. Her only child, a daughter, left for an out-of-state university. A lifelong friend and confidante moved to another community. Her husband, a successful dentist, had become more involved in various men's organizations than he had been in the past.

A sedating antidepressant was prescribed and a second appointment was made for 1 month later. At the second appointment, which lasted 1 hour, she said, "My sleep patterns have improved." She was able to articulate that she felt unneeded, incompetent, and old.

As a caregiver, how would you assess Mrs. D.'s case?

14 Alterations in Cognitive Systems, Cerebral Hemodynamics and Motor Function

FOUNDATIONAL OBJECTIVES

a. Describe the reticular activating system (RAS) as a modulator of consciousness.
Review page 279; refer to Figure 12.5.

MEMORY CHECK!

- *The RAS maintains wakefulness.* It ascends from the lower brain stem and projects throughout the cerebral cortex. The ability to respond to stimuli or arousal depends on an intact RAS in the brain stem and the ability to respond to the environment. Cognition relies on an intact cerebral cortex. Therefore, consciousness or responsiveness requires functioning from the reticular formation in the brain stem to the cerebral cortex.

b. Identify the structural and functional components of the brain.
Review pages 299, 301, 303, and 304; refer to Figures 12-5 through 12-9; and Table 12-3.

MEMORY CHECK!

- The central nervous system (CNS) consists of the **brain** and **spinal cord** encased within the meninges and bathed in cerebrospinal fluid (CSF). The brain is divided into several areas, including the cerebrum, midbrain, cerebellum, pons, and medulla oblongata. The midbrain, the medulla, and the pons compose the brain stem.
- The outer covering of the cerebrum is the *cortex*. The entire cerebrum is divided into two halves, or hemispheres, connected by a neural bridge, the *corpus callosum,* that coordinates activities between hemispheres. The cortex is concerned with thinking and sensory perception. Emotional responses and control of body temperature, water and food intake, and sex drive have their origin in the midbrain area. The *cerebellum* primarily integrates muscular movements to produce coordination in walking, talking, and other complex muscular activities. The *medulla* oblongata controls vital functions such as respiration, heart rate, and blood pressure, although these functions are modified by higher brain centers.
- Within the cerebral hemispheres are subdivisions, or lobes. The frontal lobe is located in the anterior portion of each hemisphere. The temporal lobe is located in the lower middle region of each hemisphere. The parietal lobe is the upper, rear portion. The occipital lobe is the lower, rear portion of each hemisphere.
- The *basal ganglia* are a collection of cell bodies in several areas of the brain's gray matter, including the caudate nucleus, globus pallidus, putamen, and substantia nigra. The function of the *basal ganglia* is thought to involve the *planning and programming of movement.*

c. Identify the parts of the CNS that control voluntary muscle movement.
Refer to Figures 12-7 and 12-8.

MEMORY CHECK!

- The cerebral cortex plays a major role in controlling precise, voluntary muscular movements. Motor output to skeletal muscles travels down the spinal cord in two types of descending tracts, the *pyramidal tracts* and the *extrapyramidal tracts.* The *pyramidal tracts* originate in the motor cortex and terminate in the brain stem. They *cross* to the opposite side at the medulla–spinal cord junction. Fibers of the tracts on the left cross to the right side and the pyramidal tracts convey impulses that cause precise, voluntary movements of skeletal muscles. The extrapyramidal tracts arise from the cortex and project to innervate the motor neurons; they do not cross to the opposite side. Extrapyramidal tracts convey nerve impulses that program fine repetitive motor movements.

LEARNING OBJECTIVES

After studying this chapter, the learner will be able to do the following and characterize rostral caudal progression of nonresponsiveness.

1. **Describe the outcomes for alterations in arousal.**
   Study pages 347 and 348; refer to Tables 14-1 and 14-2.

Possible causes of an **altered level of arousal** may be separated into structural and metabolic. *Structural causes* are divided according to whether the original pathologic condition is above **(supratentorial) or below (infratentorial) the tentorial plate**.

Supratentorial processes produce a decreased level of consciousness because of compression or displacement of the diencephalon or brain stem. **Infratentorial processes** produce a reduction in arousal by diseases that destroy the brain stem.

Disorders outside the brain, such as neoplasms, bleeding from trauma, and pus, can produce arousal dysfunction. Bleeding, infarcts, emboli, and neoplasms within the brain also can contribute to altered levels of arousal.

A wide spectrum of disorders or agents may produce a *metabolically* induced alteration in arousal. Hypoxia, electrolyte disturbances, hypoglycemia, drugs, and toxins alter arousal.

2. **Relate clinical manifestations to levels of consciousness and characterize rostral-caudal progression of nonresponsiveness distinguish between cerebral and brain death.**
   Study pages 348, 349, and 351-353; refer to Figures 14-1 through 14-6; and Tables 14-3 through 14-5.

The level of **consciousness** is alertness with orientation to person, place, and time. As the level decreases, there is *disorientation* first to *time,* then to *place,* and eventually to *person.* The following five categories of neurologic function are critical to identifying increasing or decreasing CNS function: (1) level of consciousness, (2) breathing patterns, (3) papillary reaction, (4) ocular-motor responses, and (5) motor responses.

An individual who is alert and oriented to time, place, and person is functioning at a high level of consciousness. From this normal level, consciousness diminishes from confusion to coma. Patterns of *breathing* respond to changes in $Paco_2$ levels. Increases in $Paco_2$ lead to *tachypnea,* which leads to *apnea* until carbon dioxide reaccumulates, stimulating tachypnea. *Pupillary changes* indicate the level of brain stem dysfunction. Severe ischemia and hypoxia usually produce *dilated* and *fixed* pupils; hyperthermia may cause *fixed* pupils. Opiates cause *pinpoint* pupils whereas barbiturate intoxication may fix pupils. Destructive or compressive injuries to the brain stem cause specific ocular motor responses. Those that involve an oculomotor nucleus or nerve cause the involved eye to deviate outward, producing a resting dysconjugate lateral eye position. *Motor responses* indicate the level of brain dysfunction and determine the side of

Rostral-Caudal Progression of Nonresponsiveness

Area Involved	Level of Consciousness	Pupils	Muscle Tone	Breathing Pattern
Diencephalon (thalamus/ hypothalamus)	Decreased concentration, agitation, dullness, lethargy, obtundation	Respond to light briskly; full-range eye movements only on "doll's eyes"—none in direction of rotation or after injection of hot or cold water in ear canal (caloric posturing)	Some purposeful movement in response to pain, combative movement Decorticate: flexion in upper extremities and extension in lower extremities	Yawning and sighing to Cheyne-Stokes
Midbrain	Stupor to coma	Midposition fixed (MPF)	Decerebrate: arms rigid, palms turned away from body	Neurogenic hyperventilation
Pons	Coma	MPF	Decerebrate	Apneustic: prolonged inspiration and expiration
Medulla	Coma	MPF	Flaccid	Ataxic: uncoordinated and irregular

*The oculocephalic and oculovestibular reflex test is used to indicate the integrity of brain stem function.

the brain that is most damaged (pyramidal neurons crossover, so the right brain affects the left body).

Brain death occurs when irreversible brain damage is so extensive that the brain can no longer maintain the body's internal respiratory and cerebral vascular functions. There is destruction of the brain stem and cerebellum.

Cerebral death, or irreversible coma, is death of the cerebral hemispheres, exclusive of the brain stem and cerebellum. The individual is permanently unable to respond in any significant way to the environment. The brain may continue to maintain internal homeostasis. Arousal returns in vegetative states, but awareness is absent. Nonresponsiveness occurs from rostral to caudal, as shown in the table at the bottom of page 86.

3. Describe alterations in awareness.
Refer to Table 14-6.

Selective attention deficit refers to the inability to select appropriately from available competing environmental stimuli for conscious processing.

Memory is the recording, retention, and retrieval of knowledge. **Retrograde amnesia** is the loss of past memories. **Anterograde amnesia** is an inability to form new memories.

Image processing is inability to categorize similarities and differences and to perform deductive reasoning.

A vigilance deficit is the inability to concentrate over time or to maintain sustained attention. In a **detection deficit**, the person is unmotivated and unable to use feedback.

Generally, the primary pathophysiologic mechanism that operates in cognitive system disorders is due directly to ischemia and hypoxia or indirectly to compression, toxins, and chemicals.

4. Describe seizure and cite conditions associated with seizure disorders.
Study pages 354-356; refer to Table 14-7.

A **seizure** is a sudden, explosive disorderly discharge of cerebral neurons and is characterized by a sudden, transient alteration in brain function, usually involving motor, sensory, autonomic, or psychic clinical manifestations and an alteration in one's level of arousal. The alteration in level of arousal is *temporary.* Among the causes of seizure activity are the following:

metabolic defects	motor syndromes
congenital malformations	infections
genetic predisposition	brain tumors
perinatal injury	vascular diseases
postnatal trauma	fever

Epilepsy, recurring, episodic seizure activity in the absence of treatment, is now believed to be caused by genetic mutations that trigger brain wiring abnormalities or chemical imbalances in brain signals or abnormal nerve connections made during attempted repair after injury.

An **epileptogenic focus** may be a group of neurons that have a *paroxysmal depolarization* shift that changes membrane potential. The *plasma membranes* of these neuronal cells appear to be *more permeable.* Greater permeability renders them more easily activated by hyperthermia, hypoxia, hypoglycemia, hyponatremia, repeated sensory stimulation, and certain sleep phases. The neural excitation spreads to the subcortical, thalamic, and brain stem areas to initiate *the tonic phase* of prolonged muscle contraction with increased muscle tore or tensions, which is followed by increased muscle tone and loss of consciousness. The *clonic phase,* consisting of *alternating* contraction and relaxation of muscles, begins as inhibitory neurons in the cortex, anterior thalamus, and basal ganglia start to inhibit the cortical excitation. This inhibition interrupts seizure discharge and produces an intermittent pattern of muscle contractions; the contractions gradually decrease and then finally cease.

5. Differentiate between partial and generalized seizures.
Refer to Tables 14-8 and 14-9.

Partial seizures (unilateral) were previously termed jacksonian or psychomotor seizures. They are now classified as simple, complex, or secondary. *Simple* are without impairment of consciousness, but have somatosensory, autonomic, psychic symptoms. *Complex seizures* have impaired consciousness with or without automatism. *Secondary* seizures evolve into generalized tonic-clonic seizures.

Generalized seizures (bilateral) were earlier termed petit-mal or grand mal. They are now classified as *absence, mycoclonic, clonic, or tonic-clonic.* An *aura* is a sensation, such as a light, a taste, warmth, or a sound, that precedes a generalized seizure. A *prodroma* is a set of early manifestations, such as malaise or headache, that may precede the onset of a seizure.

6. Define the descriptive terms of processing deficits.
Study pages 356 and 357; refer to Figure 14-7 and Tables 14-10 through 14-12.

Agnosia is a defect of *recognition of the form* and *nature of objects.* Although it most commonly is associated with cerebrovascular accidents, it may arise from any pathologic process that injures specific areas of the brain.

Dysphasia is impairment of *comprehension* or *production of language.* Comprehension or use of symbols, in either written or verbal language, is disturbed or lost. Dysphasias usually are associated with cerebrovascular accidents involving the middle cerebral artery or one of its many branches. Dysphasia results from dysfunction in the left cerebral hemisphere and usually involves the frontotemporal region. Dysphasia may be nonfluent; the individual cannot find words to express thoughts and exhibits difficulty in writing. Dysphasia also may be fluent; uttered verbal language is meaningless; the individual uses inappropriate words.

Acute confusional states result from cerebral dysfunction secondary to drug intoxication or nervous system disease. These states may begin either suddenly or gradually, depending on the amount of toxin exposure. The predominant feature of an acute confusional state is *impaired* or *lost vigilance.* The individual is unable to concentrate on incoming sensory information or on any one particular mental or motor task.

7. Describe features of dementia and Alzheimer disease.

Study pages 357-361; refer to Figure 14-8 and Tables 14-13 through 14-15.

The **dementias** are characterized by the loss of more than one cognitive or intellectual function. There may be a decrease in orientation, general knowledge and information, vigilance, recent memory, remote memory, concept formation, abstraction, reasoning, and language. Causes of dementia include degeneration, cerebrovascular accidents, compression, toxins, metabolic disorders, biochemical imbalance, demyelinization, and infections. Symptoms of dementia may be categorized as cortical, subcortical, or both. Cortical dementia manifests as *amnesic dementia (loss of recent memory) or cognitive dementia (loss of remote memory).* Subcortical dementia exhibits *slowed thought processes, personality changes,* and *loss of motor function.*

Alzheimer disease (AD) is one of the most common causes of severe cognitive dysfunction in older people. *Early-onset FAD includes gene defects on chromosomes 21 (abnormal amyloid precursor protein), 14 (abnormal presenilin 1), and 1 (abnormal presenilin 2). Late-onset FAD is linked to defects on chromosome 19* involved with the *apolipoprotein E gene-allele 4.* Pathologic alterations in the brain include formation of *neuritic plaques* containing a core of *amyloid-beta protein;* formation of *neurofibrillary tangles;* and degeneration of basal forebrain cholinergic neurons with *loss of acetylcholine.* The plaques and tangles are concentrated in the cerebral cortex and the hippocampus. Loss of acetylcholine contributes to loss of cognition.

In addition to cognitive dysfunctions, **dyspraxias**, or the *inability to perform coordinated acts,* may appear. Motor changes may occur if the posterior frontal lobes are involved. The affected individual may exhibit rigidity with flexion posturing, propulsion, and retropulsion. There is great variability in age of onset, intensity and sequence of symptoms, and location and extent of brain pathology among individuals with the disease.

Pharmacotherapy includes cholinesterase inhibitors to enhance cholinergic transmission. They have a modest effect in mild to moderate AD. An *N*-methyl-D-aspartate receptor antagonist blocks glutamate activity and may slow progression of disease in moderate to severe AD. Treatment of AD also is directed to decreasing the need for cognitive function by using memory aids, maintaining cognitive functions that are not impaired, and improving the general state of hygiene, nutrition, and health.

8. Characterize the stages of increased intracranial pressure, herniation syndrome, and cerebral edema.

Study pages 361-363; refer to Figures 14-9 through 14-11 and Box 14-2.

Increased intracranial pressure may result from an increase in intracranial content, which occurs with tumor growth, edema, excess CSF, or hemorrhage. *A rise in intracranial pressure from one component requires an equal reduction in volume of other components.* The most readily displaced content of the cranial vault is CSF.

When brain tissue is injured, management of increased intracranial pressure and cerebral oxygenation are issues; cerebral oxygenation is most critical. Cerebral oxygenation depends on cerebral blood volume, blood flow, and perfusion pressure. Increased intracranial pressure may result from an increase in intracranial content that occurs with tumor growth, edema, excess CSF, or hemorrhage. Because the cranial vault is a nonflexible encasement around the brain and its extracellular fluid, a rise in intracranial pressure from one component requires an equal reduction in volume of other components. The most readily displaced content of the cranial vault is CSF.

In *stage 1* of intracranial hypertension, vasoconstriction and external compression of the venous system occur in an attempt to further reduce the intracranial pressure following CSF displacement from the cranial vault. Clinical manifestations at this stage are subtle and transient and include confusion, drowsiness, and slight pupillary and breathing changes.

With continued expansion of the intracranial content, the resulting increase in intracranial pressure may exceed the brain's compensatory capacity to adjust to the increasing pressure. This is *stage 2,* and the pressure begins to compromise neuronal oxygenation. Systemic arterial vasoconstriction occurs to elevate the systemic blood pressure sufficiently to overcome the increased intracranial pressure.

Intracranial pressure begins to approach arterial pressure, and the brain tissues begin to experience hypoxia and hypercapnia. Cheyne-Stokes respiration occurs, the pupils become sluggish and dilated, pulse pressure widens, and bradycardia develops. Accumulating CO_2 causes vasodilation at the local tissue level. The hydrostatic pressure in the vessels drops, and blood volume increases. The brain volume increases, and intracranial pressure continues to rise. This is *stage 3* of intracranial hypertension. Cerebral perfusion pressure falls, and cerebral perfusion slows dramatically; the brain tissues experience severe hypoxia and acidosis.

In the last stage of intracranial hypertension, *stage 4,* brain tissue shifts or **herniates** from the compartment of greater pressure to a compartment of lesser pressure. The herniated brain tissues increase the content volume within the lower-pressure compartment, thereby exerting pressure on the brain tissue that normally occupies that compartment; now, both the herniated and lower, displaced tissue blood supply are impaired. Mean systolic arterial pressure soon equals intracranial pressure, and cerebral blood flow ceases.

The three types of cerebral edema are: (1) vasogenic edema, (2) cytotoxic (metabolic) edema, and (3) interstitial edema.

Vasogenic edema is clinically the most important type. It is caused by the *increased permeability of the capillary endothelium* of the brain after injury to the vascular structure. Plasma proteins leak into the extracellular spaces, drawing water to them, so *the water content of the brain parenchyma increases*. Vasogenic edema starts in the area of injury and spreads with preferential accumulation in the *white matter* of the ipsilateral side because the parallel myelinated fibers separate more easily.

In **cytotoxic (metabolic) edema**, *toxic factors directly affect* the neuronal, glial, and endothelial *cells*, causing failure of the active transport systems. The cells lose their potassium and gain larger amounts of sodium. Water follows by osmosis into the cells, causing the *cells* to *swell*. Cytotoxic edema occurs principally in the *gray matter*.

Interstitial edema is caused by movement of *cerebrospinal fluid* from the ventricles *into the extracellular spaces* of the brain tissues. The brain fluid volume is mostly increased around the ventricles; the increased pressure is within the *white matter*.

9. Describe hydrocephalus.
Study pages 363 and 364; refer to Table 14-16.

Hydrocephalus refers to various conditions characterized by excess fluid in the cranial vault, subarachnoid space, or both. It occurs because of interference with CSF flow due to increased fluid production, obstruction within the ventricular system, or defective reabsorption of the fluid.

Hydrocephalus may develop from infancy through adulthood. Congenital hydrocephalus is rare. *Noncommunicating,* or internal, hydrocephalus, in which the flow from the ventricles is obstructed, is seen more often in children, and the *communicating* type without obstruction but defective resorption of CSF, is seen more often in adults.

Obstructed CSF is under pressure and causes atrophy of the cerebral cortex and degeneration of the white matter tracts. *There is selective preservation of gray matter.*

Acute hydrocephalus manifests signs of rapidly developing increased intracranial pressure. If not promptly treated, the individual quickly becomes comatose. Normal-pressure hydrocephalus develops slowly, with declining memory and cognitive function. In infancy, head enlargement is predominant before cranial suture closure.

The diagnosis is based on results of physical examination, computed tomography, and magnetic resonance imaging. Hydrocephalus can be treated by surgery to resect cysts, neoplasms, or hematomas. Ventricular bypass into the normal intracranial channel or into an extracranial compartment by a shunt is also used therapeutically.

10. Define terms that describe alterations in motor functions.
Study pages 364-368; refer to Figures 14-12 through 14-17, and Tables 14-17 and 14-18.

Hypotonia is decreased muscle tone, shown by passive movement of a muscle against resistance. It likely is caused by decreased muscle spindle activity secondary to reduced excitability of neurons. Hypotonia is caused by cerebellar damage or, in rare cases, by pyramidal tract damage.

Hypertonia is increased muscle tone, shown by passive movement of a muscle with resistance. *Spasticity,* a type of hypertonia, is a gradual increase in tone. *Paratonia* is resistance to passive movement. *Dystonia* is sustained involuntary twisting movement. *Rigidity* is resistance to passive movement of a rigid limb.

Paraparesis/paraplegia refers to weakness/paralysis of the lower extremities. **Quadriparesis/quadriplegia** refers to paresis/paralysis of all four extremities. Both paraparesis/paraplegia and quadriparesis/quadriplegia may be caused by dysfunction of the spinal cord. **Paresis** is partial paralysis with diminished muscle power. **Paralysis** is loss of muscle function so that the muscle is unable to overcome gravity.

When the pyramidal system is destroyed below the level of the pons, **spinal shock** occurs. This is the complete cessation of spinal cord functions below the lesion. Spinal shock is characterized by complete *flaccid paralysis,* absence of reflexes, and marked disturbances in bowel and bladder function.

11. Describe amyotrophies.
Study pages 368 and 369.

Lower motor syndromes originating in the anterior horn cells or the motor nuclei of the cranial nerves are called amyotrophies. Paralytic poliomyelitis is the prototype of these disorders. In the **amyotrophies**, muscle strength, muscle tone, and muscle bulk are affected in the muscles innervated by the involved motor neurons.

Several brain stem syndromes involve damage to one or more of the cranial nerve nuclei. These are called **nuclear palsies** and may be caused by vascular occlusion, tumor, aneurysm, tuberculosis, or hemorrhage. **Bulbar palsies** involve cranial nerves IX, X, and XII. **Hyperkinesia** is excessive movement, whereas **dyskinesias** are abnormal, involuntary movements. **Hypokinesia**, or decreased movement, is a loss of voluntary movement despite consciousness and normal peripheral nerve and muscle function. In hypokinesia, the normal, habitually associated movements that provide skill, grace, and balance to voluntary movements are lost. An expressionless face, a statuesque posture, and absence of both speech inflection and spontaneous gestures are exhibited as well.

Akinesia is a decrease in associated and voluntary movements. It is related to dysfunction of the extrapyramidal system. Pathogenesis is related to either a deficiency of dopamine or a defect of the postsynaptic dopamine receptors. **Bradykinesia** is slowness of voluntary movements.

12. Compare Huntington disease to Parkinson disease.
Study pages 369, 371, and 372; refer to Figures 14-18 and 14-19. (See the following table.)

Comparison of Parkinson Disease and Huntington Disease

	Parkinson Disease	Huntington Disease
Lesion site	Basal ganglia, degeneration of dopaminergic receptors	Basal ganglia, frontal cortex
Etiology	Imbalance between dopaminergic and cholinergic activity, dopamine deficiency, trauma, viral infection, neoplasms, drugs, toxins	Autosomal dominant, chromosome 4, GABA depletion
Onset	>40 years, peak in 60s	30s and 50s
Manifestations	Resting tremor, stiffness, akinesis, flexed-forward leaning, no paralysis, depression, possible late-stage dementia	Dementia, delusions, depression, chorea-type movement
Treatment	Symptomatic, dopaminergic drugs, possible fetal cell transplant possible recombinant	No known treatment, genes

13. Describe disorders of posture-stance.
Study page 372.

Dystonia is the maintenance of abnormal posture through muscular contractions. **Decorticate posture** is characterized by upper extremities that are flexed at the elbows and held close to the body and lower extremities that are externally rotated and extended. Decorticate posture is thought to occur when the brain stem is not inhibited by the motor function of the cerebral cortex. **Decerebrate posture** refers to a position of extended and internally rotated arms with the legs extended and feet in plantar flexion. The decerebrate posture is caused by severe injury to the brain and brain stem. **Basal ganglion posture** refers to a stooped, hyperflexed posture with a narrow-based, short-stepped gait. **Senile posture** is characterized by an increasingly flexed posture similar to a basal ganglion posture. The posture is associated with frontal lobe dysfunction.

14. Describe disorders of gait.
Study page 372.

A **spastic gait** is associated with unilateral, pyramidal injury and manifests as a shuffling gait with the leg extended and held stiff. This gait causes a scraping of the foot over the walking surface. A scissors gait is associated with bilateral pyramidal injury and spasticity. The legs are abducted so they touch each other. A **cerebellar gait** manifests as a wide-based gait with the feet apart and often turned outward and inward for greater stability. Cerebellar dysfunction accounts for this particular gait. A **basal ganglion gait** is a broad-based gait. The individual takes small steps, and there is a decreased arm swing during walking. The individual's head and body are flexed and the arms are semiflexed and abducted, whereas the legs are flexed and rigid in more advanced states. Basal ganglion and frontal lobe dysfunction, respectively, account for these two gaits.

15. Describe disorders of expression.
Study page 373; refer to Figure 14-20.

Hypermimesis, a disorder of expression, is most commonly manifested as pathologic laughter or crying. Pathologic laughter is associated with right hemisphere injury, whereas pathologic crying is associated with left hemisphere injury. **Hypomimesis** is manifested as *aprosody,* or the loss of emotional language. Aprosody involves an inability to understand or express emotion in speech and facial expression. Aprosody is associated with right hemisphere damage.

Dyspraxia/apraxia is the inability to perform purposeful or skilled motor acts in the absence of paralysis, sensory loss, abnormal posture and tone, abnormal involuntary movement, incoordination, or inattentiveness. Dyspraxias arise when the connecting pathways between the left and right cortical areas are interrupted; conceptualization and execution of complex motor acts are impaired.

16. Show the relationships between pyramidal (upper) and extrapyramidal (lower) motor syndromes.

Refer to Figures 14-15 through 14-17 and Table 14-20.

Disturbances in motor function are classified as either upper or lower motor neuron disorders. Amyotrophic lateral sclerosis can involve both upper and lower neuron structures. Upper motor neuron disorders include cerebral palsies, cerebrovascular accidents, multiple sclerosis, and Parkinson disease. Lower motor neuron disorders include poliomyelitis, muscular dystrophies, myasthenia gravis, and polymyositis. (See flowchart.)

Motor Syndrome Types

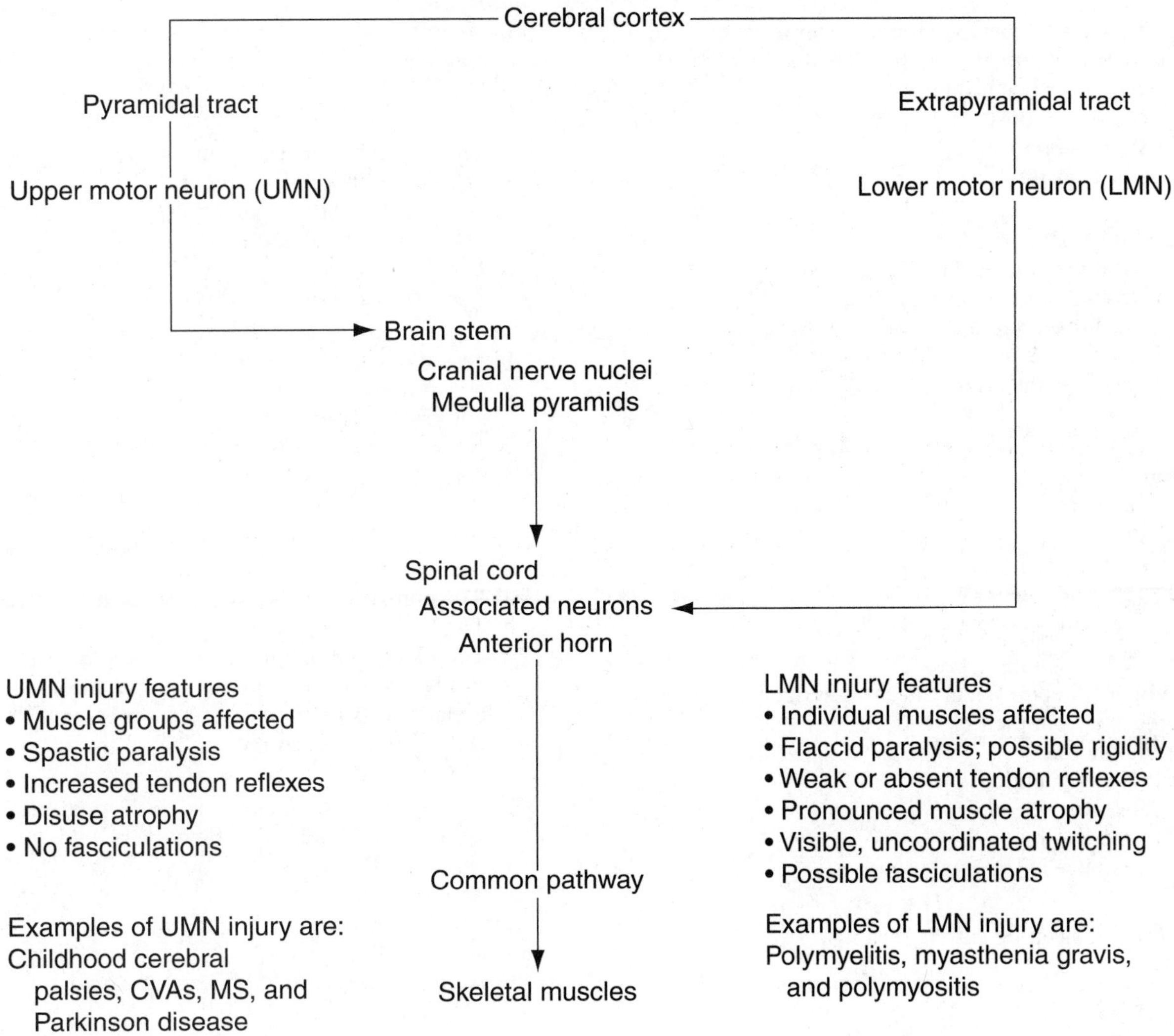

PRACTICE EXAMINATION

Multiple Choice

Circle the correct answer for each question:

1. Supratentorial processes reduce arousal by:
   a. destroying the reticular activating system.
   b. displacement of the brain stem.
   c. destroying the brain stem.
   d. Both a and c are correct.
   e. None of the above is correct.

2. An individual shows flexion in upper extremities and extension in lower extremities. This is:
   a. decorticate posturing.
   b. decerebrate posturing.
   c. excitation posturing.
   d. caloric posturing.

3. Cerebral death:
   a. is death of the cerebellum.
   b. permits normal internal homeostasis.
   c. means that respiratory and cardiovascular functions are no longer maintained.
   d. is death of the brain stem.

4. Precipitating causes of seizure include all of the following except:
   a. meningitis.
   b. stroke.
   c. hyperglycemia.
   d. hyperthermia.
   e. All of the above are correct.

5. Which epileptic seizure is characterized by temporal lobe spikes in the EEG?
   a. autonomic
   b. status epilepticus
   c. absence
   d. simple
   e. complex

6. Postictal sleeping can be seen in ______________________ seizures.
   a. partial
   b. unilateral
   c. absence
   d. tonic-clonic
   e. psychomotor

7. Alzheimer disease:
   a. can be caused by increased cerebral levels of acetylcholine.
   b. is most prevalent as a late-onset dementia.
   c. manifests as nerve cell tangles.
   d. manifests as neuron senile plaques.
   e. All of the above are correct.

8. Dystonia is:
   a. abnormal posture maintained by muscular contractions.
   b. flexed posture.
   c. stooped, hyperflexed posture.
   d. a spastic gait.

9. An individual with increased intracranial pressure from a head injury shows small and reactive pupils, widened pulse pressure, and slowed breathing. Which stage of ICP is present?
   a. stage 1
   b. stage 2
   c. stage 3
   d. stage 4

10. Infratentorial herniation occurs with:
    a. shifting of the mesencephalon.
    b. shifting of the diencephalon.
    c. shifting of the cerebellum.
    d. Both a and b are correct.
    e. None of the above is correct.

11. In cerebral vasogenic edema:
    a. active transport fails.
    b. autodigestion occurs.
    c. plasma proteins leak into extracellular spaces.
    d. cerebrospinal fluid leaves the ventricles.

12. Which statement is *not* true regarding increasing intracranial pressures?
    a. Accumulating CO_2 causes vasoconstriction.
    b. The brain volume increases.
    c. The blood volume in the vessels increases.
    d. Brain tissue shifts from the compartment of greater pressure to one of lesser pressure.
    e. Both b and c are correct.

13. Intellectual function is impaired in the dementing process. Which intellectual function is *not* impaired?
    a. anterograde memory
    b. retrograde memory
    c. abstraction
    d. language deficits
    e. All of the above functions are impaired.

Matching

Match the level of consciousness with its characteristic:

_______ 14. Confusion

_______ 15. Coma

a. orientation to person, time, and place
b. slow vocalization, decreased oculomotor activity
c. inability to think clearly
d. vocalization in response to pain stimuli
e. no arousal

Match the term with its definition:

_______ 16. Cortical dementia

_______ 17. Agnosia

_______ 18. Subcortical dementia

a. inability to understand relationships
b. inability to verify and correct input
c. inability to control motor function
d. inability to recognize sound
e. inability to remember

Match the term with its characteristic:

_______ 19. Huntington disease

_______ 20. Rigidity

_______ 21. Parkinson disease

_______ 22. Akinesia

_______ 23. Senile posture

_______ 24. Dyspraxia

_______ 25. Lower motor neuron syndrome

a. paralysis of both upper and lower extremities
b. decreased spontaneous and voluntary movements
c. absence of spontaneous gestures
d. abnormal posture maintained through muscular contractions
e. frontal lobe dysfunction
f. impaired execution of coordinated/complex acts
g. individual muscles affected
h. involuntary writing movements
i. organically caused impairment of intellectual functions
j. increased muscle tone
k. tonic reflex activity
l. flexed forward leaning

Complete the following table identifying descending levels of consciousness:

Altered Levels of Consciousness

State	Definition
Confusion	
Disorientation	
Lethargy	
Obtundation	
Stupor	
Coma	No vocalization or movement to any stimulus

CASE STUDY 1

A 12-year-old boy complained to his mother, "I am seeing blue, flashing lights, do you see them? I feel funny!" He then lost consciousness and had a major tonic-clonic seizure. His parents rushed him to the emergency department of a local hospital. On arrival at the hospital, he appeared to be asleep.

Studies at the hospital showed routine laboratory work within normal limits (WNL), lumbar puncture (CSF) was WNL, no evidence of skull fracture on x-ray study was revealed, and an electroencephalograph (EEG) showed no abnormalities.

How would you interpret the episode and findings?

CASE STUDY 2

L.B. is a 78-year-old widow living in her own home with a caretaker. Her son, who resides 300 miles away, visits regularly. He has been aware of his mother's progressing signs of cognitive/perceptual dysfunction since his father's death 2 years earlier and believes she has Alzheimer disease. On a Sunday morning visit, his mother offered to take him to lunch at McDonald's. She insisted on paying for both lunches at the ordering counter. When the cashier stated the cost, she objected saying, "You overcharged me 23 cents." The son tried to convince his mother that the cashier was correct, but she insisted she was correct. L.B. had summed the cost of the items in her head, multiplied that sum by the tax rate, and added the tax to the sum for a new total bill and was becoming angry at the young lady for overcharging her. The manager and her son concluded that L.B. was correct. When mother and son arrived home, L.B. was anxious, confused, and asked her son, "When are you going to take me home?" When told that she was home, she said, "It's all right. I'll stay here tonight but you must take me home tomorrow." The next day, Monday, her son took her to a trusted physician who knew that L.B. had asthma and had been treated with an inhaler and low-dose steroid for more than 40 years.

Why the contrast between math reasoning and confusion when returning home? What do you expect the physician to do?

15 Disorders of the Central and Peripheral Nervous Systems and the Neuromuscular Junction

FOUNDATIONAL OBJECTIVES

a. Identify the protective structures of the central nervous system (CNS).
Review pages 307-309; refer to Figures 12-15 through 12-17 and Table 12-4.

MEMORY CHECK!

- The cranium is composed of eight bones that fuse early in childhood. The cranial vault encloses and protects the brain and its associated structures. The floor of the cranial vault is irregular and contains many foramina or openings for cranial nerves, blood vessels, and the spinal cord to exit. The foramen magnum is large enough for the spinal cord to exit. Surrounding the brain and spinal cord are three protective membranes called the *meninges*: the dura mater, the arachnoid membrane, and the pia mater.
- The *dura mater* is composed of two layers and has venous sinuses between the layers. The outermost dural layer forms the periosteum of the skull. The inner dural meningeal layer forms the rigid plates that support and separate various brain structures.
- One of these membranous plates, the falx cerebri, transverses between the two cerebral hemispheres and anchors the base of the brain to the ethmoid bone. The tentorium cerebelli is a membrane that surrounds the brain stem and separates the cerebellum from the cerebral structures.
- Below the dura mater lies the *arachnoid membrane*, which is characterized by its spongy, weblike structure. The space between the dura and arachnoid membrane is the *subdural space*. Many small bridging veins traverse the subdural space. The *subarachnoid space* between the arachnoid membrane and the pia mater contains *cerebrospinal fluid (CSF)*. The delicate *pia mater* provides support for blood vessels serving the brain tissue. The choroid plexuses, structures that produce CSF, arise from the pial membrane. The spinal cord is anchored to the vertebrae by extension of the meninges. Between the dura mater and skull is a potential space, the *epidural space*.
- *CSF* is a clear, colorless fluid similar to blood plasma and interstitial fluid. The CNS's soft tissues are cushioned from traumatic jolts and blows because of the CSF's buoyant properties. The choroid plexuses in the lateral, third, and fourth ventricles produce the major portion of the CSF.

b. Describe the blood supply to the brain.
Review pages 310-313; refer to Figures 12-18 through 12-23 and Table 12-5.

MEMORY CHECK!

- The brain receives approximately 20% of the cardiac output, or 800 mL to 1000 mL of blood flow per minute. *Carbon dioxide* is a potent *vasodilator* in the CNS and *ensures* an adequate *cerebral blood supply*. The brain derives its arterial supply from two systems: the internal carotid arteries and the vertebral arteries.
- The internal carotid arteries originate from the common carotid arteries, enter the cranium through the base of the skull, and pass through the cavernous sinus. After giving off some small branches, they divide into the anterior and middle cerebral arteries. The vertebral arteries originate at the subclavian arteries and pass through the transverse foramina of the cervical vertebrae and enter the cranium through the foramen magnum. They join to form the basilar artery. The basilar artery divides at the level of the midbrain to form paired posterior cerebral arteries. Superficial arteries supply small branches that project into the brain. The *circle of Willis* is a structure with the ability to provide *collateral blood flow*. It is formed by many communicating arteries that extend to various brain structures.
- The venous drainage of the brain stem and cerebellum parallels the arterial supply; the venous drainage of the cerebrum does not. The cerebral veins are classified as superficial and deep. The veins drain into venous plexuses and dural sinuses and eventually drain into the internal jugular veins at the base of the skull. The *blood-brain barrier* selectively inhibits certain substances in the blood from entering the interstitial spaces of the brain or CSE. It is believed that the supporting cells and tight junctions between endothelial cells are involved in the formation of the blood-brain barrier and are responsible for its *selective impermeability*.

c. State the functions of the parts and associated structures of the brain.
Review pages 299, 301, 303, and 304; refer to Figures 12-5 through 12-9 and Table 12-3.

MEMORY CHECK!

Structural Functions of the Brain

Structure	Function
Brain stem	Performs sensory, motor, and reflex functions; controls cardiac, vasomotor, and respiratory centers; cranial nerve reflex
Cerebellum	Coordinates the activities of groups of muscles, maintains equilibrium, controls posture
Diencephalon:	
Thalamus	Conscious recognition of crude pain, temperature, and touch; relays sensory impulses except smell to cerebrum; emotions; arousal mechanism; complex reflex movements
Hypothalamus	Links nervous system to endocrine system; coordinates ANS; controls body temperature, hunger, thirst, and sleep
Cerebrum:	
Cerebral cortex lobes:	
Frontal	Voluntary control of skeletal muscles, unconscious skeletal muscle movement, speaking and writing
Temporal	Interpretation of odor and sound
Parietal	General body sensations
Occipital	Interpretation of sight
All lobes	Memory, emotions, reasoning, and intelligence
Left hemisphere	Language, numerical skills, motor control of right side of body
Right hemisphere	Musical and artistic awareness, space and pattern perception, insight, motor control of left side of body

LEARNING OBJECTIVES

After studying this chapter, the learner will be able to do the following:

1. Differentiate between focal and diffuse brain trauma.
Study pages 377-382; refer to Figures 15-1 and 15-2 and Tables 15-1 and 15-2.

Head injuries are caused by *blunt* or *closed* trauma and *penetrating* or *open* trauma. In blunt trauma, the head strikes a hard surface or a rapidly moving object strikes the head. The *dura remains intact*, and *brain tissues are not exposed* to the environment. When *a break in the dura exposes the cranial contents to the environment,* open trauma has occurred. Three types of injury produce brain damage: primary, secondary, and tertiary. *Primary* injury is caused by the impact and involves neural injury, primary glial injury, and vascular responses. *Secondary* injury consists of indirect consequences of the primary injury and includes altered cerebral blood flow, hypoxia, ischemia, inflammation, cerebral edema, increased intracranial pressure, and herniation; these effects cause further neural injury or death. *Tertiary* injury develops days or months later as consequences of primary or secondary injury.

Focal brain injury involves specific, grossly observable brain lesions seen in cortical contusions, epidural hemorrhage, subdural hematoma, and intracerebral hematoma. The smaller the area of impact, the greater the severity of injury because the force is concentrated into a smaller area. The focal injury may be coup or contrecoup. **Coup** is the *direct impact* area. **Contrecoup** lies *opposite the line of force*; the lesions occur where the brain strikes hard tissue on the side opposite the force.

Smaller forces of impact typically produce **contusions**, or bruises, on the brain. The contusion, in turn, can produce other focal injuries: epidural hemorrhage, subdural hematomas, and intracerebral hematomas. Contusion and bleeding occur because of small tears in blood vessels resulting from these forces. The clinical manifestations of a contusion may include immediate loss of consciousness, loss of reflexes, transient cessation of respiration, a brief period of bradycardia, and a fall in blood pressure. Vital signs may stabilize in a few seconds. Reflexes return next, and the person begins to regain consciousness. Returning to full alertness takes variable periods from minutes to days.

Large contusions and lacerations with hemorrhage may be surgically excised. Otherwise, treatment is directed at controlling intracranial pressure and managing symptoms.

Extradural hematomas, which are also called epidural hematomas or epidural hemorrhages, most often have an *artery* as the source of bleeding. Extradural hemorrhages may result in herniation through the foramen magnum.

Individuals with classic temporal extradural hematomas lose consciousness at the time of injury; some lucid periods follow. As the hematoma mass accumulates, a headache of increasing severity, vomiting, drowsiness, confusion, seizure, and hemiparesis may develop. The level of consciousness declines rapidly as the temporal lobe herniation begins. Clinical manifestations of temporal lobe herniation also include ipsilateral pupillary dilation and contralateral hemiparesis. Surgical therapy evacuates the hematoma through burr holes followed by ligation of the bleeding vessel(s).

Tearing of the *bridging veins* is the major cause of rapidly developing and subacutely developing **subdural hematomas.** However, torn cortical veins or venous sinuses and contused tissue may be the source of the bleeding. The subdural space gradually fills with blood, and herniation can result.

An acute subdural hematoma classically begins with headache, drowsiness, restlessness or agitation, slowed cognition, and confusion. These symptoms worsen over time and progress to loss of consciousness, respiratory pattern changes, and pupillary dilation. Most people with chronic subdural hematomas appear to have a progressive dementia accompanied by generalized rigidity. Chronic subdural hematomas require craniotomy to evacuate the gelatinous blood.

In **intracerebral hematomas** (intraparenchymal hemorrhages), *small blood vessels* are traumatized by shearing forces. The intracerebral hematoma expands, increases intracranial pressure, and compresses brain tissues.

In individuals with intracerebral hematomas, as the intracranial pressure rises, clinical manifestations of temporal lobe herniation may appear. Delayed intracerebral hematoma results in sudden, rapidly progressive decreases in levels of consciousness with pupillary dilatation, breathing pattern changes, hemiplegia, and bilateral presence of Babinski reflexes. Evacuation of a singular intracerebral hematoma is occasionally helpful for subcortical white matter hematomas. Otherwise, treatment is directed at reducing the intracranial pressure and allowing the hematoma to be reabsorbed slowly.

Diffuse brain injury or diffuse axonal injury (DAI) results from the inertial force to the head; it is *associated with high levels of acceleration, deceleration, and rotation.* The severity of the diffuse injury correlates with how much shearing force is applied to the brain stem. DAI often results in increased intravascular blood within the brain, vasodilation, and increased cerebral blood volume. Several categories of diffuse brain injury exist: mild concussion, classic concussion, mild DAI, moderate DAI, and severe DAI.

Mild concussion involves temporary axonal disturbances. Cerebral cortical dysfunction related to attentional and memory systems results, and *the individual does not lose consciousness.* The initial confusional state lasts for one to several minutes.

Classic cerebral concussion causes reflexes to fail transiently. Confusional states last for hours or days. *Loss of consciousness lasts more than 6 hours.*

In **mild DAI**, 30% of individuals display some *decerebrate or decorticate posturing.* They may experience prolonged stupor or restlessness.

In **moderate DAI**, widespread physiologic impairment exists throughout the cerebral cortex and diencephalon. Some *axons* in both hemispheres actually *tear.* Prolonged *unconsciousness* lasts longer than 24 hours, sometimes for weeks to months. Recovery is often incomplete in surviving individuals.

Severe DAI, formerly called *primary brain stem injury* or *brain stem contusion*, involves severe mechanical disruption of many axons in *both cerebral hemispheres* as well as axons extending to the diencephalon and brain stem. Profound sensorimotor and cognitive deficits are present. *Increased intracranial pressure* appears 4 to 6 days after injury.

Secondary brain trauma results from systemic and intracranial responses to primary brain trauma. Systemic hypotension, hypoxia, anemia, and hypercapnia and hypocapnia contribute to secondary brain insults. Secondary brain trauma management requires removal of hematomas and management of hypotension, hypoxemia, anemia, intracranial pressure, fluid selection, temperature, and ventilation.

2. Discuss the pathogenesis and manifestations of spinal cord injuries.

Study pages 382, 383, and 385-387; refer to Figures 15-3 through 15-7 and Tables 15-3 through 15-6.

Spinal cord injuries occur most often as a result of vertebral injuries. Traumatic forces injure the vertebral or neural tissues by compressing the tissue, pulling or exerting traction on the tissue, or shearing tissues so that they slide into one another.

Vertebral injuries occur most often at the first to second *cervical,* fourth to seventh *cervical*, and twelfth *thoracic* to second *lumbar vertebrae.* These are the most *mobile portions* of the vertebral column. The cord occupies most of the vertebral canal in these areas, and its size makes it more easily injured. Within a few minutes after injury, microscopic hemorrhages appear in the central gray matter and pia-arachnoid. Edema progresses into the white matter, impairing the microcirculation of the cord with reduced vascular perfusion and development of metabolic changes in spinal cord tissues, including lactate, and increasing concentrations of norepinephrine. The elevated norepinephrine values may produce further ischemia, vascular damage, and necrosis of tissue. Cord swelling increases the individual's degree of dysfunction. In the cervical region cord, swelling may be life threatening because of *impairment of diaphragm function*. Acellular collagenous tissue replaces the traumatized cord, usually in 3 to 4 weeks. Meninges thicken as part of the scarring process.

Normal activity of the spinal cord cells at and below the level of injury ceases because of the lack of continuous tonic discharges from the brain or brain stem and inhibition of suprasegmental impulses immediately after cord injury. This causes **spinal shock**, which is characterized by a complete *loss of reflex function in all segments below the level of the lesion*. This condition involves all skeletal muscles; bladder, bowel, and sexual function; and autonomic control.

Spinal shock may last for 7 to 20 days following onset; it may persist as long as 3 months. Indications that spinal shock is terminating include the reappearance of reflex activity, hyperreflexia, spasticity, and reflex emptying of the bladder. Loss of motor function and sensory function depends on the level and degree of injury. Paraplegia or quadriplegia can result. Return of spinal neuron excitability occurs slowly. Motor, sensory, reflex, and autonomic functions return to normal, or autonomic neural activity develops in the isolated segment.

Autonomic hyperreflexia (dysreflexia) is a syndrome that may occur at any time after spinal shock resolves. The syndrome is associated with a *massive, uncompensated cardiovascular response to stimulation of the sympathetic nervous system*. Individuals most likely to be affected have lesions at the T6 level or above. Hyperreflexia involves the stimulation of sensory receptors below the level of the cord injury. The intact autonomic nervous system reflexively responds with an arteriolar spasm that increases blood pressure. Baroreceptors in the cerebral vessels, the carotid sinus, and the aorta sense the hypertension and stimulate the parasympathetic system. The heart rate decreases, but the visceral and peripheral vessels do not dilate because efferent impulses cannot pass through the cord, and cardiovascular compensation is incomplete. The most common precipitating cause is a distended bladder or rectum, but any sensory stimulation can elicit autonomic hyperreflexia.

For a suspected or confirmed vertebral fracture or dislocation, the immediate intervention is immobilization of the spine to prevent further injury. Decompression and surgical fixation may be necessary. Corticosteroids are given to decrease secondary cord injury. In cases of autonomic hyperreflexia, intervention must be prompt because a cerebrovascular accident is possible. The head of the bed should be elevated, and the injurious stimulus should be found and removed. Medications may be used if these measures do not effectively reduce blood pressure.

3. Describe degenerative disorders of the spine.
Study pages 387 and 388; refer to Figures 15-8 and 15-9.

The etiology for **degenerative disk disease** (DDD) includes biochemical and biomechanical alterations of the tissue that comprise the intervertebral disk. *Fibrocartilage* replaces the *gelatinous mucoid material* of the nucleus pulposus as the disk changes with aging; the narrowing disk results in variable segmental instability. The pathologic findings in DDD include disk protrusion, spondylolysis, and/or subluxation and degeneration of vertebrae (spondylolisthesis) and spinal stenosis.

Spondylolysis is a structural defect that involves the *lamina* (neural arch of the vertebra). The most common site where this occurs is the *lumbar spine*. Heredity plays a significant role, and spondylolysis is associated with other congenital spinal defects. As a result of torsional and rotational stress, microfractures occur at the affected site and eventually cause dissolution of the pars interarticularis. **Spondylolisthesis** is caused when a vertebra *slides forward* in relation to an inferior vertebra; this commonly occurs at *L5-S1*. Spinal stenosis may represent several conditions ranging from entrapment of a single nerve root in the lateral recess to diffuse central stenosis involving many roots.

The local processes involved in **low back pain** include tension caused by tumors or disk prolapse, bursitis, synovitis, degenerative joint disease, abnormal bone pressures, spinal immobility, and inflammation caused by osteomyelitis, bony fractures, or ligamentous strains. Pain may be referred from viscera or the posterior peritoneum. General processes resulting in low back pain include bone diseases such as osteoporosis and osteomalacia seen in hyperparathyroidism

Most individuals with acute low back pain benefit from bed rest, analgesic medications, exercises, physical therapy, and education. Surgical treatments include diskectomy and spinal fusions. Individuals with chronic low back pain can be treated with anti-inflammatory and muscle relaxant medications and exercise programs. Spinal surgery has a limited role in curing chronic low back pain.

Herniation of an intervertebral disk is a *protrusion* of part *of the nucleus pulposus* through a tear in the fibrous capsule enclosing the gelatinous center of the disk. Rupture of intervertebral disks is usually caused by trauma, degenerative disease, or both. Lifting with the trunk flexed and sudden straining when the back is in an unstable position are the most common causes; males are more affected than females. Most commonly affected are the lumbosacral disks; disk herniation occasionally occurs in the cervical area. The symptoms may be immediate or occur within a few hours, or they may take months to years to develop. The pain of a herniated disk in the lumbosacral area radiates along the sciatic nerve over the buttock and into the calf or ankle. With the herniation of a lower cervical disk, paresthesia and pain are present in the upper arm, forearm, and hand, according to the affected nerve root distribution.

The conservative therapeutic approach, not likely effective, comprises traction, bed rest, heat and ice to the affected areas, and an effective analgesic regimen. The surgical approach is indicated if there is weakness and decreased deep tendon reflexes and bladder/bowel reflexes or if the conservative approach is unsuccessful.

4. Compare and contrast cerebrovascular accidents (stroke syndromes).
Study pages 388-390.

Cerebrovascular accidents are classified as ischemic (thrombotic, embolic) or hemorrhagic. These *accidents are vascular in origin but are manifested neurologically.*

The following are risk factors for cerebrovascular occlusive disease:

Hypertension	Polycythemia vera and thrombocythemia
Cigarette smoking	Impaired cardiac function
Hyperhomocysteinemia	Atrial fibrillation
Diabetes mellitus	*Chlamydia pneumoniae* infection
Insulin resistance	

The development of a **thrombotic stroke** is caused by arteries supplying the brain and is most frequently attributed to *atherosclerosis and inflammatory disease processes that damage arterial walls. Atheromatous plaques* tend to form at branchings and curves in the cerebral circulation. Degeneration or bleeding into the vessel wall may cause endothelial damage. Platelets and fibrin adhere to the damaged wall, and delicate thrombi form. Small thrombi collect over time and gradual occlusion of the artery occurs. Once the artery is occluded, the thrombus may enlarge lengthwise in the vessel.

In thrombotic strokes, treatment is directed at supportive management to control cerebral edema and increased intracranial pressure. Intervention to restore blood supply may be indicated. Arresting the disease process by controlling risk factors is critical. Drugs that achieve defibrinogenation to permit local blood flow are useful.

The new definition for **transient ischemic attack (TIA)** is a *brief episode* of neurologic dysfunction caused by a focal disturbance of brain or retinal ischemia with clinical symptoms typically lasting more than an hour, *no evidence of infarction, and complete clinical recovery.* Thrombotic particles cause an intermittent blockage of circulation.

An **embolic stroke** involves *fragments that break from a thrombus that was formed outside the brain.* Common sites are in the heart, aorta, common carotid artery, or thorax. The embolus usually involves small vessels and obstructs a bifurcation or other narrowing to cause ischemia. Conditions associated with an embolic stroke include atrial fibrillation, myocardial infarction, endocarditis, rheumatic heart disease, valvular prostheses, atrial septal defects, and disorders of the aorta, carotid arteries, or vertebral-basilar circulation. In individuals who experience an embolic stroke, usually a *second stroke follows at some point,* because the source of emboli continues to exist. Emboli usually lodge in the distribution of the middle cerebral artery. Treatment of embolic strokes is directed at preventing further embolization by instituting anticoagulation therapy and correcting the primary problem. Rehabilitation is indicated in both thrombotic and embolic strokes.

The most common causes of **hemorrhagic stroke** are hypertension, ruptured aneurysms, arteriovenous malformation, and hemorrhage associated with bleeding disorders. Hypertensive hemorrhage is associated with a significant increase in systolic-diastolic pressure over several years and usually occurs within the brain tissue. A mass of blood forms as its volume increases; adjacent *brain tissue is displaced and compressed.* Rupture or seepage into the ventricular system occurs in many of the cases. The most common sites for hypertensive hemorrhages are in the putamen of the basal ganglia and the hypothalamus.

Lacunar strokes (lacunar infarcts) are very small and *involve the small arteries,* predominantly in the basal ganglia, internal capsules, and brain stem. Because of the subcortical location and small area of infarction, these strokes may cause motor and sensory deficits.

Treatment of an intracranial stroke, regardless of cause, is focused on stopping or reducing the bleeding, controlling the increased intracranial pressure, preventing another hemorrhagic episode, and preventing vasospasm. At times, an attempt is made to evacuate or aspirate the blood.

Cerebral infarction results when an area *of the brain loses blood.* The symptoms depend on the blood vessel involved. Essentially, if the internal carotid artery branches are involved, there is confusion, inability to plan, aphasia, perception disorders, paralysis, or blindness. If the vertebral artery branches are involved, there is diplopia, ataxia, vertigo, dysphagia, and dysphonia.

Aspirin, systemic anticoagulation, and thrombolysis improve outcomes in individuals with ischemic stroke. Antiplatelet therapy and statins decrease recurrence. Endarterectomy may be effective.

5. Describe intracranial aneurysm and vascular malformations.
Study pages 390-392; refer to Figures 15-10 and 15-11 and Table 15-7.

Intracranial aneurysms may result from arteriosclerosis, congenital abnormality, trauma, inflammation, or infection. Cocaine has also been linked to aneurysm formation. Aneurysm *development is attributed to hemodynamic stress and is believed to be exacerbated by hypertension and certain connective tissue disorders.*

Aneurysms may be classified on the basis of shape and form. **Saccular aneurysms** (berry aneurysms) occur in approximately 2% of the population and are probably the result of congenital abnormalities in the media of the arterial wall. **Fusiform aneurysms** (giant aneurysms) are larger than 25 mm in diameter and occur as a result of diffuse arteriosclerotic changes. They are found most commonly in the basilar arteries or terminal portions of the internal carotid arteries.

Aneurysms are frequently asymptomatic. Clinical manifestations may arise from cranial nerve compression, but the signs vary according to the location and size of the aneurysm. The treatment of choice for an aneurysm is surgical management before rupture occurs. The location and size of the aneurysm and the person's clinical status determine whether invasive therapy is feasible.

Arteriovenous malformation (AVM) is a tangled *mass of dilated blood vessels.* Although sometimes present at birth, AVM exhibits a delayed age of onset, most commonly occurring before 30 years of age. Fifty percent of individuals with this condition experience a hemorrhage. Clinical manifestations of AVM range from headache and dementia to seizures and intracerebral or subarachnoid hemorrhage.

A **subarachnoid hemorrhage** occurs when blood escapes from defective or injured vasculature into the subarachnoid space. Individuals at risk are those with aneurysm, vascular malformations, and head injuries. When a vessel tears, blood under pressure is pumped into the subarachnoid space and produces an inflammatory reaction in these tissues.

Clinical manifestations of a subarachnoid hemorrhage include headache, changes in mental status, transient motor weakness, nausea or vomiting, visual or speech disturbances, cranial nerve palsies, and stiff neck. A **Kernig sign** is present if pain in the back and neck is produced when the knee is straightened with hip and hip in flexed position. In the **Brudzinski sign,** neck pain and increased rigidity occur with passive flexion of the neck. Vasospasm and delayed cerebral ischemia are serious complications. Treatment of vasospasm includes use of calcium channel blockers and augmentation of cerebral perfusion by volume expansion and hemodilution.

6. Describe chronic, recurring headaches.

Study pages 392 and 393; refer to Table 15-8.

Headache is a common neurologic disorder and is *usually a benign symptom.* However, it can be associated with brain tumors, meningitis, and giant cell arteritis. Migraine, cluster, paroxysmal hemicrania, and tension headaches are chronic, recurring types that are not associated with structural abnormalities or systemic disease.

Prevalence of **migraine headache** is higher in women, is highest in patients between 25 and 55 years of age, and the rate in women remains higher than that in men into older age. Migraine headaches are *episodic and repeating and last 4 to 72 hours.* Three phases are present in migraine headache: premonitory, migraine aura, and headache. It is diagnosed when any two of the following occur: unilateral pain, worsening with movement; photophobia or phonophobia; throbbing; moderate to severe nausea; and vomiting. Migraines are caused *by multiple genetic and environmental factors.* Trigger factors include stress, hunger, weather changes, sunlight, noise, jet lag, menstruation, and alcohol or nitrates. The pathogenesis of migraine headaches includes a vascular theory, depression, and serotonergic and other neurotransmitter alterations.

Avoidance of triggers, adequate sleep, regular eating habits, and daily relaxation and meditation can create a headache-protective environment. With the onset of acute migraine, *a dark room, ice, and sleep can provide relief.* Drug considerations include antiemetics, ergotamine and dihydroergotamine, and 5-HT (serotonin) antagonists.

Cluster headaches *occur primarily (eight times more commonly) in men* between 20 and 50 years of age. Several attacks can occur during the day for a period of days followed by long periods of remission. Cluster headache has an episodic and chronic form.

The headache attack usually begins without warning and is characterized by severe, burning, *periorbital*, and retrobulbar or temporal pain that lasts 30 minutes to 2 hours. The *same side is affected in subsequent episodes.* Associated symptoms include lacrimation, reddening of the eye, nasal stuffiness, eyelid ptosis, and nausea. Pain often is referred to the midface and the teeth. If the attacks occur more frequently without sustained spontaneous remission, they are classified as chronic cluster headaches. Alcohol can stimulate an attack in about 50% to 70% of cases, but it is not a triggering factor during remission.

Pathogenic mechanisms may include vascular alterations, neurogenic or neuroimmunologic dysregulation of the hypothalamus, dysregulation of the parasympathetic ganglia, sympathetic deficit, and stimulation of the trigeminal nucleus. The rhythmicity of attacks is probably related to disorders of the hypothalamus.

Prophylactic drugs are used to treat cluster headaches. The most effective are prednisone, lithium, methysergide, calcium channel antagonists, and valproate. Acute attacks are managed with oxygen inhalation, sumatriptan, and inhaled ergotamine.

Chronic paroxysmal hemicrania is a *cluster type of headache that occurs with more daily frequency but with shorter duration.* The attacks are more common in women, usually after pregnancy. The pathophysiology involves a disorder of sympathetic hyperactivity, but the mechanism is different from that in cluster headache, because there is effective relief of symptoms with indomethacin.

Tension headache is the most common type of headache. Age of onset is during the second decade of life. It is a mild to moderate *bilateral headache with a sensation of a tight band or pressure around the head. The onset of pain is usually gradual.* The headache occurs in episodes and may last for several hours or several days. It is not aggravated by physical activity.

Both a central mechanism and a peripheral mechanism cause tension headaches. The central mechanism probably involves hypersensitivity of pain fibers from the trigeminal nerve. The peripheral mechanism is probably related to contraction of jaw and neck muscles.

Meningitis and Encephalitis

	Bacterial Meningitis	Aseptic Meningitis (Viral)	Encephalitis
Site	Pia mater, arachnoid, subarachnoid space, CSF, ventricles	Meninges	Meninges
Infectious agents	*Neisseria meningitidis, Streptococcus pneumonia*	Several viruses	Arthropod-borne viruses, herpes simplex virus type 1, complications of systemic viral infection
Lesion	Meningeal vessels become hyperemic and permeable	Similar to bacterial	Nerve cell degeneration
Manifestations	Throbbing headache, photophobia, flexion of legs and thighs, stiff neck, projectile vomiting, confusion	Mild but similar symptoms to those of bacterial meningitis	Fever, delirium, confusion, coma, seizure, cranial paresis and paralysis
CSF	Increased pressure, bacteria, elevated protein values; decreases in glucose levels and neutrophils and monocyte content	Increased pressure, normal glucose levels and lymphocyte content	Same as aseptic meningitis
Treatment	Antibiotics	Antiviral agents and steroids	Herpes infections—antiviral agents, control of intracranial pressure

Note: Fungal meningitis is a chronic, much less common infection than bacterial or viral meningitis.

Mild headaches are treated with ice, and more severe forms are treated with aspirin or nonsteroidal anti-inflammatory drugs. Chronic tension headaches are best managed with a tricyclic antidepressant.

7. Compare meningitis to encephalitis.
Study pages 394-396; refer to Figure 15-12 and Table 15-9.

8. Characterize CNS abscesses.
Study pages 394 and 395; refer to Figure 15-13.

Abscesses are *localized collections of pus within the parenchyma or functioning cells of the brain and spinal cord.* Abscesses occur following open trauma and during neurosurgery; from foci of infection such as the middle ear, mastoid cells, nasal cavity, and nasal sinuses; and through metastatic or hematogenous spread from distant foci. Streptococci, staphylococci, and *Bacteroides* in combination with anaerobes are the most common bacteria that cause abscesses. However, yeast and fungi have also been found in CNS abscesses.

Initially, a localized inflammatory process surrounding a necrotic core leads to cerebral edema, hyperemia, softening, and petechial hemorrhage. After a few days, fibroblasts and capillaries deposit collagen fibers that contain and encapsulate the purulent focus.

Clinical manifestations of **brain abscesses** include fever, headache, nausea, vomiting, decreasing cognitive abilities, paresis, and seizures. These signs and symptoms develop because of the infection and expanding mass. Clinical manifestations of **spinal cord abscesses** are spinal discomfort, root pain accompanied by spasms of the back muscles and limited vertebral movement because of pain and spasm, weakness that results from progressive cord compression, and paralysis.

Aspiration or excision accompanied by antibiotic therapy is the recommended, but somewhat controversial, treatment for brain abscesses. Intracranial pressure must be managed. Spinal cord abscesses are treated with surgical excision or aspiration because decompression is necessary. Antibiotic and supportive therapies are also required.

9. Identify the neurologic complications of AIDS.
Study pages 396 and 397.

Approximately 40% to 60% of all people with AIDS experience neurologic complications. The most common neurologic disorder is HIV-associated cognitive dysfunction. Other common neurologic disorders are peripheral neuropathies, vacuolar myelopathy, opportunistic infection of the CNS, and neoplasms.

HIV-associated dementia is characterized by insidious onset and unpredictable but progressive cognitive dysfunction in conjunction with motor and behavioral alterations. Later, cognitive dysfunction is accompanied by psychomotor slowing, loss of balance, ataxia, spastic paralysis or paraparesis, and generalized hyperreflexia. HIV cognitive dysfunction is likely the result of direct brain tissue infection by the virus. HIV is mostly found in white matter subcortical areas.

Vacuolar myelopathy and multinucleated giant cell encephalitis involving diffuse degeneration of the spinal cord may occur in people with AIDS. A progressive spastic paraparesis with ataxia is the predominant clinical manifestation. Leg weakness, upper motor neuron signs, incontinence, and posterior column sensory loss may be present.

Peripheral neuropathy, which is an HIV neuropathy, is a sensory neuropathy. Individuals experience painful dysthesias and paresthesias in the extremities. Weakness and decrease or absence of distal reflexes may be seen.

Some individuals demonstrate acute **aseptic meningitis** at approximately the time of seroconversion to positive HIV status. Headache, fever, and meningismus with cranial nerve involvement, especially of cranial nerves V and VII, may appear.

Opportunistic viral infections may cause nervous system disease. Papovavirus may produce a demyelinating disorder called progressive multifocal leukoencephalopathy, which causes sensory and motor deficits, aphasia, and apraxia. People with cytomegalovirus encephalitis experience nystagmus and cranial nerve deficits.

Opportunistic nonviral infections are the most common CNS disorders associated with AIDS. Clinical manifestations of CNS toxoplasmosis, which is a common AIDS disorder, are highly variable and include clumsiness, hemiplegia, aphasia, seizures, ataxia, and cognitive changes.

CNS neoplasms associated with AIDS include CNS lymphoma, systemic non-Hodgkin lymphoma, and metastatic Kaposi sarcoma

Demyelinating CNS Diseases

	Multiple Sclerosis	ALS
Lesion site	Irreversible CNS axonal demyelination and sclerosis	Scarring/sclerosis of corticospinal tract in lateral column of spinal cord—upper and lower motor neurons
Etiology	Immunogenetic—viral/genetic/environmental, T cells become autoreactive to myelin, B cells produce autoantibodies and inflammatory cytokines against myelins	Genetics, defective superoxide dismutase gene
Onset	Between 20 and 50 years of age	40s, peaks in early 50s
Manifestations	Remissions and exacerbations but progressive paresthesia, diplopia, cerebellar incoordination, urinary dysfunction	Progressive muscle weakness and atrophy, respiratory failure, paralysis, normal intellectual and sensory function until death
Treatment	Steroids to shorten exacerbations, drugs to reduce relapses, supportive and rehabilitative management	Antiglutamates may reduce excitotoxicity and lengthen time before need for ventilation assistance

10. Distinguish between the demyelinating disorders multiple sclerosis and amyotrophic lateral sclerosis (ALS).
Study pages 397 and 398; refer to Figure 15-14.

11. Describe myasthenia gravis.
Study pages 399 and 400.

Myasthenia gravis is a disorder of voluntary or striated muscles characterized by muscle weakness and fatigability due to a defect in nerve impulse transmission at the neuromuscular junction. Between 70% and 80% of persons with myasthenia gravis have pathologic changes in the *thymus;* this disorder is an *autoimmune disease*. Different types of myasthenia gravis exist. **Ocular myasthenia**, which is more common in males, involves muscle weakness confined to the eye muscles. **Generalized autoimmune myasthenia** involves the proximal musculature throughout the body and exhibits varying rates of progression with possible remissions.

In myasthenia gravis, postsynaptic acetylcholine receptors on the muscle cell's plasma membrane are no longer recognized as "self." Therefore, *IgG antibody is secreted against the acetylcholine receptors*. These antibodies fix onto the receptor sites and block the binding of acetylcholine. Eventually, the antibody action causes the destruction of receptor sites and the diminished transmission of the nerve impulse across the neuromuscular junction.

The muscles of the eyes, face, mouth, throat, and neck *are usually affected first*. Manifestations include diplopia, ptosis, and ocular palsies; facial droop and an expressionless face; difficulty chewing and swallowing; drooling, episodes of choking, and aspirations; and a nasal, low-volume but high-pitched monotonous speech pattern. The muscles of the neck, shoulder girdle, and hip flexor are less often affected.

Myasthenic crisis occurs when severe muscle weakness causes extreme quadriparesis or quadriplegia, respiratory insufficiency that can lead to *respiratory arrest*, and extreme difficulty in swallowing. **Cholinergic crisis** is caused by the muscle hyperactivity secondary to excessive accumulation of acetylcholine at the neuromuscular junctions and excessive parasympathetic activity. As in myasthenic crisis, the individual is in danger of respiratory arrest.

Anticholinesterase drugs, steroids, and immunosuppressant drugs are used to treat myasthenia gravis and myasthenic crisis. Treatment of individuals with cholinergic crisis involves withholding anticholinergic drugs until blood levels fall out of the toxic range while providing ventilatory support.

12. Describe the pathophysiology, manifestations, and treatment of CNS tumors; classify common brain tumors.

Study pages 400 and 402-404; refer to Figures 15-15 and 15-16; and Tables 15-11 and 15-12.

Cranial tumors can be either primary or metastatic. **Primary intracerebral tumors** originate from brain substance, neuroglia, neurons, cells of the blood vessels, and connective tissue. They include astrocytomas, oligodendrogliomas and ependymomas. **Primary extracerebral tumors** originate outside the substance of the brain and include meningiomas, and neurofibromas. **Metastatic tumors** can be found inside or outside the brain substance.

Cranial tumors have local and generalized clinical manifestations. The local effects are caused by the destructive action of a particular site in the brain and by compression that reduces cerebral blood flow. The effects are varied and include seizures, visual disturbances, unstable gait, and cranial nerve dysfunction. The generalized effects result from increased intracranial pressure.

Intracranial brain tumors do not metastasize as readily as tumors in other organs because there are no lymphatic channels within the brain substance. If metastasis does occur, it is usually through seeding of cerebral blood or CSF, during cranial surgery, or through artificial shunts.

The principal treatment for cerebral neoplasms is surgical or radiosurgical excision or surgical decompression if total excision is not possible. Chemotherapy and radiotherapy may also be used. Supportive treatment is directed at reducing edema.

In an estimated 25% of *persons with cancer, metastasis to the brain develops*. One third of metastatic brain tumors arise from the *lung*, approximately one sixth from the breast, and a lesser number from the gastrointestinal tract and kidney. Other tumors metastasize less often. Carcinomas are disseminated to the brain by the circulation. Metastatic brain tumors carry a poor prognosis. If a solitary tumor is found, surgery or radiation therapy is used; but if multiple tumors exist, only symptomatic relief is pursued.

Neurofibromas (benign nerve sheath tumors) are a group of autosomal dominant disorders. *Neurofibromatosis type 1* causes multiple cutaneous neurofibromas, café au-lait spots and freckles, and, less commonly, bone and soft tissue tumors. Inactivation of the *NF1* gene results in loss of function of neurofibromin in Schwann cells and promotes tumorigenesis. In about 50% of cases, *learning disabilities* are present.

Neurofibromamatosis type 2 is rare. Mutations of the *NF2* gene promote development of CNS schwannomas. Most commonly affect individuals in their 20s and 30s. The *vestibular division of cranial nerve VIII is most commonly affected* and can cause hearing loss or deafness.

Spinal cord tumors are classified as **intramedullary tumors**, those originating within the neural tissues, or **extramedullary tumors**, those originating from tissues outside the spinal cord. Intramedullary tumors have the same cellular origins as brain tumors. Extramedullary tumors arise from the meninges, epidural tissue, or vertebral structure. The most common primary extramedullary spinal cord tumors are neurofibromas and meningiomas.

The acute onset of clinical manifestations of spinal cord tumor suggests a vascular occlusion of vessels supplying the spinal cord. In the **compressive syndrome**,

Classification of Common Primary Brain Tumors

Type	Frequency	Age Group	Feature(s)
Astrocytoma	50% (brain/spinal cord)	Adults	Slow-growing, invasive, infiltrative
Oligodendroglioma	10%-15% (brain)	Adults	Slow-growing
Ependymoma	6%-10% (brain ventricles)	All ages	Variable growth rate, invasive
Meningioma	30% (brain)	All ages	Slow-growing, circumscribed

the motor dysfunction and sensory manifestations occur as the tumor grows. Pain develops.

The **irritative syndrome** combines the clinical manifestations of a cord compression with radicular pain. This pain is in the sensory root distribution and indicates root irritation. Sensory changes include paresthesia and impaired pain and touch perception; motor disturbances include cramps, atrophy, fasciculation, and decrease or absence of deep tendon reflexes.

PRACTICE EXAMINATION

Multiple Choice

Circle the correct answer for each question:

1. In blunt head trauma:
   a. brain tissues are exposed.
   b. only focal injury occurs.
   c. the dura is severed.
   d. the dura remains intact.

2. In an automobile accident, an individual's forehead struck the windshield. The coup/contrecoup injury would be in the:
   a. frontal/parietal region.
   b. frontal/occipital region.
   c. parietal/occipital region.
   d. occipital/frontal region.

3. In moderate diffuse axonal injury:
   a. coma lasts more than 24 hours.
   b. coma lasts less than 24 hours.
   c. axons in cerebral hemispheres and those extending into the diencephalon and brain stem are disrupted.
   d. tearing of axons in the cerebral hemisphere occurs.
   e. Both a and d are correct.

4. Most spinal cord injuries occur in the:
   a. cervical and thoracic regions.
   b. cervical and lumbar regions.
   c. thoracic and lumbar regions.
   d. lumbar and sacral regions.

5. Injury of the cervical cord may be life threatening because of:
   a. increased intracranial pressure.
   b. disrupted reflexes.
   c. spinal shock.
   d. loss of bladder and rectal control.
   e. diaphragmatic impairment.

6. Autonomic hyperreflexia is characterized by all of the following *except:*
   a. hypotension.
   b. slower heart rate.
   c. stimulation of sensory receptors below the level of the cord lesion.
   d. precipitation because of a distended bladder or rectum.

7. Intervertebral disk herniation:
   a. usually occurs at the thoracic level.
   b. in the lumbosacral area causes pain over the gluteal region and into the calf or ankle.
   c. is infrequent in the lumbosacral disks.
   d. Both b and c are correct.
   e. a, b, and c are correct.

8. TIAs are:
   a. unilateral neurologic deficits that slowly resolve.
   b. generalized neurologic deficits that occur a few seconds every hour.
   c. focal neurologic deficits that develop suddenly, last more than an hour, and clear without evidence of infarction.
   d. neurologic deficits that slowly evolve or develop.

9. Which is a risk factor for the development of CVAs?
   a. polycythemia vera
   b. hypertension
   c. diabetes mellitus
   d. hyperhomocysteinemia
   e. All of the above are risk factors.

10. Which most typically characterizes the victims of a cerebral embolic stroke?
    a. individuals older than 65 years with a history of hypertension
    b. individuals with a long history of TIAs
    c. middle-aged individuals with a history of heart disease
    d. individuals with gradually occurring symptoms that then rapidly disappear

11. Ruptured aneurysms are most likely in which of the following cerebrovascular accidents.
    a. TIA
    b. thrombotic
    c. embolic
    d. hemorrhagic

12. Which is *not* a primary intracerebral neoplasm?
    a. astrocytoma
    b. meningioma
    c. oligodendroglioma
    d. ependymoma

13. In bacterial meningitis, the CSF has:
    a. normal glucose levels.
    b. an elevated number of lymphocytes.
    c. neutrophilic infiltration.
    d. None of the above is correct.
    e. a, b, and c are correct.

14. Multiple sclerosis involves:
    a. degeneration of dopaminergic receptors.
    b. activation of T cells autoreactive to myelin.
    c. depletion of GABA.
    d. lower motor neuron muscle wasting.

15. Manifestations of subarachnoid hemorrhage include which of the following? (More than one answer may be correct.)
    a. a stiff neck
    b. muscle flaccidity
    c. Kernig sign
    d. a delayed age of onset

Matching
Match the injury with its characteristic:

_______ 16. Concussion
_______ 17. Contusion
_______ 18. Extradural hematoma
_______ 19. Subdural hematoma
_______ 20. Intracerebral hematoma

a. bleeding into the brain's parenchyma
b. bruising of part of the brain
c. violent displacement of brain tissue resulting from rotation, acceleration, or deceleration
d. arterial bleeding
e. venous bleeding

Match the disease with its site of dysfunction:

_______ 21. Spondylolysis
_______ 22. Myasthenia gravis
_______ 23. Multiple sclerosis
_______ 24. Guillain-Barré syndrome
_______ 25. Amyotrophic lateral sclerosis

a. cerebral cortex
b. neural arch of vertebra
c. peripheral nerve myelin
d. neuromuscular junction
e. ventricular system of brain
f. corticospinal tracts
g. CNS myelin
h. muscles

Fill in the Blank

Complete the following table comparing focal to diffuse traumatic brain injury:

Focal and Diffuse Traumatic Brain Injuries

Type of Injury	Characteristics
Focal	
Contusion	
Coup/contrecoup	
Extradural hematoma	Arterial bleeding, immediate to delayed loss of consciousness, possible herniation
Subdural hematoma	
Delayed intracerebral hematoma	
Diffuse	
Mild concussion	
Classic cerebral concussion	
Mild DAI	
Moderate DAI	
Severe DAI	Axonal tears in both hemispheres, diencephalon, and brain stem; sensory and cognitive deficits; increased intracranial pressure

CASE STUDY

Mrs. B. is an overweight 71-year-old white female who slurred to her daughter, "My right head hurts. Can you understand me?" Upon hospital admission, she exhibited some severe right-handed numbness with a weak left hand grip. Her smile was asymmetrical with right-sided facial weakness that had persisted for 48 hours. Mrs. B. has a history of smoking moderately for 50 years. Her mother had adult-onset diabetes and died of breast cancer at age 62; one sister died of a subarachnoid hemorrhage at age 63; and another sister is hemiparetic because of a CVA. One brother is hypertensive, and three other, younger siblings are apparently healthy.

Vital signs showed a normal temperature, elevated heart rate, and normal respirations, but a severely elevated blood pressure. CSF obtained by lumbar puncture tested negative for blood with normal protein and glucose levels. Electrocardiogram findings were normal. An electroencephalogram showed localized activity in the left hemisphere. A CT scan showed increased density on the left. Blood chemistry results were normal except for elevated glucose.

How would you assess Mrs. B.'s history, her family history, and her symptoms and signs?

Complete the following table to differentiate types of cerebrovascular accidents:

Cerebrovascular Accidents

Type	Thrombotic	Embolic	Hemorrhagic	Ischemic	Lacunar
Involved sites					
Risk factors					
Causes					

16 Alterations of Neurologic Function in Children

FOUNDATIONAL OBJECTIVES

a. Identify the features of neural growth and development.
Review pages 409 and 410; refer to Figure 16-1.

MEMORY CHECK!

- The nervous system develops from embryonic ectoderm. Stages include: (1) formation of the neural tube (3-4 weeks of gestation); (2) forebrain development from neural tube (2-3 months of gestation); (3) neuronal proliferation and migration (3-5 months of gestation); (4) formation of network connections and synapses (5 months of gestation to many years postnatal); and (5) myelination (birth to many years postnatal). Environmental factors have a significant effect on neural development.
- The growth and development of the brain occur rapidly during the 15th and 29th weeks of gestation and again at 30 weeks of gestation through the first year of life, reflecting the development and multiplication of neurons. *One half of postnatal brain growth occurs in the first year and is 90% complete by age 6 years.* The cortex thickens with maturation, and the sulci deepen as cortical functions develop. Cerebral blood flow and oxygen consumption are about twice those of the adult brain during these years. The bones of the infant's skull are separated at the suture line to form anterior and posterior fontanelles, or "soft spots." The posterior fontanelle may be open until 2 to 3 months of age, whereas the anterior fontanel normally closes by 18 months.

b. Identify the normal infant neurologic reflexes.
Refer to Table 16-1.

MEMORY CHECK!

- Many *reflex* patterns are mediated by the brain stem and spinal cord at birth. As the infant matures, the neonatal reflexes disappear in a predictable order as voluntary motor functions replace them during infancy. If these reflexes persist, developmental delays or central motor lesions are likely.

LEARNING OBJECTIVES

After studying this chapter, the learner will be able to do the following:

1. Describe the major forms of central nervous system(CNS) malformation.
Study pages 410-416; refer to Figures 16-2 through 16-5 and Tables 16-2 and 16-3.

Neural tube defects are caused by an arrest in development of the brain and spinal cord. A strong association with fetal death obscures the actual incidence somewhat. These defects can be subdivided into *posterior defects (anencephaly), the myelodysplasias (defects of the vertebral column and spinal cord)*, and the less frequent anterior midline defects. Maternal ingestion of the daily allowance of folic acid before conception or early in pregnancy reduces the risks for neural tube defects.

Anencephaly is the absence of the skull and parts of the brain that results from early *closure of the anterior neural tube*. It is a relatively common disorder that is fatal.

Encephalocele is *the herniation of the brain and meninges* through a midline defect in the skull. An encephalocele may be located in the nasopharynx, in which case no obvious deformity is noted, but the defect may cause nasal congestion. CNS tissue may be seen on nasal examination. This type of defect has a good prognosis for surgical repair. Size, location, and timing of the development of encephalocele determine the potential outcome for the child's development and cognition.

Meningocele is the *protrusion of meninges through a vertebral defect*. The spinal cord is not involved. The meningocele is present at birth as a protruding sac at the level of the defect. It can occur in the cervical, thoracic, or lumbar area.

Myelomeningocele, or spina bifida cystica, is a *herniation* of the meninges, spinal fluid, a portion of the spinal cord, and nerves through a vertebral defect; 80% are located in the lumbosacral region. The *Arnold-Chiari malformation* is a serious association with myelomeningoceles that displaces the cerebellar tonsils downward and can result in cysts within the spinal cord.

Spina bifida occulta is a less serious form of myelomeningocele, with the defect occurring in the lumbar or sacral area of the spine because of *incomplete fusion of the vertebral laminae*. Spina bifida occulta is more common than myelomeningocele and usually causes no neurologic deficits; it may occur in 10% to 25% of infants. Physical findings include abnormal hair growth along the spine, a midline sacral dimple with or without a sinus tract, angioma over the defect, and an overlying subcutaneous mass.

Craniosynostosis is the *premature closure of cranial sutures* during the first 20 months of life. Asymmetry of the skull or interference with brain growth may result if multiple sutures are involved.

Microcephaly is a defect in brain growth as a whole. *Primary* microcephaly may be caused by an autosomal recessive genetic disorder or a chromosomal deficit. *Secondary* microcephaly may be caused by toxin, radiation, or chemical exposure during periods of induction and major cell migration. It may be caused by various insults during the third trimester.

Congenital hydrocephalus is characterized by an *increase in the volume of cerebrospinal fluid (CSF)* that may be caused by overproduction, a defect in reabsorption, or blockage of the ventricular drainage system. Before fusion of the sutures, the skull is able to accommodate the increased fluid, which preserves neuronal function. *Dandy-Walker* deformity is causes by cystic dilation of the fourth ventricle and aqueductal compression, which obstructs CSF flow.

2. Describe the static encephalopathic processes.
Study pages 415-417; refer to Figure 16-6 and Table 16-4.

Cerebral palsy (CP) is a *static* encephalopathy, meaning that *the resulting damage does not change over time*. Clinical manifestations, however, may change as the child continues to develop. CP can be classified according to the neurologic symptoms produced. These include spasticity, ataxia, dyskinesia, and a combination of all three. CP can be caused by prenatal cerebral hypoxia or perinatal trauma. Symptoms include increased motor tone and reflexes, loss of fine motor coordination, mental retardation, seizure disorders, and developmental disabilities.

Phenylketonuria (PKU) is an encephalopathy caused by an inherited metabolic disorder and is progressive in nature. *Phenylalanine hydroxylase deficiency* prevents the conversion of the amino acid phenylalanine to tyrosine so *phenylalanine accumulates in the serum*. A high level of phenylalanine causes insufficient amounts of other amino acids to enter the brain, resulting in malformation, *defective myelination,* or cystic degeneration of the white and gray matter. Diagnosis is usually made by nonselective newborn screening. Treatment is to restrict phenylalanine in the diet, which generally results in normal growth and development.

Tay-Sachs disease is a *fatal autosomal recessive disorder* caused by impairment of the lysosomal enzyme *hexosaminidase A*. Approximately 80% of the individuals affected are of Jewish ancestry. In Tay-Sachs disease, the pathologic changes predominate in the CNS. With time, neurons become distorted and balloon; and microglial cells, which also are swollen and filled with large granules, proliferate. Cystic degeneration of the cerebral white matter and atrophy of the cerebellar hemispheres often occur. Changes in the spinal cord, particularly in the motor cells, result in hypotonia, hyporeflexia, and overall weakness. Onset of the disease occurs when the infant is 4 to 6 months old, and death usually occurs by 5 years of age.

3. Characterize childhood seizures.
Study page 417; refer to Table 16-5.

Seizures during infancy and childhood may be the result of asphyxia, intracranial bleeding, CNS infection, fever, electrolyte imbalance, or inborn errors of metabolism. Febrile seizures between ages 6 months and 5 years are usually benign. Many seizure disorders are idiopathic, having no known cause. *Epilepsy* is a neurologic condition characterized by a predisposition to recurrent seizures. The incidence of epilepsy varies greatly with age and likely occurs during infancy or childhood in 0.5% to 1% of children; the incidence decreases with age.

4. Describe the acute encephalopathic processes.
Study page 418; refer to Table 16-6.

Reye syndrome is an acute encephalopathy caused by an *interaction of nonsteroidal antiinflammatory drugs (NSAIDs), salicylate, viruses*, and *liver dysfunction.* It is the result of a toxin interfering with mitochondrial function. Clinical manifestations begin with vomiting and lethargy *(stage 1)* and progress to disorientation, delirium, central neurologic hyperventilation, and stupor *(stage 2)*. Obtundation, coma, and decorticate rigidity ensue *(stage 3)*, followed by rapidly developing seizures, flaccidity, and respiratory arrest *(stage 4)*. Avoiding NSAIDs and salicylates during viral illnesses in children is the widely accepted preventive measure. Treatment is supportive in early stages to highly complicated neurointensive care in later stages.

Drug-induced encephalopathies appear in a child with unexplained neurologic changes. Such encephalopathies may result from accidental ingestion, therapeutic or intentional overdose, or ingestion of *environmental toxins*. High blood levels of *lead,* if not treated, lead to encephalopathy that causes serious and irreversible neurologic damage. Children at the greatest risk are those prone to the practice of *pica*. Pica is the habitual, purposeful, and compulsive ingestion of nonfood substances, such as clay, dirt, and *paint chips*.

Bacterial meningitis refers to inflammation of the meningeal coverings of the brain and spinal cord. The origin of the inflammation and acute encephalopathy also can be viral. Sixty percent of all pediatric cases are caused by *Neisseria meningitidis. Streptococcus pneumoniae* is the second most common microorganism found in children older than 4 years. *Escherichia coli* and group B beta-hemolytic streptococci are the most common causes of meningitis in the newborn.

The hallmark of **viral meningitis** consists of a *mononuclear* response in the CSF instead of a *neutrophilic response* seen in bacterial meningitis and normal glucose levels instead of the *decreased glucose* levels seen in bacterial meningitis. The symptoms are similar to, but milder than, those seen in bacterial meningitis. Malaise, fever, headache, nuchal and spinal rigidity, nausea, and vomiting are common.

5. Describe cerebrovascular disease in children.
Study page 419.

Occlusive cerebrovascular disease in children is rare but may result from embolism, sinovenous thrombosis, or congenital or iatrogenic narrowing of vessels, which *decreases blood flow and oxygen to the brain.* **Stroke** is among the top ten causes of death in children. Risk factors include cardiac disease, hematologic and vascular disorders, and infection. **Moyamoya disease** is a rare, chronic, progressive vascular *stenosis of the circle of Willis* that obstructs arterial flow to the brain. The vascularity may be a congenital anomaly or it can develop as a result of cranial radiation therapy. Treatment is surgical bypass of the occluded region.

6. Describe the types of brain tumors in children and characterize their presentation.
Study pages 419 and 421-423; refer to Figures 16-7 through 16-9; and Tables 16-7 and 16-8.

Brain tumors are the most common solid tumors in childhood and the second most common neoplasms in children. Genetic, environmental, and immune factors are all implicated in causation. Most childhood brain tumors arise from *glial tissue*, with two thirds of tumors found in the posterior fossa **(the infratentorial area)**. One third are found in the anterior fossa (**the supratentorial area**).

Brain tumors are unique in their presentation by virtue of their locations. *Infratentorial tumors* often cause increased intracranial pressure because of a mass blockage of the fourth ventricle. Signs include early morning vomiting with neither nausea nor headache, lethargy, and irritability. *Supratentorial tumors* frequently cause localized neurologic symptoms, such as truncal ataxia, impaired coordination, gait anomalies, and loss of balance. Diagnosis is confirmed by radiologic imaging.

The most common brain tumors in childhood are *medulloblastoma, ependymoma, astrocytoma, brainstem glioma, and optic nerve glioma.*

Neuroblastoma is an *embryonal neoplasm of the sympathetic nervous system* and can be located anywhere there is nervous tissue. Causes of neuroblastoma have a familial basis. More than 90% of children with neuroblastoma have increased catecholamines in their urine.

Retinoblastoma is *a rare congenital eye neoplasm* that has both hereditary and nonhereditary forms. Approximately 40% of retinoblastomas are inherited as an autosomal dominant disorder; the others are acquired. The primary sign of a retinoblastoma is a white pupillary reflex called a *cat's eye reflex* that is caused by the mass behind the lens.

PRACTICE EXAMINATION

True/False

1. An 11-month-old infant who displays a strong asymmetrical tonic neck is probably just "slow" in development and should be assumed to have normal neurologic function.
2. Ninety percent of neural tube defects are anencephaly.
3. Anencephaly is the result of premature closure of the sutures of the skull.
4. Environmental influences play an important role in neural tube defects.
5. Encephalocele is the result of herniation of the brain and meninges through a defect of the lower vertebrae.
6. The cause of most childhood bacterial meningitis is *Neisseria meningitidis.*
7. The prognosis for an individual with meningomyelocele depends on the level and extent of the defect.
8. Hydrocephaly may be caused by the overproduction of CSF, blockage of CSF flow, or inhibition of reabsorption.
9. Hydrocephaly is almost *never* a neural tube defect, because such defects usually permit leakage of the CSF out of the defect.
10. Seizure disorders in children are usually static and resolve naturally because the neurons and the neuronal pathways are constantly maturing.
11. An obvious "sac" on the back of a newborn should be thoroughly probed and examined to determine where it is attached to underlying structures.

Fill in the Blanks

12. Aspirin administration during a viral illness has been associated with ______________________ syndrome, which is considered to be a(n) ______________________ encephalopathy.
13. Early morning vomiting without associated nausea may be indicative of a(n) ______________________ fossa brain tumor.
14. Focal neurologic findings such as ataxia may be associated with a(n) ______________________ fossa brain tumor.
15. A child becoming significantly more ill with symptoms of headache, lethargy, and stiff neck after several days of treatment for otitis media may be showing findings consistent with ______________________.
16. ______________________ is a disease associated with premature closure of the sutures of the skull.

Matching

Match the description with the alteration:

_______ 17. May restrict brain growth

_______ 18. May result from increased CSF

_______ 19. Protrusion of the meninges through a vertebral defect

_______ 20. May require cesarean section for delivery

_______ 21. Static disease in which findings change over time

_______ 22. Defect in metabolism of an amino acid with severe neurologic involvement

_______ 23. Associated with ingestion of aspirin during an upper respiratory infection

_______ 24. Very small head

_______ 25. Infectious process that may cause profound damage to cranial nerves

a. meningitis
b. microcephaly
c. Reye syndrome
d. PKU
e. cerebral palsy
f. hydrocephaly
g. meningocele
h. congenital hydrocephaly
i. craniosynostosis

Complete the following table identifying the type and characteristics of most childhood brain tumors:

Common Brain Tumors in Children

Type	Frequency	Usual site
Astrocytoma		
Optic nerve glioma	6%	
Medulloblastoma		
Brain stem glioma		
Ependymoma		Ependymal cells lining ventricles

CASE STUDY

Allen S. is an 11-year-old white boy who presents to the pediatric nurse practitioner's office for a school physical. His past medical history is unremarkable, and the family history also is benign. After the examination has started, his mother requests that the practitioner pay particular attention to her son's lower back. She explains, "He has an area down there that is extremely tender and that has been tender as long as I can remember." The problem worsened this year when Allen was hit from behind while playing sandlot football and was paralyzed and numb from the hips down for approximately 15 minutes. When asked why he was not taken to the emergency department for this injury, his mother said, "I never sought care for him because his symptoms went away within a few minutes and he seemed fine!"

As the physical examination continues, the nurse practitioner notes that Allen has an extremely tender area over the lower lumbar spine and that palpation causes pain in both legs. He has a very deep, dime-sized sacral dimple and highly fissured skin over his lower sacral spine. Deep tendon reflexes, strength, and sensation are all within normal limits. Bowel and bladder function are normal as well. Spinal radiographs are ordered.

What would you expect the radiographs to reveal, and what would be the next step/s?

17 Mechanisms of Hormonal Regulation

FOUNDATIONAL OBJECTIVES

After reviewing this chapter, the learner will be able to do the following:

1. **Identify the functions of the endocrine system, and describe the regulation of hormone secretion.**
   Review pages 426-428; refer to Figure 17-2, and Tables 17.1 and 17.2.

2. **Classify the types of hormones, their receptors, and proposed mechanisms of action.**
   Review pages 428-431; refer to Figures 17-3 through 17-6, and Table 17-3.

3. **State the relationship between the hypothalamus and the pituitary; identify the hormones of the anterior pituitary and posterior pituitary, their target organs, and their functions.**
   Review pages 431 and 433-435; refer to Figures 17-7 through 17-10, and Tables 17-4 and 17-5.

4. **Identify the thyroid hormones and state their functions.**
   Review pages 435; refer to Figures 17-11 and 17-12, and Table 17-6.

5. **Cite the physiologic effects of parathyroid hormone and the variables that affect its secretion.**
   Review page 437.

6. **Identify the production sites of pancreatic somatostatin, insulin, and glucagon, and state their roles in metabolism.**
   Review pages 437 and 439; refer to Figures 17-13 and 17-14, and Table 17-7.

7. **Describe the effects of the adrenal cortical glucocorticoids, mineralocorticoids, and gonadotropins; note the adrenal medullary secretions and their roles.**
   Review pages 439-441 and 443; refer to Figures 17-15 through 17-18.

PRACTICE EXAMINATION

Multiple Choice

Circle the correct answer for each question:

1. Organs that respond to a particular hormone are called:
   a. target organs.
   b. integrated organs.
   c. responder organs.
   d. hormone attack organs.
   e. None of the above is correct.

2. A major feature of the "plasma membrane receptor" mechanism of hormonal action is:
   a. action of cyclic AMP.
   b. increased lysosomal activity.
   c. requirement of a second messenger.
   d. All of the above are correct.
   e. Both a and c are correct.

3. A major feature of the "activation of genes" mechanism of hormonal action is:
   a. a second messenger is used.
   b. a hormone–Golgi complex is used.
   c. the hormone enters the cell.
   d. lysosomal activity increases.
   e. All of the above are correct.

4. A hormone having an antidiuretic effect similar to that of antidiuretic hormone (ADH) is:
   a. insulin.
   b. oxytocin.
   c. hGH.
   d. aldosterone.
   e. adrenocorticotropic hormone (ACTH).

5. The hypothalamus controls the adenohypophysis by direct involvement of:
   a. nerve impulses.
   b. prostaglandins.
   c. cerebrocortical controlling factors (CCCFs).
   d. regulating hormones.
   e. None of the above is correct.

6. Hormones convey regulatory information by:
   a. endocrine signaling.
   b. paracrine signaling.
   c. autocrine signaling.
   d. synaptic signaling.
   e. All of the above are correct.

7. If calcium levels in the blood are too high, thyrocalcitonin (calcitonin) concentrations in the blood should:
   a. increase, thereby inhibiting osteoclasts.
   b. increase, thereby stimulating osteoclasts.
   c. increase, but this change would not affect osteoclasts.
   d. decrease, thereby inhibiting osteoclasts.
   e. decrease, thereby stimulating osteoclasts.

8. In the negative feedback mechanism controlling thyroid hormone secretion, which is the nonregulatory hormone?
   a. thyrotropin-releasing hormone (TRH)
   b. thyroid-stimulating hormone (TSH)
   c. thyroxine
   d. All of the above are regulatory for thyroid hormone secretion.

9. The control of parathyroid hormone is most accurately described as:
   a. negative feedback controlled by the hypothalamus.
   b. positive feedback controlled by the pituitary.
   c. negative feedback involving the pituitary.
   d. negative feedback not involving the pituitary.
   e. Both a and c are correct.

10. The renin-angiotensin-aldosterone system begins to function when renin is secreted by the:
   a. adrenal cortex.
   b. adrenal medulla.
   c. pancreas.
   d. kidneys.
   e. None of the above is correct.

11. The effects of adrenal medullary hormones and the effects of sympathetic stimulation can be described as:
   a. opposites in all respects.
   b. overlapping in some respects.
   c. opposites in some respects.
   d. variable depending on the sex involved.
   e. overlapping in most respects.

12. Which best describes the respective effects of insulin and glucagon on blood glucose?
   a. Insulin raises blood glucose; glucagon lowers it.
   b. Both raise blood glucose.
   c. Insulin lowers blood glucose; glucagon raises it.
   d. Both lower blood glucose.
   e. None of the above is correct.

13. The releasing hormones produced in the hypothalamus travel to the anterior pituitary via the:
   a. stem neurons.
   b. infundibular stem.
   c. hypophyseal stalk.
   d. hypophysial portal system.

14. Which anabolic hormone increases muscle protein synthesis?
   a. T_4
   b. aldosterone
   c. FSH
   d. insulin

15. Aldosterone maintains electrolyte balance by:
   a. retention of potassium.
   b. elimination of sodium.
   c. retention of both Na^+ and K^+.
   d. Both a and b are correct.
   e. None of the above is correct.

Matching

Match the group of adrenocortical hormones with its function:

_______ 16. Mineralocorticoids

_______ 17. Glucocorticoids

a. blood cell formation
b. antiinflammatory
c. conserve sodium
d. usually no function
e. bone mineralization

Match the hormone with its target organ:

_______ 18. ACTH

_______ 19. TSH

_______ 20. TRF

_______ 21. prolactin

a. mammary glands
b. adrenal cortex
c. adrenal medulla
d. thyroid gland
e. adenohypophysis

Match the hormone with its role:

_______ 22. Epinephrine

_______ 23. Glucocorticoids

_______ 24. Mineralocorticoids

_______ 25. Gonadocorticoids

a. influence(s) inflammatory response
b. inhibit(s) growth
c. cause(s) fight-or-flight response
d. control(s) Na^+, H^+, and K^+ levels
e. act(s) as minor sex hormone(s)
f. stimulate(s) skin pigmentation

Fill in the Blank

Complete the following table identifying the origins and effects of hormones:

Site of Origin and Effects of Hormones

Site	Hormone	Effect
Hypothalamus	Releasing hormones	
Posterior pituitary	Antidiuretic hormone (ADH)	
	Oxytocin	
Anterior pituitary	Adrenocorticotropic hormone (ACTH)	
	Melanocyte-stimulating hormone (MSH)	
	Growth hormone (GH)	
	Thyroid-stimulating hormone (TSH)	
	Follicle-stimulating hormone (FSH)	
	Prolactin	
	Luteinizing hormone (LH)	
Thyroid	Thyroxine (T_3, T_4)	
	Calcitonin	
Parathyroid	Parathyroid hormone (PTH)	
Pancreatic islets of Langerhans	Insulin	
	Amylin	
	Glucagon	
Adrenal cortex	Glucocorticoids, mostly cortisol	
	Mineralocorticoids, mostly aldosterone	
	Androgens and estrogens	
Adrenal medulla	Catecholamines (epinephrine and norepinephrine)	
Pineal gland	Melatonin	

18 Alterations of Hormonal Regulation

FOUNDATIONAL OBJECTIVES

a. Diagram the negative feedback system of hormone secretion.
Review page 427; refer to Figure 17-2.

MEMORY CHECK!

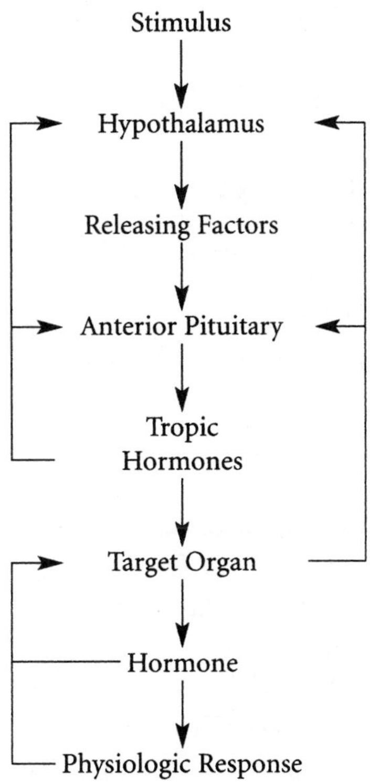

***Note:* This example applies to the thyroid gland. Negative feedback is a corrective mechanism that reverses or reduces a stimulus.**

b. Describe hormone receptors as recognizing and signaling mechanisms for hormonal action.
Refer to Figures 17-3 through 17-6 and Table 17-3.

MEMORY CHECK!

- Hormone receptors are located on the plasma membrane or in the intracellular compartment of a target cell. *Water-soluble hormones*, which include the protein hormones and epinephrine or norepinephrine, cannot cross the cell membrane and interact or bind with receptors located in or on the cell membrane. *Fat-soluble hormones*, steroids, vitamin D, and thyroid hormones (THs) diffuse freely across the plasma and nuclear membranes to bind primarily with nuclear receptors.
- In the *plasma membrane model,* the hormones are called "first messengers." The *receptors* for the water-soluble hormones first recognize the hormone on the plasma membrane and then bind with the hormone. Once recognition and binding have occurred, the hormone-receptor complex initiates the transmission of an intracellular signal by a "second messenger"; the second messenger relays the message inside the cell where a response can occur.

Continued

MEMORY CHECK!—Cont'd

The best-known second messenger is cyclic adenosine monophosphate (cAMP), although other substances are known as second messengers.

- For cells having cAMP as a second messenger, the purpose of these interactions is to activate the intracellular cyclic nucleotides, such as adenylate cyclase. This enzyme converts adenosine triphosphate (ATP) to cAMP. Elevated levels of cAMP alter cell function in specific ways. An example of the function of cAMP as a second messenger can be seen in the action of epinephrine. The epinephrine-receptor complex interaction increases the synthesis of cAMP. *Cyclic AMP*, in turn, activates an elaborate enzyme cascade in which inactive enzymes are converted in sequence to *active enzymes* that *lead to glycogen breakdown into glucose.*
- In the *lipid-soluble hormonal model*, relatively small hydrophobic molecules cross the plasma membrane by simple diffusion. Once inside the cytosol, *some hormones bind to receptor molecules in the cytoplasm and then diffuse into the nucleus.* Hormones without cytoplasmic receptors diffuse directly into the nucleus and bind with an acceptor molecule. Once activated by hormones, the first messengers, the receptor likely *binds* to specific sites on the chromatin of the target cell. This step causes RNA transcription and *increased synthesis of specific proteins.*

MEMORY CHECK!

SITE OF ORIGIN AND EFFECTS OF HORMONES

Site	Hormone	Effect
Hypothalamus	Releasing hormones	Act on anterior pituitary to release specific hormones
Posterior pituitary	Antidiuretic hormone (ADH)	Causes conservation of body water by promoting water resorption by renal tubules
	Oxytocin	Stimulates uterine contraction and lactation
Anterior pituitary	Adrenocorticotropic hormone (ACTH)	Stimulates production of glucocorticoids by adrenal cortex
	Melanocyte-stimulating hormone (MSH)	Stimulates pigment production in skin
	Growth hormone (GH)	Promotes growth of body tissues
	Thyroid-stimulating hormone (TSH)	Stimulates production and release of THs
	Follicle-stimulating hormone (FSH)	Initiates maturation of ovarian follicles; stimulates spermatogenesis
	Prolactin	Stimulates secretion of breast milk
	Luteinizing hormone (LH)	Causes ovulation and stimulates ovary to produce estrogen and progesterone; stimulates androgen production by interstitial cells of testes
Thyroid	Thyroxine (T_3, T_4)	Increases rate of cellular metabolism
	Calcitonin	Osteoblastic—lowers serum calcium
Parathyroid	Parathyroid hormone (PTH)	Osteoclastic—raises serum calcium

Continued

Pancreatic islets of Langerhans	Insulin	Promotes utilization of glucose; lowers serum glucose
	Amylin	Delays nutrient uptake and suppresses glucagon after meals
	Glucagon	Promotes utilization of glycogen; raises serum glucose
Adrenal cortex	Glucocorticoids, mostly cortisol	Antagonizes effects of insulin; inhibits inflammatory response and fibroblastic activity
	Mineralocorticoid, mostly aldosterone	Promotes retention of sodium by renal tubules
	Androgens and estrogens	Promotes secondary sex characteristics
Adrenal medulla	Catecholamines (epinephrine and norepinephrine)	Regulates blood pressure by effects on vascular smooth muscle and heart

LEARNING OBJECTIVES

After studying this chapter, the learner will be able to do the following:

1. Identify the mechanisms causing hormonal alterations.
Study pages 447 and 448; refer to Figure 18-1 and Table 18.1.

Any significantly elevated or depressed hormone values have a variety of causes. Two major mechanisms are responsible for these alterations: (1) **inappropriate amounts of hormones delivered to the target cells** and (2) **inappropriate response by the target cell.** *Failure of feedback systems* occurs when positive feedback is not recognized, so hormone synthesis is inadequate, or when negative feedback is recognized, so there is excessive synthesis. *Hormone inactivity* exists when there is inadequate free hormone because of hormone degradation or circulating inhibitors such as antibodies. *Dysfunctional delivery* occurs if there is inadequate blood supply, carrier proteins, or ectopic production of hormones. Inappropriate target cell response occurs if the number of *cell receptors decreases*, their *receptor/hormone affinity* is impaired; *antibodies against receptors* are present; or there is *unusual receptor expression. Intracellular disorders* develop if there is *inadequate synthesis of second messengers*, acquired defects in *postreceptor signaling, altered synthesis of intracellular proteins of enzymes, or nuclear co-regulator dysfunction.*

2. Distinguish between syndrome of inappropriate ADH secretion (SIADH) and diabetes insipidus.
Study pages 449-450 and Table 18.2.

Diseases of the posterior pituitary are rare, but when they occur, they are usually related to abnormal antidiuretic hormone (ADH/vasopressin) secretion. **SIADH** is characterized by high levels of ADH without normal physiologic stimuli for its release.

SIADH is associated with several forms of cancer because of the *ectopic secretion of ADH by tumor cells.* Tumors associated with SIADH include oat cell adenocarcinoma of the lung, carcinoma of the duodenum and pancreas, leukemia, lymphoma, and Hodgkin lymphoma. *Transient SIADH* may follow pituitary surgery as stored ADH is released in an unregulated fashion. SIADH may be seen in infectious pulmonary diseases because of the ectopic production of ADH by infected lung tissue or by increased posterior pituitary secretion of ADH in response to hypoxia. SIADH also may be associated with psychiatric disease and may occur after treatment with a variety of drugs that stimulate ADH release.

The main features of SIADH are *water retention* and *solute loss*, particularly of sodium. This state leads to serum hyponatremia and hyposmolality. As ADH is released continually, water retention results from the normal action of ADH on the renal tubules and collecting ducts. This action increases their permeability to water through the action of *aquaporin,* which is a water channel protein. Hyponatremia suppresses renin and aldosterone secretion, thus decreasing proximal tubule reabsorption of sodium.

Thirst, impaired taste, anorexia, dyspnea on exertion, fatigue, and dulled consciousness occur when the serum sodium level falls from 140 to 130 mEq/L. Vomiting and abdominal cramps occur with a drop in sodium level from 130 to 120 mEq/L. With a serum sodium level below 113 mEq/L, confusion, lethargy, muscle twitching, and seizures may occur. Symptoms usually resolve with correction of hyponatremia.

The treatment of SIADH involves the correction of any underlying casual problems, correction of severe hyponatremia by administration of hypertonic saline, and careful fluid restriction. Resistant or chronic SIADH may be treated with demeclocycline, which causes development of tubular resistance to ADH.

Diabetes insipidus is related to an *insufficiency of ADH leading to polyuria and polydipsia.* There are three forms of diabetes insipidus: a neurogenic or central form, a nephrogenic form, and a psychogenic form. **The neurogenic form of diabetes insipidus** occurs when any organic lesion of the hypothalamus, infundibular stem, or posterior pituitary interferes with ADH synthesis, transport, or release, resulting in too little ADH. **Nephrogenic diabetes insipidus** is an insensitivity of the renal tubule to ADH, particularly the collecting tubules. This diabetes is generally related to disorders and drugs that damage the renal tubules or inhibit the generation of cAMP in the tubules. The **psychogenic form** is caused by an extremely large volume of fluid intake.

The clinical manifestations of diabetes insipidus are caused by the absence of ADH. These signs and symptoms include polyuria, nocturia, continuous thirst, polydipsia, low urine osmolality, and high-normal plasma osmolality. Individuals with long-standing diabetes insipidus develop a large bladder capacity and hydronephrosis.

Individuals who have excessive urine output and low urine osmolality after a dehydration or water restriction test may require ADH replacement with a synthetic vasopressin analog. Drugs that potentiate the action of otherwise insufficient amounts of endogenous ADH may be used to stimulate ADH release from the hypothalamus in less severely affected individuals.

3. Describe the disorders of the anterior pituitary as either hypofunctions or hyperfunctions of the gland.

Study pages 450-453; refer to Figures 18-2 through 18-4.

Anterior pituitary hypofunction may develop from infarction of the gland, removal or destruction of the gland, vasospasm of the artery supplying the gland, or autoimmune hypophysitis. **Hyperfunction of the anterior pituitary** generally involves an *adenoma* composed of secretory pituitary cells. An adenoma may cause *hypersecretion of the hormone it produces* and hyposecretion of another hormone because of the compressive effects of the tumor.

The pituitary gland is extremely vascular and is therefore extremely vulnerable to infarction and subsequent **hypopituitarism**. The pituitary gland may be *susceptible to necrosis* because its blood supply through the *portal system is already partially deoxygenated.* The likelihood of infarction increases during pregnancy. The primary pathologic mechanism in postpartum pituitary infarction, or **Sheehan syndrome**, is *vasospasm of the artery* supplying the anterior pituitary. Following tissue necrosis, edema occurs, which expands the pituitary within the fixed confines of the sella turcica. This expansion further impedes blood supply to the pituitary and promotes *hypofunction.*

The signs and symptoms of hypofunction of the anterior pituitary are highly variable and depend on which hormones are affected. If all hormones are absent, a condition termed **panhypopituitarism** develops. The affected individual suffers from cortisol deficiency because of lack of ACTH, thyroid deficiency from lack of TSH, diabetes insipidus from lack of ADH, and gonadal failure and loss of secondary sex characteristics from absence of FSH and LH. GH and somatomedin levels are low and may affect children. These deficiencies do not generally develop in adults.

When there is a GH deficiency in children, **hypopituitary dwarfism** infrequently occurs. A dwarf has a normal face with *normal proportions* of head, trunk, and limbs; a dwarf also has normal intelligence. In adult GH deficiency, there is social withdrawal, fatigue, loss of motivation, osteoporosis, and reduced lean body mass.

In cases of hypopituitarism, the underlying disorder should be corrected as quickly as possible. Thyroid and cortisol replacement therapy may need to be initiated and maintained. Sex steroid replacement may be required, depending on the needs and desires of the individual.

Pituitary adenomas that cause **hyperpituitarism** are usually benign, slow-growing tumors. Effects from an increase in tumor size include nonspecific complaints of headache, fatigue, neck pain or stiffness, and seizures. Visual changes produced by pressure on the optic chiasma include visual field impairments. If the tumor infiltrates other cranial nerves, various neuromuscular functions are affected. Hypersecretion of hormones secreted by the adenoma leads to symptoms associated with the particular hormone that is affected.

Acromegaly occurs in adults who are exposed to continuously excessive levels of *GH*. Acromegaly is uncommon. The most common cause of acromegaly is a primary autonomous GH-secreting pituitary *adenoma*. Acromegaly occurs in adults *after epiphyseal closure has occurred* and is a slowly progressive disease. In the adult, increased amounts of GH and somatomedins cause increases in connective tissue and cytoplasm. If untreated, acromegaly is associated with a decreased life expectancy because of a greater occurrence of hypertension, congestive heart failure, diabetes mellitus, and colon or lung cancer.

In the individual with acromegaly, bony proliferation involves *periosteal vertebral growth* and enlargement of the *facial bones* and the bones of the hands and feet. The associated growth results in protrusion of the lower jaw and forehead. Because somatomedins stimulate cartilaginous growth, ribs elongate at the bone-cartilage junction, causing a barrel-chested appearance and increased proliferation of cartilage in joints. Because of bony and soft tissue overgrowth, nerves may be entrapped and damaged, which may be manifested by weakness, muscular atrophy, foot drop, and sensory changes in the hands. Because of a space-occupying lesion, central nervous system signs and symptoms such as headache, seizure activity, and visual disturbances may develop. The metabolic effects of GH hypersecretion include impaired carbohydrate tolerance and increased metabolic rate. Diabetes mellitus occurs when the pancreas is unable to secrete enough insulin to offset the effects of GH.

In children and adolescents whose *epiphyseal plates have not yet closed*, the effect of increased GH levels is **giantism.** Giantism is very rare because of early recognition and treatment of the adenoma. It occurs when the epiphyses are not fused and high levels of somatomedins stimulate excessive skeletal growth.

The goals of treatment are to protect the individual from the effects of tumor growth and to control hormone hypersecretion while minimizing damage to appropriately secreting portions of the pituitary. Surgery and radiation therapy are used, depending on the extent of tumor growth.

Prolactinomas are the most common hormonally active pituitary tumors. Pathologic elevated prolactin *in women* results in amenorrhea, galactorrhea, hirsutism, and osteopenia because of estrogen deficiency. *In men,* hyperprolactinemia causes hypogonadism and erectile dysfunction. Dopaminergic agonists are the treatment of choice for prolactinomas.

4. Describe the disorders of hyperthyroidism; note the progressive states of severity.

Study pages 453-456; refer to Figures 18-5 through 18-8.

Whenever THs from any source exert greater-than-normal responses, **thyrotoxicosis** exists. **Hyperthyroidism** is a form of thyrotoxicosis in which excess THs are secreted by the thyroid gland. Specific diseases of *primary* hyperthyroidism include Graves disease, toxic multinodular goiter, and solitary toxic adenoma. *Secondary* hyperthyroidism is less common and is caused by TSH-secreting pituitary adenoma. Thyrotoxicosis not associated with hyperthyroidism is seen in subacute thyroiditis, increased TSH secretion,

Manifestations of Hypothyroid and Hyperthyroid States

Characteristic	Hypothyroidism	Hyperthyroidism
Basal metabolic rate	Decreased	Increased
Sympathetic response	Decreased	Increased
Weight	Gain	Loss
Temperature tolerance	Cold intolerance	Heat intolerance
	Decreased sweating	Increased sweating
Gastrointestinal function	Constipation	Diarrhea
	Decreased appetite	Increased appetite
Cardiovascular function	Decreased cardiac output	Increased cardiac output
	Bradycardia	Tachycardia and palpitations
Respiratory function	Hypoventilation	Dyspnea, tachypnea
Muscle tone and reflexes	Decreased	Increased
General appearance	Myxedematous	Exophthalmos
	Deep voice	Lid lag
	Impaired growth (child)	Decreased blinking
		Enlarged thyroid gland
General behavior	Mental retardation (infant)	Restlessness, irritability, anxiety
	Mental and physical sluggishness	Hyperkinesis
	Somnolence	Wakefulness

Note: Hypothyroidism is more common than hyperthyroidism.

ectopic thyroid tissue, and ingestion of excessive TH. All forms of thyrotoxicosis share some common characteristics because of increased circulating levels of THs. The major types of therapy used to control the elevated levels of TH include drug therapy, radioactive iodine therapy, and surgery.

Graves disease, a form of *type II hypersensitivity,* is the most common form of hyperthyroidism and is likely associated with *autoantibodies* against the TSH receptor. The antibody binds to the plasma membrane and initiates thyroid hyperplasia of the gland (goiter), vascularity, and hypersecretion of hormone. Ophthalmopathy is characterized by edema of the orbital contents, exophthalmos, and extraocular muscle weakness that sometimes leads to diplopia and pain, lacrimation, photophobia, and blurred vision. Treatment consists of a combination of radioactive iodine, surgery, or antithyroid drugs.

Thyrotoxic crisis (thyroid storm) is a rare but a dangerous worsening of the thyrotoxic state; death can occur within 48 hours without appropriate treatment. This condition occurs most often in individuals who have undiagnosed or partially treated severe *hyperthyroidism and* who are subjected to *excessive stress* from other causes. The systemic symptoms of thyrotoxic crisis include hyperthermia, tachycardia, high-output heart failure, agitation or delirium, and nausea, vomiting, or diarrhea contributing to fluid depletion. The symptoms may be attributed to increased β-adrenergic receptors and catecholamines. The treatment is to reduce circulating TH levels by blocking TH synthesis.

5. Describe the disorders of hypothyroidism; describe thyroid cancer.
Study pages 456 and 457; refer to Figures 18-9 and 18-10.

Deficient production of TH by the thyroid gland results in **hypothyroidism,** which may be either primary or secondary. *Primary causes* include congenital defects or loss of thyroid tissue following treatment for hyperthyroidism and defective hormone synthesis resulting from antithyroid antibodies or endemic iodine deficiency. Autoimmune thyroiditis, or **Hashimoto disease,** results in destruction of thyroid tissue by circulating thyroid antibodies and infiltration of lymphocytes. Causes of the less common *secondary* hypothyroidism are insufficient pituitary stimulation of the normal gland and peripheral resistance to TH. The individual develops a low metabolic rate with this disorder.

The characteristic sign of severe hypothyroidism is *myxedema*. It is characterized by swelling of the hand, face, feet, and periorbital tissues.

Myxedema coma is a medical emergency associated with severe hypothyroidism. Symptoms include hypothermia without shivering, hypoventilation, hypotension, hypoglycemia, and lactic acidosis. Older patients with severe vascular disease and with moderate or untreated hypothyroidism are particularly at risk for development of myxedema coma. It also may occur after overuse of narcotics or sedatives or after an acute illness in hypothyroid individuals.

Hypothyroidism in infants occurs because of absence of thyroid tissue and hereditary defects in TH synthesis. Signs may not be evident for at least 4 months after birth but include abdominal protrusion, umbilical hernia, subnormal temperature, lethargy, excessive sleeping, and slow pulse. Skeletal growth is stunted and the child will be dwarfed with short limbs if not treated. These signs constitute **cretinism.** *Mental retardation* in cretins is a function of the severity of hypothyroidism and the delay before initiation of thyroxine treatment.

Hypothyroidism is difficult to identify at birth, but high birth weight, hypothermia, delay in passing meconium, and neonatal jaundice may suggest this condition. There is a high probability of normal growth and intellectual function if treatment is started immediately after birth.

Thyroid carcinoma is the most common endocrine malignancy but is still relatively rare. The most consistent causal risk factor for the development of thyroid cancer is exposure to ionizing radiation. Changes in voice and swallowing and difficulty in breathing are related to impingement of tumor growth on the esophagus or trachea. Treatment for this rare entity may include partial or total thyroidectomy, TSH suppressive therapy, radioactive iodine therapy, postoperative radiation therapy, and chemotherapy.

6. Distinguish between primary and secondary hyperparathyroidism and hypoparathyroidism.
Study pages 457 and 458.

Approximately 80% of **primary hyperparathyroidism** disorders result from a chief cell adenoma with an increased secretion of PTH. This causes hypercalcemia and decreased serum phosphate levels.

Secondary hyperparathyroidism may be a compensatory response of the parathyroid glands to chronic hypocalcemia. Loss of calcium by failing kidneys leads to increased secretion of PTH.

Hypersecretion of PTH causes excessive osteoclastic and osteolytic activity resulting in *bone resorption.* Pathologic fractures, kyphosis of the dorsal spine, and compression fractures of the vertebral bodies may occur. Chronic hypercalcemia may be associated with kidney stones, gastrointestinal disturbances, and muscle weakness and lethargy.

Long-term management of hypercalcemia uses drugs that decrease resorption of calcium from bone. Definitive treatment requires the surgical removal of the hyperplastic parathyroid glands.

Hypoparathyroidism is most commonly caused by *damage to the parathyroid glands during thyroid surgery.* In the absence of PTH, the ability to resorb calcium from bone and to regulate calcium reabsorption from the renal tubules is impaired. Hypocalcemia lowers the threshold for nerve and muscle excitation. Muscle spasms, hyperreflexia, clonic-tonic seizures, laryngeal spasms, and, in severe cases, death from asphyxiation are seen with hypocalcemia.

The treatment of hypoparathyroidism involves administration of calcium and vitamin D. Hypoplastic dentition, cataracts, bone deformities, and basal ganglia calcifications do not respond to the correction of hypocalcemia, but the other symptoms of hypocalcemia are reversible.

7. Describe the similarities and differences between insulin-dependent (type 1) and non–insulin-dependent (type 2) diabetes mellitus; note other types of diabetes mellitus.

Study pages 458, 459 and 461-464; refer to Figures 18-11 and 18-12, and Tables 18-3 through 18-6.

The four major categories of **diabetes mellitus** are absolute insulin deficiency (type 1 diabetes mellitus), insulin resistance with an insulin secretory deficit (type 2 diabetes mellitus), other types of diabetes mellitus, and gestational diabetes mellitus (GDM). Types 1 and 2 are the most common.

Note: The normal fasting plasma glucose (FPG) is 70-110 mg/dL when there has been no caloric intake for at least 8 hr. Diabetic conditions exist whenever: (1) FGP = 100-125 mg/dL, (2) 2 hr FGP = 75-199 mg/dL during oral glucose tolerance testing (OGTT), or (3) glycosylated hemoglobin (HbA) is 5.7% to 6.4%. Whenever these diabetic conditions are present, there is increased risk of cardiovascular disease and premature death.

The diagnosis of diabetes is based on several observations: (1) more than one elevated fasting plasma glucose value; (2) elevated plasma glucose values in response to an oral glucose tolerance test; and (3) the classic symptoms of polydipsia, polyphagia, and polyuria. In individuals with poorly controlled diabetes, increases in the quantities of *glycosylated hemoglobins are seen.* Once a hemoglobin molecule is glycosylated, it remains that way.

Other signs and symptoms are weight loss, fatigue, prolonged wound healing, visual changes, neuropathies, and formation of atherosclerosis.

The treatment of individuals with either type 1 or type 2 diabetes requires appropriate meal planning to restrict intake of total calories, cholesterol, and saturated fats. Oral medication may be needed for optimal management of hyperglycemia. *Insulin is required in type 1 diabetes* and also may be required in the treatment of some individuals with type 2 diabetes. Exercise is an important aspect of treatment for the individual with type 2 diabetes. *Exercise reduces after-meal blood glucose levels and diminishes insulin requirement.* Also, exercise facilitates weight loss in the overweight individual.

8. Identify the acute complications of diabetes mellitus; describe the features of each.

Study page 465; refer to Figure 18-13 and Table 18-7.

Acute complications of diabetes mellitus include hypoglycemia or insulin shock, diabetic ketoacidosis (DKA), and hyperosmolar hyperglycemic nonketotic syndrome (HHNS).

Classification of Diabetes and Glucose Intolerance States

Classification	Characteristics
Type 1 diabetes mellitus: Beta cell deficiency/destruction; immune-mediated	Long preclinical record with autoimmune T cell-mediated destruction of beta cells; ketoacidois prone; genetic-environmental etiology; insulin-dependent; ketosis-prone; individual usually not obese; develops before age 30 years
Type 2 diabetes mellitus: Resistant to insulin with an insulin secretory deficiency	Usually some insulin production; decreased islet cells; not ketosis-prone; frequently abdominally obese; strong familial pattern; rapidly increasing in children; usually develops after age 40 years; often related to hypertension and dyslipidemia
Other forms: Secondary diabetes; maturity-onset diabetes of the young (MODY)	Mutation in gene responsible for insulin secretion or action; mutation in enzymes involved in beta cell function; diagnosis similar to that of type 2
Gestational diabetes mellitus (GDM)	Glucose intolerance develops during pregnancy (third trimester); usually women were previously undiagnosed with type 1 or type 2; increased risk of development within 15 years after parturition

Acute Complications of Diabetes Mellitus

Variable	Hypoglycemia/Insulin Shock	DKA	HHNS
Onset	Rapid	Slow	Slowest
Symptoms	Weak, anxious, confused, tachycardic	Nausea, vomiting, polyuria, polyphagia polydipsia, headache, irritable, comatose, fruity breath odor, shortness of breath	Similar to those of DKA; stuporous, hypotensive, dehydrated
Skin	Perspiring	Hot, flushed, dry	Very dry
Mucous membranes	Normal	Dry	Extremely dry
Respiration	Normal	Hyperventilation, "fruity" or acetone odor to breath	Normal
Those at risk	Type 1 and 2 DM, fluctuating blood glucose levels, insufficient food intake, excessive exercise, excessive oral insulin	Type 1 DM, stressful situation, insulin omission	Elderly, young type 2 DM, high carbohydrate diets, diuresis, hyperosmolar dialysis
Blood sugar/dL	30 mg/dL or less in newborns, 60 mg/dL or less in adults	Greater than 250 mg /dL	Greater than 600 mg/dL
Treatment	Fast-acting carbohydrate, intravenous glucose, subcutaneous glucagon	Low-dose insulin, electrolyte and fluid replacement	Fluid replacement with crystalloids and colloids

Note: The *Somogyi effect* occurs if an overdose of insulin induces hypoglycemia followed by rebound hyperglycemia because of release of hormones that stimulate lipolysis gluconeogenesis and glycogenolysis leading to elevated serum glucose. The *Dawn phenomenon* is an early-morning hyperglycemia caused by nocturnal elevation of GH.

9. Describe the chronic complication of diabetes mellitus.
Study pages 465-468; refer to Figure 18-14 and Table 18-8.

Chronic Complications of Diabetes Mellitus

Chronic Hyperglycemia			
Involves Nonenzymatic glycosylation Shunting of glucose to polyol pathway Activation of protein kinase C all of which lead to the chronic complications of diabetes mellitus			
Diabetic Neuropathies	**Microvascular Disease**	**Macrovascular Disease**	**Infection**
Somatic and peripheral nerve cell damage results in neuropathy—more sensory than motor deficits	Retinopathy*	Coronary heart disease*	Sensory impairment, atherosclerosis—ischemia, hypoxia, leukocytic and immunity impairment, delayed wound healing, increased risk for sepsis, more bacterial infection because of more glucose

	Nephropathy*		
	Capillary basement membrane thickening decreased tissue or ischemia, perfusion hypertension	CVA*	
		Peripheral vascular disease*	
		Proliferation of fibrous plaques, atherosclerosis because of high serum lipids, ischemia	

*Major consequences.

10. Describe the etiology, pathogenesis, and manifestations of hyperfunction and hypofunction of the adrenal cortex.
Study pages 469-472; refer to Figures 18-15 through 18-17.

Cushing disease refers specifically to pituitary-dependent *hypercortisolism.* Cushing-like syndrome also may develop as a result of the *exogenous administration of cortisone.* Elevations of pituitary ACTH and adrenal neoplasms account for many cases of hypercorticoadrenalism. **Cushing syndrome** (chronic hypercortisolism) refers to excessive levels of *circulating cortisol* caused by hyperfunction of the adrenal cortex with or without pituitary involvement.

Two observations consistently apply to individuals with Cushing syndrome: (1) they lack diurnal or circadian secretion patterns of ACTH and cortisol and (2) they do not increase ACTH and cortisol secretion in response to a stressor.

Most of the clinical signs and symptoms of Cushing are caused by hypercortisolism. The most common feature is the accumulation of adipose tissue in the trunk, facial, and cervical areas. These have been described as *"truncal obesity," "moon face," and "buffalo hump."* Protein wasting is commonly observed in hypercortisolism and is caused by the catabolic effects of cortisol on peripheral tissues. *Muscle wasting* is especially obvious in the muscles of the extremities. Loss of the protein matrix in bone leads to *osteoporosis* and accompanying pathologic fractures, vertebral compression fractures, bone and back pain, kyphosis, and reduced height. Loss of collagen also leads to thin, *weakened integumentary tissues* through which capillaries are more visible. This accounts for the characteristic purple striae observed in the trunk area. Loss of collagenous support around small vessels makes them susceptible to rupture and easy bruising.

With elevated cortisol values, vascular sensitivity to catecholamines increases significantly, leading to vasoconstriction and hypertension. Chronically elevated cortisol values also cause suppression of the immune system and increased susceptibility to infections.

Hyperaldosteronism is characterized by excessive aldosterone secretion by the adrenal glands. An aldosterone-secreting adenoma or excessive stimulation of the normal adrenal cortex by substances such as angiotensin, ACTH, and elevated serum potassium may cause hypersecretion.

Conn disease, or **primary hyperaldosteronism**, presents a clinical picture of hypertension, hypokalemia, renal potassium wasting, and neuromuscular manifestations. The most common cause of primary aldosteronism is the benign, single *adrenal adenoma,* followed by multiple tumors and idiopathic hyperplasia of the adrenals.

Because aldosterone secretion is normally stimulated by the renin-angiotensin system, **secondary hyperaldosteronism** can result from sustained elevated renin release and activation of angiotensin. Increased renin-angiotensin secretion occurs with decreased circulating blood volume and reduced delivery of blood to the kidneys.

Hypertension and hypokalemia are the essential manifestations of hyperaldosteronism. Hypertension usually results from increased intravascular volume and altered serum sodium concentrations. If hypertension is sustained, left ventricular hypertrophy and progressive arteriosclerosis develop. Aldosterone-stimulated potassium loss can result in the typical manifestations of hypokalemia—namely, paralytic ileus, dysrhythmias, and metabolic alkalosis.

Treatment of hypertension and hypokalemia consists of correction of any underlying causal abnormalities. If an aldosterone-secreting adenoma is present, it must be surgically removed.

Hypersecretion of adrenal **androgens** and **estrogens** may be caused by benign or malignant adrenal tumors, Cushing syndrome, or defects in steroid synthesis. The clinical manifestations depend on the hormone secreted, the sex of the individual, and the age at which the hypersecretion occurs. Hypersecretion of estrogens causes **feminization**, or the development of female sex characteristics. Hypersecretion of androgens causes **virilization**, or the development of male sex characteristics.

The effects of an *estrogen-secreting tumor* are most evident in *males* and cause gynecomastia, testicular atrophy, and decreased libido. In female children, such tumors may lead to the early development of secondary sex characteristics. *Androgen-secreting tumor* changes are more easily observed in *females* and include excessive face and body hair growth or hirsutism, clitoral enlargement, deepening of the voice, amenorrhea, acne, and breast atrophy. In children, virilizing tumors promote precocious sexual development and bone aging. Treatment of androgen-secreting tumors usually involves surgical excision.

Hypocortisolism develops either because of *inadequate stimulation* of the adrenal glands by *ACTH* or because of an inability of the adrenals to produce and secrete the *adrenal cortical hormones.* Hypofunction of the adrenal cortex may affect glucocorticoid or mineralocorticoid secretion or a combination of both. Primary adrenal insufficiency is termed **Addison disease**, a relatively rare adult disorder.

Addison disease is characterized by elevated serum ACTH values with inadequate corticosteroid synthesis and output. The most common cause is idiopathic organ-specific autoimmune disease. The symptoms of Addison disease are primarily a result of hypocortisolism and hypoaldosteronism. They include weakness, gastrointestinal disturbances, hypoglycemia, hyperpigmentation from increased ACTH secretion, and hypotension.

The treatment of Addison disease involves glucocorticoid and possibly mineralocorticoid replacement therapy and dietary modifications to include adequate sodium. Hypocortisolism requires long-term daily glucocorticoid replacement therapy, and additional cortisol must be administered during acute stress.

11. Characterize adrenal medulla hyperfunction.
Study page 472.

The most prominent cause of adrenal medulla hypersecretion is a **pheochromocytoma (chromaffin cell tumor).** Fewer than 10% of these rare tumors metastasize; if they do, they are usually found in the lungs, liver, bones, or paraaortic lymph glands. Pheochromocytoma causes *excessive production of epinephrine and norepinephrine* because of the autonomous functioning of the tumor.

The clinical manifestations of a pheochromocytoma include persistent hypertension associated with flushing, diaphoresis, tachycardia, palpitations, and constipation. Headaches appear because of sudden changes in catecholamines in the blood that affect cerebral blood flow. Hypermetabolism may develop because of stimulation of the thyroid gland by the catecholamines. Glucose intolerance may occur because of catecholamine-induced inhibition of insulin release by the pancreas.

The usual treatment of pheochromocytoma is surgical excision of the tumor. Medical therapy with adrenergic blocking agents is used to stabilize blood pressure prior to surgery.

PRACTICE EXAMINATION

Multiple Choice

Circle the correct answer for each question:

1. Which laboratory values would be expected in an individual with SIADH?
   a. serum sodium = 150 mEq/L and urine hypoosmolality
   b. serum potassium = 5 mEq/L and serum hypoosmolality
   c. serum sodium = 120 mEq/L and urine hypoosmolality
   d. serum potassium = 3 mEq/L and serum hyperosmolality

2. Hypopituitarism in an adult male likely includes all of the following *except:*
   a. dwarfism.
   b. impotence.
   c. muscular mass decrease.
   d. skin pallor.

3. Excessive secretion of GH in an adult may cause:
   a. acromegaly.
   b. giantism.
   c. hypoglycemia.
   d. decreased metabolic rate.

4. A manifestation shared by both diabetes mellitus and diabetes insipidus is:
   a. elevated blood and urine glucose values.
   b. inability to produce ADH.
   c. inability to produce insulin.
   d. polyuria.
   e. elevated blood urine and ketone body values.

5. The manifestations of hyperthyroidism include all of the following *except:*
   a. diarrhea.
   b. constipation.
   c. heat intolerance.
   d. weight loss.
   e. wakefulness.

6. Hypothyroidism crisis is:
   a. myxedema coma.
   b. Addison disease.
   c. Cushing disease.
   d. Graves disease.
   e. cretinism.

7. Graves disease is:
   a. hyperthyroidism.
   b. associated with autoimmunity.
   c. manifested by ophthalmopathy.
   d. All of the above are correct.

8. Inadequate levels of THs at birth may cause:
   a. mental retardation.
   b. immediate death.
   c. thyroid crisis.
   d. myxedema.
   e. dwarfism.

9. Hyperparathyroidism causes:
   a. increased osteoclastic activity.
   b. decreased plasma calcium.
   c. increased absorption of phosphorus from the GI tract.
   d. hypocalcemia.

10. A manifestation of hypocalcemia is:
    a. myopathy.
    b. lethargy.
    c. hypertension.
    d. tetany.
    e. bone cysts.

11. What is the most common cause of acromegaly?
    a. anterior pituitary adenoma
    b. overproduction of ACTH
    c. overproduction of TSH
    d. pituitary atrophy

12. If a 19-year-old woman were suffering from shortness of breath, weight loss, excessive sweating, exophthalmos, and irritability, which hormone would you expect to find elevated in her serum?
    a. cortisol
    b. thyroxine
    c. ACTH
    d. 17-ketosteroid

13. A 24-year-old woman with a history of "juvenile-onset" diabetes is found in a stuporous state. She is hypotensive and has cold, clammy skin. What is the likely etiology of her condition?
    a. hyperglycemia
    b. insulin shock
    c. renal failure
    d. peripheral neuropathy

14. A 10-year-old boy was brought into the emergency room comatose, suffering from metabolic acidosis with a blood glucose level of 800 mg/dL. The most probable disease causing his condition is:
    a. cretinism.
    b. type 1 diabetes mellitus.
    c. type 2 diabetes mellitus.
    d. GDM.

15. Your neighbor, not previously diagnosed as a diabetic, has gained 80 pounds in the past year and is able to produce some insulin. Her fasting blood glucose value is always elevated. She is being treated with oral insulin-stimulating drugs. Your neighbor is most likely suffering from:
    a. diabetes insipidus.
    b. type 1 diabetes mellitus.
    c. type 2 diabetes mellitus.
    d. GDM.

16. Common symptoms and signs of diabetes mellitus include all of the following except:
    a. hyperglycemia.
    b. blurred vision.
    c. increased muscle anabolism.
    d. persistent infection.
    e. polyuria.

17. Which laboratory finding is inconsistent with a diagnosis of absolute insulin deficiency?
    a. FBS (fasting blood sugar) of 90 mg/dL
    b. ketonuria
    c. blood glucose level of 210 mg/dL after 1 hour following ingestion of 100 g glucose
    d. decreased serum insulin level
    e. All of the above are consistent with type 1 diabetes mellitus.

18. Common complications of diabetes mellitus include all of the following except:
    a. retinopathy.
    b. peripheral neuropathy.
    c. nephropathy (kidney disease).
    d. None of the above is common.
    e. All of the above are common.

19. An individual with type 1 diabetes mellitus experiences hunger, lightheadedness, headache, confusion, and tachycardia while performing cross-country running. The likely cause of these manifestations is:
    a. hyperglycemia.
    b. eating a snack before running.
    c. hypoglycemia because of running.
    d. Both a and b are correct.
    e. None of the above is correct.

20. Which is/are expected during hyperinsulinism?
    a. excess insulin
    b. high serum glucose
    c. epinephrine release
    d. All of the above are correct.
    e. Both a and c are correct.

21. Long-term corticosteroid therapy may cause which of the following? (More than one answer may be correct.)
    a. delayed wound healing
    b. osteoporosis
    c. peptic ulcers
    d. hyperkalemia

22. Which electrolyte alteration occurs in Addison disease?
    a. hypokalemia
    b. hypernatremia
    c. hyponatremia
    d. hypocalcemia

23. A benign tumor of adrenal glands that causes hypersecretion of aldosterone is:
    a. Addison disease.
    b. pheochromocytoma.
    c. Gushing disease.
    d. Cushing syndrome.
    e. Conn disease.

Matching

Match the hypersecretion with the consequence:

_______ 24. Hypersecretion of aldosterone

_______ 25. Hypersecretion of glucocorticoids

a. decreased cardiac output
b. hyperglycemia or osteoporosis
c. BMR (basal metabolic rate) increases
d. hypernatremia
e. hyponatremia

Fill in the Blank

Complete the following table comparing SIADH to diabetes insipidus:

SIADH and Diabetes Insipidus

	Cause	Manifestations
SIADH		
Diabetes insipidus		

Complete the following table of comparative manifestations for hypercortisolism and hypocortisolism:

Hypercortisolism/Hypocortisolism

Hypercortisolism	Hypocortisolism

Complete the following table by matching general alterations with specific endocrine disorders:

Manifestations/Effects of Endocrine Disorders

Effect	Examples
Fluid and electrolyte imbalances	
Cardiovascular dysfunction	
General growth alterations	Dwarfism, giantism, acromegaly
Reproductive irregularities	
Altered glucose metabolism	
Metabolic rate abnormalities	Hyperthyroidism, hypothyroidism, cretinism, myxedema

CASE STUDY 1

Scott, a 17-year-old high school football player, was brought to the hospital emergency department in a coma. According to his mother, "He has lost weight during the past month in spite of eating large amounts of food." Besides losing weight, she also said, "He was excessively thirsty and had frequently awakened his younger brother as he noisily urinated several times during the night." Physical findings were not significant except for tachycardia and hyperpnea.

Laboratory serum studies revealed the following:

Glucose on admission = 1000 mg/dL
pH = 7.25 (low)
pco_2 = 30 mm Hg (low)
HCO_3^- = 12 mEq/L (low)
Glycosylated hemoglobin = 9% (high)

What do you think Scott's symptoms, signs, and diagnostic studies suggest?

CASE STUDY 2

A 49-year-old short, overweight Native American woman seeking care at a clinic was diagnosed with type 2 diabetes several years ago. She ignored recommendations for care and is now complaining of weakness in her right foot. The patient says, "My foot has been weak for a long time, it is hard to bend, and it feels numb." She denies any other problems except being thirsty and having to get out of bed at night to urinate, but she admits to gaining about 20 pounds lately.

Notable findings on physical examination reveal a weight of 198 pounds and a blood pressure of 166/101. Her retina shows mild arteriolar narrowing. Right limb strength is less than half that of left limb strength, and sensory perception to light touch on the soles of both feet is diminished.

What laboratory tests would you order now and after fasting? Interpret the laboratory reports. What treatment would you recommend?

19 Structure and Function of the Hematologic System

FOUNDATIONAL OBJECTIVES

After reviewing this chapter, the learner will be able to do the following:

1. **Identify the components of blood plasma.**

   Review pages 477, 478 and 480; refer to Figure 19-1 and Table 19-1.

2. **Identify the structural characteristics, normal values, functions, and life span of the cellular components of blood.**

   Review pages 480 and 481; refer to Figures 19-2 through 19-4 and Table 19-2.

3. **Describe lymphoid organs and the mononuclear phagocyte system (MPS).**

   Review pages 482 and 483; refer to Figures 19-5 and 19-6 and Table 19-3.

4. **Describe the development of erythrocytes, leukocytes, and platelets; identify the CSFs and the nutritional requirements necessary for these developmental processes.**

   Review pages 483-489; refer to Figures 19-7 through 19-14 and Table 19-4.

5. **Describe the mechanisms and the sequence of events in hemostasis; note the blood tests for hematologic disorders.**

   Review pages 489-492; refer to Figures 19-15 though 19-18 and Table 19-5.

6. **Diagram the fibrinolytic system.**

   Review page 493; refer to Figure 19-18.

7. **Identify various hematologic tests and value changes for different age groups.**

   Refer to Tables 19-6 and 19-7.

PRACTICE EXAMINATION

Multiple Choice

Circle the correct answer for each question:

1. Which is *not* a plasma component?
   a. colloids
   b. electrolytes
   c. gases
   d. glucose
   e. platelets

2. Which is the most abundant protein in blood plasma?
   a. fibrinogen
   b. albumins
   c. globulins
   d. immunoglobulins
   e. hormones

3. Eosinophils:
   a. can phagocytize.
   b. ingest antigen-antibody complexes.
   c. can be induced to attack parasites.
   d. Only a and c are correct.
   e. a, b, and c are correct.

4. The precursor of granulocytes is the:
   a. monoblast.
   b. megakaryoblast.
   c. M-CSF.
   d. myeloblast.

5. Identify the correct sequence in the differentiation of erythrocytes.
   a. proerythroblast, normoblast, reticulocyte
   b. normoblast, reticulocyte, erythroblast
   c. normoblast, proerythroblast, reticulocyte
   d. normoblast, erythroblast, reticulocyte

6. A differential count of WBCs includes all of the following *except:*
   a. 54% to 67% neutrophils.
   b. 5% to 10% natural killer cells.
   c. 3% reticulocytes.
   d. 3% to 8% monocytes and macrophages.
   e. 25% to 36% lymphocytes.

7. The purpose of erythropoietin is to:
   a. decrease maturation of erythroblasts.
   b. detect hypoxia.
   c. control erythrocyte production.
   d. control the size of platelets.

8. The main regulator of platelet circulating mass is:
   a. GP11b/111a complex.
   b. ADP.
   c. thrombopoietin.
   d. thromboxane.

9. About how many times more RBCs than WBCs are there in 1 mm^3 of blood?
   a. 15
   b. 90
   c. 100
   d. 1000
   e. None of the above is correct.

10. If the total leukocyte count of an individual was 7000/mm^3, about how many neutrophils would normally be present in 1 mm^3 of blood?
    a. 400
    b. 700
    c. 2100
    d. 3000
    e. 4200

11. Which granulocyte function is similar to that of tissue mast cells?
    a. lymphocytes
    b. monocytes
    c. neutrophils
    d. basophils
    e. eosinophils

12. Erythropoietin:
    a. is secreted by the kidney.
    b. production is stimulated by tissue hypoxia.
    c. causes recycling of iron for production of RBCs.
    d. is released by the kidney to stimulate erythrocyte and platelet formation.
    e. Both a and b are correct.

13. Which is *not* an agranulocyte?
    a. mast cell
    b. lymphocyte
    c. monocyte
    d. reticulocyte
    e. Both a and d are correct.

14. Which are the most effective phagocytes?
    a. neutrophils and basophils
    b. lymphocytes and eosinophils
    c. basophils and monocytes
    d. neutrophils and monocytes
    e. None of the above is correct.

15. Which vitamins are needed for erythropoiesis?
    a. C and E
    b. B2 and B12
    c. A and D
    d. Both a and b are correct.
    e. a, b, and c are correct.

16. Kupffer's cells are found in the:
    a. liver.
    b. kidney.
    c. bone marrow.
    d. spleen and lymph nodes.

17. Which test reflects bone marrow activity?
    a. reticulocyte count
    b. hemoglobin mean
    c. hematocrit mean
    d. g/dL

18. As an individual ages:
    a. the erythrocyte life span shortens.
    b. lymphocytic function decreases.
    c. platelet numbers decrease.
    d. All of the above are correct.

19. Hemostasis involves all of the following *except:*
    a. vasoconstriction.
    b. platelet plug formation.
    c. intrinsic pathway activities.
    d. clot formation.
    e. prostacyclin I.

20. When a blood vessel is damaged:
    a. subendothelial collagen is exposed.
    b. platelets are attracted to collagen.
    c. platelets degranulate.
    d. Both a and b are correct.
    e. a, b, and c are correct.

21. The biochemical mediators released by adhering platelets cause:
    a. vasodilation of the injured vessel.
    b. vasoconstriction of the injured vessel.
    c. the inflammatory process to proceed.
    d. All of the above are correct.

22. Which is the correct sequence in coagulation?
    a. X, tissue thromboplastin, XA
    b. prothrombin activator complex, X, XA
    c. fibrinogen, thrombin, stabilizer fibrin
    d. damaged tissue, VII, prothrombin

23. Which is the correct sequence in fibrinolysis?
    a. fibrin, plasminogen
    b. FDP, fibrinogen
    c. plasminogen, XIIa
    d. plasmin, FDP

Matching

Match the colony-stimulating factor with the cells that are stimulated:

_______ 24. IL-3

_______ 25. GM

a. erythrocytes
b. macrophage, neutrophil
c. eosinophil
d. normoblast
e. erythroblast

Complete the following table identifying the normal values, functions, and life span of the cells in the blood:

Cellular Components of the Blood

Cell	Normal Amounts	Function	Life Span

20 Alterations of Hematologic Function

FOUNDATIONAL OBJECTIVES

a. Identify the differentiation sequence, function, and normal values for erythrocytes.
Review pages 485-488; refer to Figures 19-9 through 19-13 and Table 19-4.

MEMORY CHECK!

DIFFERENTIATION OF ERYTHROCYTES

Uncommitted Pluripotential Stem Cell

↓ ← Erythropoietin

Committed Proerythroblast (Large nucleus)

↓

Normoblast
(The nucleus shrinks and undergoes reabsorption)

↓

Reticulocyte
(No nucleus; enters vascular circulation from the bone marrow)

↓

Erythrocyte
(Loses capacity for hemoglobin synthesis, disk shape and size achieved)

- The function of erythrocytes is to transport gas to and from the tissue cells and lungs. The normal adult ranges of indices for circulating erythrocytes* in the blood are as follows:

  Number = 4.2-6.2 million/mm^3
  Hematocrit = 42%-48%
  Hemoglobin = 12-16.5 g/dL

- The rate of *erythropoiesis* or formation of RBCs is measured by the *reticulocyte count*. A low count may indicate the inability of bone marrow to respond. A high count may indicate a good marrow response to low numbers of RBCs. *Erythropoietin* is secreted by the kidney in response to tissue hypoxia from anemia, high altitude, or pulmonary disease. Erythropoietin stimulates the proliferation of stem cells in the marrow and accelerates maturation of erythroblasts.

**Note:* Reticulocytes normally constitute less than 1% of the RBCs found in blood and 1 mm^3 equals 1 μL, or one-millionth of a liter.

b. Identify the differentiation sequence for granulocytes, agranulocytes, and platelets.
Refer to Figure 19-7.

MEMORY CHECK!

DIFFERENTIATION OF WHITE BLOOD CELLS (WBCs) AND PLATELETS

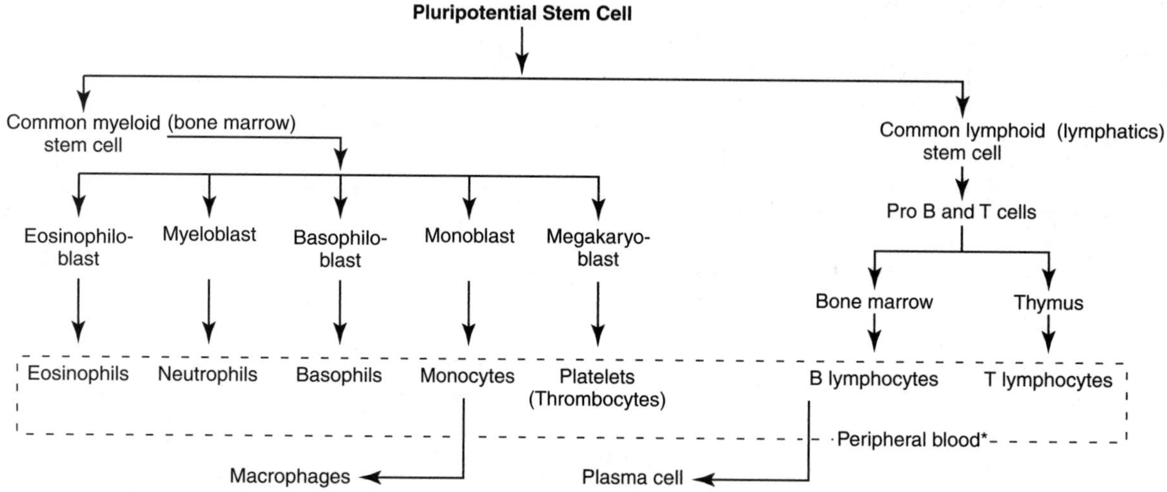

The granulocytes, agranulocytes, and platelets circulate in the peripheral blood.
Specific colony-stimulating factors (CSFs) secreted by cells control at specific sequential sites the production, maturation, function, and development of blood cells.

c. Briefly diagram the blood-clotting mechanisms and the fibrinolytic system.
Refer to Figures 19-15 through 19-18.

MEMORY CHECK!

BLOOD CLOTTING CASCADE

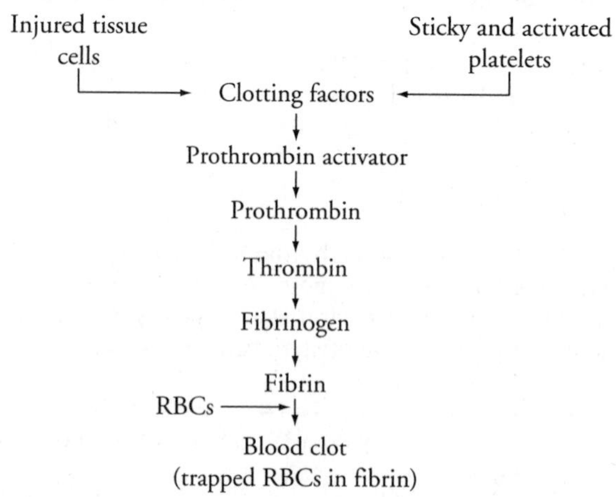

* Note: Various coagulation factors from the intrinsic and extrinsic pathways participate.
FVIIa complex initiates clotting by activating factors X and IX. Alternatively, factor XI can activate IXa. Factors Va:Xa, known as the prothrombinase complex, activate prothrombin. Thrombin activates several other proteases and cofactors. Clot formation finally occurs when thrombin cleaves fibrinogen to soluble fibrinogen monomers (SFMs), which are cross-linked by factor XIIIa, and with activation of protease-activated receptors (PARs) on platelets.

MEMORY CHECK!

FIBRINOLYTIC SYSTEM

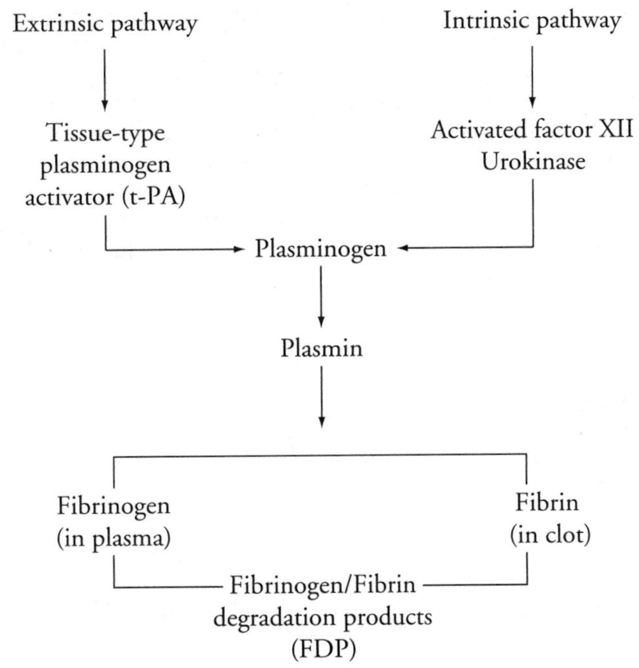

LEARNING OBJECTIVES

After studying this chapter, the learner will be able to do the following:

1. Define and classify anemia.
Study pages 500 and 501; refer to Table 20-1.

Anemia is a reduction in the total number of circulating erythrocytes or a decrease in the quality or quantity of hemoglobin. Whether there is *decreased/defective production or destruction of erythrocytes*, anemias are classified according to either their **etiologic basis** or the **morphologic appearance** of the erythrocytes. Descriptions of anemias based on erythrocyte cellular structure refer to the cell's size and hemoglobin content. The morphologic classification is widely used. Terms that refer to cellular size end with *-cytic*. Terms that describe hemoglobin content end with *-chromic*. An erythrocyte can be macrocytic, meaning abnormally large, or microcytic, meaning abnormally small, and hyperchromic, containing an unusually high concentration of hemoglobin within its cytoplasm, or hypochromic, containing an abnormally low concentration of hemoglobin. For comparison, cells of normal size are termed normocytic and cells with normal amounts of hemoglobin are termed normochromic. In some anemias, the erythrocytes take on various sizes or have various shapes; these states are anisocytosis and poikilocytosis, respectively.

2. Describe the pathophysiology of the clinical manifestations of anemias.
Study pages 501 and 502; refer to Figure 20-1.

Compensation for reduced oxygen-carrying capacity of the blood *requires the cardiovascular and respiratory systems to respond.* A reduction in the number of circulating erythrocytes after hemorrhage affects the consistency and volume of the blood. To compensate for reduced blood volume, fluids from the interstitium move into the blood vessels and plasma volume expands. The thinner, less viscous blood flows faster and more turbulently than normal blood. Increased blood flow within the heart can cause ventricular dysfunction, cardiac dilation, and heart valve insufficiency.

Hypoxemia of anemia causes arterioles, capillaries, and venules to dilate, speeding blood flow even more. As venous return to the heart increases, *the heart must pump harder and faster* to meet normal oxygen demand and to prevent cardiopulmonary congestion. Congestive heart failure can develop.

Tissue hypoxia also causes the rate and *depth of breathing* to increase in an attempt to make more oxygen available to the remaining erythrocytes. When anemia is severe or sudden in onset, *peripheral blood vessels constrict to direct available blood flow to the vital organs.* A number of systemic symptoms occur subsequent to this shunting of blood.

Decreased blood flow is sensed by the kidneys, and in an effort to improve kidney perfusion, the *renal renin-angiotensin response is activated.* This results in salt and water retention, causing increased workload for the heart. The individual experiences shortness of breath or dyspnea, a rapid pounding heartbeat, dizziness, and fatigue, even when at rest.

The skin, mucous membranes, lips, nail beds, and conjunctivae become *pale* because of reduced hemoglobin concentration or *yellowish* as a result of an accumulation in the skin of products of RBC breakdown or hemolysis. Decreased oxygen delivery to the skin results in *impaired healing* and loss of elasticity. Thinning and early graying of the hair can occur.

If the anemia is caused by vitamin B12 deficiency, the nervous system is affected. *Myelin degeneration* may occur with *loss of nerve fibers* in the spinal cord. Paresthesias, gait disturbances, extreme weakness, spasticity, and reflex abnormalities may then result.

Decreased oxygen supply to the gastrointestinal tract often produces abdominal pain, nausea, vomiting, and anorexia. Low-grade fever, less than 101° F, occurs in some anemic individuals and may be the result of the release of *leukocytic pyrogens from ischemic tissues.* Therapeutic intervention for any anemic condition requires treatment of the underlying disorder and palliation of symptoms. Therapies for anemia include transfusions, dietary corrections, and the administration of supplemental vitamins or iron.

3. Develop a comparative table of the macrocytic-normochromic, microcytic-hypochromic, and normocytic-normochromic anemias.
Study pages 502-506; refer to Figures 20-2 through 20-5 and Tables 20-1 and 20-2.

Anemias

Anemia	Etiology	High-Risk Groups	Symptoms
Macrocytic-Normochromic			
Pernicious	Insufficient influence of vitamin B_{12} on developing cells because of deficient IF; antibodies develop against parietal cells gastrectomy or ileectomy therapies; chronic gastritis	Anglo-Saxon and Scandinavian populations	Typical*; digestive symptoms from lack of HCl and enzymes; glossitis; peripheral neuropathy: tingling, numbness, loss of vibratory sense
Folate (folic acid)	Inhibition of DNA synthesis by dietary deficiency	Alcoholics; chronically malnourished persons	Typical*; similar to those of pernicious anemia except no neurologic disorders
Microcytic-Hypochromic			
Iron deficiency (IDA)	Excessive bleeding, which depletes iron; poor diet; no meat; possible *Helicobacter pylori* infection	Pregnant women; adolescents, children, elderly; those with chronic blood loss	Typical*
Sideroblastic (SA)	Dysfunctional iron uptake by erythroblasts; decreased heme synthesis, enzymes etc.; genetic factors	Acquired from drugs: ethanol, lead chloramphenicol; hereditary via recessive X-linked transmission	Typical*; mild hepatomegaly and splenomegaly; erythropoietic hemochromatosis
Normocytic-Normochromic			
Aplastic (AA)	Radiation; drugs; lesions within red bone marrow immune response that halt erythropoiesis (Fanconi anemia)	Anyone	Typical*; petechiae; ecchymosis; bleeding; infection; pancytopenia
Posthemorrhagic	Sudden and acute blood loss	Surgery; trauma	Shock; acidosis

Anemias—Cont'd

Anemia	Etiology	High-Risk Groups	Symptoms
Hemolytic	Premature dysfunction or destruction of mature erythrocytes in circulation genetics, resulting in fragile cells; acquired from infections, drugs, autoimmunity, warm immunoglobulin G (IgG) or cold IgM antibodies	Anyone	Splenomegaly; jaundice
Anemia of chronic inflammation	Bacterial toxins; cytokines from activated macrophages and lymphocytes; suppressed progenitor cells; reduced iron in blood	Acquired immunodeficiency syndrome (AIDS), autoimmunity, neoplasms	Mild because of disability or disease (ACD) caused by a chronic condition

*Typical signs and symptoms: fatigue, weakness, dyspnea, and pallor.

Treatment: Removing cause, if possible, and replacing the deficient element; marrow transplants; or immunosuppression.

4. Describe the types, causes, manifestations, and treatment of polycythemia.
Review pages 506-508; refer to Table 20-3.

Polycythemia is an unusual disease—considered a myeloproliferative, nonmalignant disease—that causes excessively large numbers of erythrocytes in the blood. It is typically accompanied by increased circulating platelets and granulocytes. There are essentially two types of polycythemia: (1) primary and secondary absolute and (2) relative. *Relative polycythemia* results from *hemoconcentration* of blood associated with *dehydration.* The primary form of absolute polycythemia is relatively rare and tends to occur in men between the ages of 40 and 60 years of Jewish or European ancestry. Rarely is polycythemia found in children or multiple members of a single family. *Secondary polycythemia*, the more common form, is essentially a physiologic *response to hypoxia*. It is not uncommon to find an increased RBC count in individuals living at high altitudes, in smokers, and in individuals with congestive heart failure or chronic obstructive pulmonary disease.

The clinical signs of polycythemia include ruddy, red color of the face, hands, feet, ears, and mucous membranes; engorgement of retinal and sublingual veins; elevated blood pressure; splenomegaly; and hepatomegaly. Symptoms include headache, a feeling of fullness in the head, dizziness, weakness, itching, sweating, epigastric distress, fatigue on exertion, backache, and visual disturbances. The clinical manifestations of vascular disease likely predominate. Angina pectoris, calf pain associated with vasospasms during walking, thrombosis, and cerebral insufficiency can occur.

Treatment for polycythemia consists of reducing erythrocytosis and blood volume, controlling symptoms, and preventing thrombosis. Erythrocytosis and blood volume are reduced by phlebotomy, wherein a vein is opened and blood is removed according to need. Radioactive phosphorus is also used to suppress erythropoiesis. Smokers should be urged to quit, and patients with congestive heart failure and chronic obstructive pulmonary disease require appropriate pharmaceutical intervention.

5. Describe terms associated with high and low leukocyte counts and the causes of the alterations.
Study pages 508 and 509; refer to Table 20-4.

Leukocytosis exists when the leukocyte count is higher than normal; **leukopenia** is a condition in which the leukocyte count is lower than normal. *Leukocytosis is a normal, protective response* to invading microorganisms, strenuous exercise, emotional changes, temperature changes, anesthesia, surgery, pregnancy, some drugs, hormones, and toxins. Malignancies and hematologic disorders also cause leukocytosis. Increased levels of circulating neutrophils, eosinophils, basophils, and monocytes are chiefly a physiologic response to infection. Elevations also can occur as a result of polycythemia and chronic myelocytic leukemia, which increase stem cell proliferation in the bone marrow.

Leukopenia is never beneficial. As the leukocyte count falls below $1000/mm^3$, the individual is at risk for infection. The risk for serious, *life-threatening infections* develops *with counts below* $500/mm^3$. Leukopenia can be caused by radiation, anaphylactic shock, systemic lupus erythematosus, and certain chemotherapeutic agents. Decreased leukocytic counts occur when infectious processes delete the circulating granulocytes and monocytes. Infectious agents draw them out of the circulation and into infected tissues faster than they can be replaced. Decreases can also be caused by disorders that suppress bone marrow function.

Granulocytosis or **neutrophilia** is prevalent in the early stages of *infection or inflammation,* when stored neutrophils from the venous sinuses are released into the circulating blood. Emptying of the venous sinuses stimulates formation of granulocytes in the marrow. When the demand for neutrophils exceeds the circulatory supply, the marrow releases immature neutrophils and other leukocytes into the blood; this is called a **shift to the left**. The shift to the left is sometimes called a *leukemoid* reaction because the morphologic findings in blood smears are similar to those in individuals with leukemia. As infection or inflammation diminishes and granulopoiesis replenishes the circulating granulocytes, a shift to the right, or back to normal, occurs. **Neutropenia**, or low neutrophilic count, may be caused by decreased or ineffective neutrophil production because the marrow is producing other formed elements. Also, autoimmunity, reduced neutrophil survival, and abnormal neutrophil distribution and sequestration in tissues lead to neutropenia. Neutropenia exists when the neutrophil count is less than 2000/mm^3. If neutrophils are reduced to below 500/mm^3 and the entire granulocyte count is extremely low, a serious condition called **agranulocytosis** results. The usual cause of agranulocytosis is *interference with hematopoiesis* in the bone marrow or increased cell *destruction* in the circulation. Chemotherapeutic agents used in the treatment of hematologic disorders and other malignancies and some drugs cause bone marrow suppression. Clinical manifestations of agranulocytosis include respiratory infection, general malaise, septicemia, fever, tachycardia, and ulcers in the mouth and colon. If untreated, sepsis due to agranulocytosis can result in death within 3 to 6 days.

Eosinophilia is an absolute increase in the total numbers of circulating eosinophils. *Allergic disorders* associated with asthma, hay fever, parasitic invasion, and drug reactions are often the cause of eosinophilia. Chemotactic factor of anaphylaxis (CTF-A) and histamine released from mast cells attract eosinophils to the area. Eosinopenia is a decrease in circulating eosinophils; generally the result of migration of eosinophils into inflammatory sites. It may also be seen in Cushing syndrome as a result of stress from surgery, shock, trauma, burns, or mental distress.

Basophilia (increased basophils) is rare and is generally seen as a response to inflammation and *hypersensitivity reactions* of the immediate antibody response type. An increase in basophils also is seen in chronic myeloid leukemia and myeloid metaplasia. **Basopenia** (decreased basophils) is seen in hyperthyroidism, acute infection, and long-term therapy with steroids, as well as during ovulation and pregnancy.

Monocytosis, an increase in monocytes, is often transient and correlates poorly with disease states. When present, it is most commonly associated with bacterial infections during the *late stages of recovery* when monocytes are needed to phagocytize any surviving microorganisms and debris. Monocytosis is seen in chronic infections, such as tuberculosis and subacute bacterial endocarditis. **Monocytopenia**, a decrease in monocytes, is rare but has been identified with hairy cell leukemia and prednisone therapy.

A **lymphocytosis** is rare in acute bacterial infections and occurs most often in acute viral infections, especially those caused by the Epstein-Barr virus (EBV). **Lymphocytopenia** may be associated with *neoplasias, immune deficiencies,* and destruction by *drugs*. It may be that the lymphocytopenia associated with heart failure and other acute illnesses is caused by elevations of cortisol. Lymphocytopenia is a major problem in AIDS. The lymphocytopenia seen with this condition is caused by the human immunodeficiency virus (HIV), which is cytopathic for helper T lymphocytes.

6. Describe the pathogenesis of infectious mononucleosis.
Study pages 511 and 512.

Infectious mononucleosis is an acute infection of B lymphocytes. The most common etiologic virus is the EBV. *Transmission of EBV usually occurs through saliva*—hence, the common name "kissing disease."

Infectious mononucleosis usually affects young adults between the ages of 15 and 35 years. The incubation period for infectious mononucleosis is approximately 30 to 50 days. The proliferation of clones of B and T cells and removal of dead and damaged leukocytes are largely responsible for the swelling of cervical lymphoid tissues. Splenomegaly occurs in affected individuals. The accompanying sore throat is caused by inflammation at the site of viral entry.

Serologic tests to determine a *heterophile antibody* response are necessary for diagnosis. These heterophilic antibodies are IgM agglutinins against nonhuman RBCs (sheep or horse).

Infectious mononucleosis is usually self-limiting with recovery occurring in a few weeks. Treatment consists of rest and alleviation of symptoms with analgesics. Streptococcal pharyngitis is treated with penicillin or erythromycin. Steroids are used when airway obstruction or other organ involvement is evident.

7. Classify, contrast, and describe the manifestations of leukemia.
Study pages 512-515; refer to Figures 20-6 through 20-8 and Tables 20-5 and 20-7.

Leukemia is a malignant disorder of the blood and blood-forming organs, exhibiting an *uncontrolled proliferation of dysfunctional leukocytes*. The excessive proliferation of leukemic cells crowds the bone marrow and causes decreased production and function of normal hematopoietic cells.

The two major forms of leukemia are acute and chronic. They are classified according to predominant cell type *(myeloid or lymphoid)* and the degree of differentiation. There are four types of leukemia: acute lymphocytic (ALL), acute myelogenous (AML), chronic lymphocytic (CLL), and chronic myelogenous (CML). Leukemias involving lymphatic vessels, lymph nodes, spleen, and thymus are lymphocytic; those involving the bone marrow are myelogenous.

Acute leukemia is characterized by undifferentiated and immature, or *blastic cells*. The onset of disease is abrupt and rapid, and the affected individual usually has a *short survival* time. In *chronic leukemia*, the predominant cell appears *mature,* but does not function normally. The onset of disease is gradual and the prolonged clinical course results in a relatively *longer survival* time. Leukemia occurs with varying frequencies at different ages and is about 10 times more common in adults than in children in the United States.

Causal risk factors acting together with a genetic predisposition can alter the nuclear DNA of a single cell, and the resulting leukemic cell proliferates. The leukemic cell is unable to mature and respond to normal regulatory mechanisms. *Abnormal chromosomes are reported in 40% to 50% of patients with acute leukemia.* Hereditary abnormalities such as Down syndrome, aplastic anemia, and immune deficiencies are also associated with an increased incidence of leukemia.

Acquired disorders that progress to acute leukemia include CML, polycythemia, Hodgkin lymphoma, multiple myeloma, ovarian cancer, CLL, and sideroblastic anemia. Large doses of *ionizing* radiation are also associated with an increased incidence in myelogenous leukemia. Drugs such as chloramphenicol and certain alkylating agents cause bone marrow depression and can also predispose an individual to leukemia. AML is the most frequently reported secondary cancer following *high doses* of chemotherapy used for some other cancers.

Signs and symptoms related to bone marrow depression include fatigue caused by anemia, bleeding due to thrombocytopenia, and fever caused by infection. Bleeding may occur in the skin, gums, mucous membranes, and gastrointestinal tract. Visible signs include petechiae and ecchymosis, hematuria, and midcycle or heavy menstrual bleeding. Neurologic manifestations include headache, vomiting, papilledema, facial palsy, blurred vision, auditory disturbances, and meningeal irritation if leukemic cells infiltrate the cerebral or spinal meninges. The presence of the *Philadelphia chromosome* is observed in about 95% of individuals with CML.

Current survival rates range from 20% for AML to 73% for CLL. *Death* is usually caused by *hemorrhage or infection.*

8. Differentiate multiple myeloma from the leukemias.

Study pages 520 and 521; refer to Figures 20-13 through 20-15.

Multiple myeloma is a B cell cancer *arising from a malignant plasma cell* that infiltrates and destroys bone marrow and aggregates into tumor masses within the skeletal system. Multiple myelomas involve chromosomal translocations, which occur in many individuals. One chromosome partner is chromosome 14, the site of immunoglobulin genes, which recombines with other chromosomal sites. This disorder likely originates in the *bone marrow and moves through the circulation to lymph nodes; then the myeloma cells return to the bone marrow or soft tissue sites.* Development of myeloma is governed by cytokines; interleukin-6 (IL-6) is likely the major osteoclastic factor.

Chemotherapy, radiation therapy, plasmapheresis, blood stem cell transplantation, and marrow transplantation have been used for treatment. With chemotherapy and aggressive management of complications, a median survival of 24 to 30 months and a 10-year survival rate of 3% are possible. After conventional chemotherapy relapse, thalidomide can be used because it suppresses tumor necrosis factor and has antiangiogenesis ability.

Multiple Myeloma and Common Leukemias

Characteristic	Multiple Myeloma	Common Leukemias
Malignant proliferation of WBCs in the bone marrow	Yes	Yes
Anemia	Yes	Yes
Bleeding	Yes	Yes
Recurrent infections	Yes	Yes
Plasma cells	Yes	No
Ineffective immunoglobulins/M-protein	Yes	No
Bence-Jones protein in urine	Yes	No
Pathologic bone fractures	Yes	No
Elevation of WBC count in blood	No	Yes
Osteocytic lesions	Yes	Possible
Elevated calcium serum	Yes	Possible
Bone pain	Yes	Possible
Renal disease	Yes	Possible

9. Compare Hodgkin to non-Hodgkin lymphomas.
Study pages 516-521 and 534 and 535; refer to Figures 20-9 through 20-12 and Tables 20-8 through 20-10.

Lymphomas are tumors of: (1) primary lymphoid tissue or the thymus and bone marrow and (2) secondary lymphoid tissue or lymph nodes, spleen, tonsils, and intestinal lymphoid tissue. Most lymphomas are neoplasms of secondary lymphoid tissue involving lymph nodes or spleen. The major types of malignant lymphomas are **Hodgkin** and **non-Hodgkin lymphomas**. *Bone marrow involvement* occurs more often in non-Hodgkin lymphoma than in Hodgkin lymphoma. Hodgkin lymphoma uses one of four histologic subtypes for classification. The subtypes are based on the appearance of the nonmalignant cells and the specific type of cytokine involved. Non-Hodgkin lymphoma lacks the *Reed-Sternberg cells* seen in Hodgkin lymphoma and features other cellular changes not characteristic of Hodgkin lymphomas. In both types of lymphoma, the *genetic alterations* involve mutation of *proto-oncogenes* and inactivation or disruption of tumor *suppressor genes.*

Malignant Lymphomas

	Hodgkin Lymphoma	Non-Hodgkin Lymphoma
Cause	No apoptosis of B cells nor rearrangement of immunoglobulin genes; EBV; Reed-Sternberg cells release cytokines	Translocations on proto-oncogenes and tumor suppression genes, cancer causing suppressor genes, cancer causing viruses, immunodeficiency, *H. pylori* infection
Cellular deviation	B cells	B cells (85%), T cells and NK cells (15%)
Nodes involved	Painless node in neck; single node or chain: cervical, inguinal, axillary, retroperitoneal	Noncontinuous nodes: cervical, axillary, inguinal, femoral
Symptoms	Mostly localized manifestations of systemic fever, night sweats, weakness, weight loss, pericardial involvement from mediastinal nodes	Similar to those of Hodgkin lymphoma plus pleural effusion, abdominal pain, splenomegaly, and hepatomegaly (generalized manifestations more likely)
Treatment	Radiotherapy or surgery for localized, chemotherapy for generalized; bone marrow or stem cell transplantation	Chemotherapy, immunotherapy, and radiotherapy; autologous stem cell transplantation
Curability	More than 75%	Long term, nodular lymphoma has better prognosis (15 years) than diffuse disease (42% for 10 years)

*Reed-Sternberg cells are malignant tissue macrophages that secrete cytokines that cause accumulation of inflammatory cells.

Note: Burkitt lymphoma is a B cell tumor involving the jaw and facial bones occurring in east-central Africa.

10. Describe thrombocytopenia and thrombocythemia.
Study pages 523-526.

Thrombocytopenia exists when the platelet count is below 100,000 platelets per mm^3 of blood. Thrombocytopenia results from either decreased platelet production, increased consumption, or both. *Hemorrhage* from minor trauma can occur with counts of 50,000/mm^3 or below. *Spontaneous bleeding* can occur with counts between 15,000 and 10,000/mm^3. *Severe bleeding* results if the count is below 10,000/mm^3. Such bleeding can be fatal if it occurs in the gastrointestinal tract, respiratory system, or central nervous system. Thrombocytopenia exists in primary and secondary forms.

Heparin-induced thrombocytopenia (HIT) is an immune-mediated, adverse drug reaction caused by IgG antibodies directed against the heparin–platelet factor 4 complex. The IgG binds to platelet receptors and activates platelet aggregation, decreasing platelet counts by 5000 to 10,000/mm^3 after heparin administration. If HIT is not treated by withdrawal of heparin and use of alternative anticoagulants, intravascular aggregation of platelets causes rapid arterial and venous thrombosis.

Immune thrombocytopenic purpura (ITP) is usually a chronic condition more prevalent in females. It is thought to be an autoimmune disorder in which an IgG autoantibody is formed that binds to and destroys the platelets. The individual most commonly presents with mucosal or skin bleeding, which often is manifested as menorrhagia, hematuria, purpura, and petechiae. Initial therapy for ITP consists of glucocorticoids to suppress the immune response. Intravenous immunoglobulin is used to prevent major bleeding. If platelet counts do not increase appropriately, splenectomy is considered to remove the site of platelet destruction.

In **thrombotic thrombocytopenia purpura (TTP),** platelets aggregate and occlude the microcirculation. Platelet aggregation occurs without activation of the coagulation cascade and is related to other thrombotic microangiopathic conditions, including hemolytic syndromes and low–platelet count syndromes. Defects in plasma ADAMTS13 result in high-molecular-weight von Willebrand factor on endothelial cell surfaces and the formation of large aggregates of platelets that form occlusions in smaller vessels. Plasma exchange with fresh frozen plasma, which replaces ADAMTS13, is the treatment of choice.

Thrombocythemia has a platelet count greater than $400,000/mm^3$ of blood. It is usually asymptomatic until the count exceeds 1 $million/mm^3$. Then, intravascular clot formation or *thrombosis, hemorrhage, or other abnormalities can occur.*

Primary or **essential thrombocythemia (ET)** is a myeloproliferative disorder in which platelet precursors in the marrow are produced in excess of $600,000/mm^3$. The thrombocythemia is secondary to increased plasma thrombopoietin. Clinical manifestations of primary thrombocytosis include thrombosis of peripheral blood vessels and, in severe cases, thrombosis of hepatic, mesenteric, or pulmonary vessels. Splenomegaly and easy bruising also occur. In individuals with thrombotic and hemorrhagic complications, the platelet count is lowered by use of chemotherapy agents. Anagrelide, the drug of choice for treatment, interferes with platelet maturation, rather than production, thus not interfering with red and white cell growth and development.

Secondary thrombocythemia occurs following splenectomy because platelets that normally would be stored in the spleen remain in circulating blood. Secondary thrombocytosis may be seen in conjunction with treatment of rheumatoid arthritis and cancers.

11. Identify the causes of coagulation disorders; characterize disseminated intravascular coagulation.

Study pages 526-530; refer to Figure 20-16.

Disorders of coagulation are usually caused by defects or *deficiencies of* one or more of the *clotting factors*. Two common inherited disorders are the **hemophilias** and **von Willebrand disease**. These are caused by deficiencies of clotting factor, hemophilia by a single clotting factor deficiency and von Willebrand disease by multiple clotting factor deficiencies.

Other coagulation defects are acquired and usually result from deficient synthesis of clotting factors by an *impaired liver.* A deficiency of vitamin K, which is necessary for normal synthesis of the clotting factors by the liver, is an acquired coagulation defect.

Disseminated intravascular coagulation (DIC) is an acquired coagulation disorder that has a variety of predisposing conditions. DIC is a paradoxical condition in which *clotting and hemorrhage occur* within the vascular system *simultaneously*. The development of DIC is generally associated with endothelial damage, exposure to tissue factor (TF), which complexes with factor VII, and direct activation of factor X. Gram-negative sepsis, septic shock, hypoxia, and low-flow states associated with cardiopulmonary arrest can damage the endothelium and precipitate DIC by activating the intrinsic clotting pathway. *Endotoxins* of gram-negative organisms activate both intrinsic and extrinsic clotting pathways.

Release of TF is associated with normal tissue breakdown. Excessive amounts of *TF* in the circulation *activate both clotting pathways.* When either system is activated, widespread, unrestricted coagulation occurs throughout the body, leading to thrombic events within the vasculature.

The amount of thrombin that enters the systemic circulation during DIC greatly exceeds the ability of the body's naturally occurring antithrombins. The obstruction that results from circulatory deposition of thrombin interferes with blood flow and causes widespread organ *hypoperfusion* that can lead to ischemia, infarction, and necrosis with manifestations of multisystem organ dysfunction. The clotting factors are consumed as widespread clotting develops. Thrombosis in the presence of hemorrhage constitutes this paradoxical alteration.

Plasmin, which is present because of overstimulation of the clotting cascade, begins to degrade fibrin before a stable clot can develop. As fibrin is broken down by plasmin, *fibrin degradation products (FDPs)* are released into the circulation; these are potent *anticoagulants*. The macrophage system likely is unable to clear the blood of FDPs because of lack of fibronectin. The clearance of particulate matter or fibrin clumps is mediated by the adhesive properties of fibronectin.

Treatment of DIC attempts to remove the underlying pathology, control ongoing thrombosis, and maintain organ viability. The treatment is nonstandarized; heparin is useful in some cases, not in others. Organ viability is treated primarily by fluid replacement to ensure adequate circulating blood volume so that optimal tissue perfusion can be maintained.

12. Characterize thromboembolic disorders.

Study page 530; refer to Figure 20-17.

Thromboembolic disease results from a *fixed (thrombus)* or *moving (embolus)* blood clot that blocks flow within a vessel, thus denying nutrients to tissues distal to the occlusion. Death can result when clots obstruct blood flow to the heart, brain, or lungs. Hypercoagulability is the result of a deficiency of anticoagulation proteins. Secondary causes are conditions that promote venous stasis. The term *Virchow triad* refers to three risk factors for thrombus formation: (1) loss of integrity of the vessel endothelium, (2) abnormalities of blood flow, and (3) alterations in the blood constituents.

PRACTICE EXAMINATION

Multiple Choice

Circle the correct answer for each question:

1. Anemia refers to a deficiency of:
   a. blood plasma.
   b. erythrocytes.
   c. platelets.
   d. hemoglobin.
   e. Both b and d are correct.

2. Morphologic classification of anemia is based on all of the following except:
   a. size.
   b. color.
   c. shape.
   d. cause.

3. Hypoxemia causes:
   a. arterioles, capillaries, and venules to dilate.
   b. the heart to contract more forcefully.
   c. the rate and depth of breathing to increase.
   d. Both a and b are correct.
   e. a, b, and c are correct.

4. Which symptoms are consistent with aplastic anemia, but not with pernicious anemia?
   a. hemorrhage into the tissues
   b. pallor
   c. fatigue
   d. hypoxia
   e. neuropathy

5. A cause of macrocytic-normochromic anemia is:
   a. iron deficiency.
   b. antibodies against parietal cells.
   c. an enzyme deficiency.
   d. inheritance of abnormal hemoglobin structure.
   e. None of the above is correct.

6. An individual with chronic gastritis and tingling in the fingers requires which of the following for treatment?
   a. oral vitamin B12
   b. vitamin B12 by intramuscular injection
   c. ferrous fumarate by intramuscular injection
   d. oral folate
   e. transfusions

7. Secondary polycythemia may be caused by:
   a. dehydration.
   b. chronic obstructive pulmonary disease.
   c. living at high altitudes.
   d. Both b and c are correct.
   e. a, b, and c are correct.

8. The symptoms of polycythemia are essentially caused by:
   a. fewer erythrocytes than normal.
   b. decreased blood volume.
   c. increased blood viscosity.
   d. increased rate of blood flow.

9. Leukocytosis is found in all of the following except:
   a. inflammatory responses.
   b. allergic responses.
   c. bacterial infections.
   d. bone marrow depression.

10. What is the most notable characteristic of infectious mononucleosis?
    a. It has a short incubation period, less than 1 week.
    b. It usually affects preteens.
    c. The presence of heterophil antibody is diagnostically helpful.
    d. Lymphocytosis persists for less than 1 week.

11. Which likely does *not* play a role in leukemia?
    a. radiation
    b. Down syndrome
    c. polycythemia
    d. chloramphenicol
    e. diet

12. CML is characterized by its:
    a. acute onset.
    b. high incidence in children.
    c. presence of the Philadelphia chromosome.
    d. survival time, which is days to months.

13. Clinical manifestations of multiple myeloma include all of the following except:
    a. bone pain.
    b. decreased serum calcium.
    c. M-protein.
    d. renal damage.
    e. pathologic fractures.

14. A thrombocytopenia with a platelet count less than 50,000/mm^3 likely will cause:
    a. hemorrhage from minor trauma.
    b. spontaneous bleeding.
    c. death.
    d. polycythemia.

15. Thromboembolic disease can be caused by all of the following except:
    a. injured vessel walls.
    b. tissue damage that releases excessive TF.
    c. obstructed blood flow.
    d. deficient dietary intake of vitamin K.
    e. polycythemia.

16. DIC is associated with:
    a. endothelial damage.
    b. activation of factor X.
    c. release of TF.
    d. Both a and c are correct.
    e. a, b, and c are correct.

Matching

Match the etiology of the anemia with RBC morphologic appearance:

_______ 17. Vitamin B12 deficiency

_______ 18. Iron deficiency

_______ 19. Folic acid deficiency

_______ 20. Excessive bleeding

a. macrocytic-normochromic
b. microcytic-hypochromic
c. normocytic-normochromic

Match the leukocytic alteration with its cause:

_______ 21. Eosinophilia

_______ 22. Leukopenia

a. pregnancy
b. allergic disorders
c. radiation
d. early stage of infection
e. surgical stress

Match the cause with the malignant lymphoma:

_______ 23. Epstein-Barr virus

_______ 24. Reed-Sternberg cell

_______ 25. More frequent extranodal involvement

a. Hodgkin lymphoma
b. non-Hodgkin lymphoma

Fill in the Blank

Complete the following table identifying conditions resulting from abnormal hematologic values:

Hematologic Values

Test	Disorder*
RBC count, hemoglobin, hematocrit	
WBC count	L: radiation, chemotherapy, anaphylactic shock, splenomegaly, immunosuppression, AIDS
	H: leukemia, allergy, bacterial and parasitic infections
Platelet count	L: hemorrhage, heparin administration, autoimmunity (ITP), (TTP); H: myeloproliferative disorder (ET), splenectomy
Prothrombin time	
Bleeding time	
Fibrin degradation products	

*L, low value; H, high value.

CASE STUDY 1

Ann is an apparently healthy 26-year-old white woman. Since the beginning of this current golf season, she has had increased shortness of breath and low levels of energy and enthusiasm. These symptoms seem worse during her menses. Today, while playing poorly in a golf tournament at a high, mountainous course, she complained to her golfing partner, "I am lightheaded and it is hard for me to breathe." She was taken to a clinic of a multispecialty medical group.

The attending physician's notes indicated a temperature of 98° F, elevated heart and respiratory rates, and low blood pressure. Ann stated, "I've had a heavy menstrual flow for 10 to 12 years, and I take 1000 mg of aspirin every 3 to 4 hours for pain for 6 days during my periods." During the summer months while playing golf, she also takes aspirin to avoid "stiffness in the joints."

Laboratory values are as follows:
Hemoglobin = 8 g/dL
Hematocrit = 32%
Erythrocyte count = $3.1 \times 10^6/mm^3$
RBC smear showed microcytic and hypochromic cells.
Reticulocyte count = 1.5%
Other laboratory values were within normal limits.

Considering the circumstances and the preliminary work-up, what type of anemia is most likely for Ann? Which clinical signs and laboratory value(s) show that her body is attempting to compensate for anemia?

CASE STUDY 2

L.L., a 9-year-old boy, was brought to his dentist for a regular preschool checkup. The dentist and mother were having a chatty conversation when L.L.'s mother stated, "My son has stopped showing interest in sports and complains of being tired all the time." During the dental examination, the dentist noted gingival bleeding whenever the tissue was lightly probed. Three nontender lymph nodes were palpable in the submandibular nodes. No other abnormalities were noted. The dentist advised the mother to take L.L. to the medical clinic next door.

The physical examination showed L.L.'s skin to be pale with ecchymoses and petechiae of the trunk. The spleen and liver were not palpable, and the remaining findings were unremarkable. A sample of blood was withdrawn.

The CBC results revealed the following:

Hemoglobin = 9.2 g/dL
Hematocrit = 30%
RBCs = $3 \times 10^6/mm^3$
WBCs = $16 \times 10^3/mm^3$
Neutrophils = $8 \times 10^3/mm^3$
Basophils = $250/mm^3$
Eosinophils = $445/mm^3$
Monocytes = $1900/mm^3$
Lymphocytes = $4500/mm^3$
Blasts = much higher than normal
Platelets = $30 \times 103/mm^3$

Considering the examinations and CBC, what would the physician likely conclude and do?

21 Alterations of Hematologic Function in Children

FOUNDATIONAL OBJECTIVE

a. Identify the postnatal changes occurring in the blood throughout childhood.
Refer to Table 19-7.

MEMORY CHECK!

- Blood cell counts tend to rise above adult levels at birth and then decline gradually throughout childhood. The immediate rise in values is the result of accelerated hematopoiesis during fetal life, the trauma of birth, and cutting of the umbilical cord. The presence of large numbers of immature erythrocytes and leukocytes in peripheral blood is found in the neonate. Within the first 2 weeks to 3 months of life, but up to age 1 year, normal values for adults are approached. Platelet counts in full-term neonates are comparable to those of adults and remain so throughout infancy and childhood. Average blood volume in the full-term neonate is slightly above that of older children and adults, 85 mL/kg of body weight compared with 75 mL/kg, respectively.

LEARNING OBJECTIVES

After studying this chapter, the learner will be able to do the following:

1. Describe the etiology of childhood iron deficiency anemia and identify appropriate diagnostic and treatment measures.
Study page 536; refer to Table 21-1.

Iron deficiency anemia, the most common childhood anemia, is caused by poor dietary iron intake, gastrointestinal blood loss, or both. Early exposure to cow's milk protein often causes hemorrhagic bowel inflammation and occult blood loss in the infant. The onset of menstruation in females also is a contributor. The incidence of iron deficiency anemia is highest between 6 months and 2 years of age and peaks again in adolescence, during rapid growth periods.

There are few symptoms in infants and young children until moderate anemia develops. General irritability, activity intolerance, and weakness are indicators of anemia. When hemoglobin falls below 5 g/dL, systolic murmurs may occur. Iron stores are best measured by serum ferritin and total iron-binding capacity measurements. Treatment for iron deficiency anemia is iron supplements; oral supplements are preferred.

2. Compare and contrast the two major causes of hemolytic disease of the newborn.
Study pages 536, 537, and 539; refer to Figure 21-1.

The two major causes of **hemolytic disease of the newborn (HDN)** are **ABO blood type incompatibility** and **Rh factor incompatibility**. Blood type incompatibility is a mild form of hemolytic disease. Rh incompatibility is potentially much more severe than blood type incompatibility. Blood type incompatibility in the mother occurs when maternal antibodies to fetal erythrocytes are formed because of a prior incompatible pregnancy or exposure of the mother to fetal erythrocytes during pregnancy. *Incompatibility in the infant* occurs when sufficient antibody, usually immunoglobulin G *(IgG), crosses the placenta* from the mother to the infant or when *maternal antibodies* attach to and *damage fetal erythrocytes*. ABO incompatibility occurs in 20% to 25% of pregnancies, with only 1 in 10 cases producing HDN. Usual causes are a type O mother with a type A or B fetus, a type A mother with a type B fetus, or a type B mother with a type A fetus. Hemolysis in the newborn is usually limited, resolves after birth, and requires limited treatment; however, mild hemolysis may contribute to hyperbilirubinemia.

Rh incompatibility occurs in less than 10% of pregnancies and is rarely a problem during the first pregnancy; the *first pregnancy initiates sensitization*. Anti-Rh antibodies are formed only in response to the presence of *incompatible (Rh-positive)* red blood cells (RBCs) to the blood of an *Rh-negative mother*. Usually this exposure occurs as fetal blood is mixed with the mother's blood at the *time of delivery*. A problem develops if the baby is Rh positive, having inherited the Rh antigens from the father. The mother's immune system responds by making *anti-Rh antibodies to the baby's Rh-positive status*. Rh incompatibility becomes a greater problem with subsequent pregnancies when maternal antibodies cross the placenta into fetal blood. It should be noted that HDN caused by Rh incompatibility occurs in only 5% of pregnancies after five or more pregnancies. In the most severe form, Rh incompatibility can lead to **hydrops fetalis** with severe anemia, edema, central nervous system (CNS) damage, and fetal death. Because the maternal antibodies remain in the neonate's circulatory system after birth, erythrocyte destruction can continue. This process causes hyperbilirubinemia, also known as **icterus neonatorum (neonatal jaundice),** shortly after birth. Without replacement transfusions, in which the child receives Rh-negative erythrocytes, the bilirubin is deposited in the brain, a condition termed kernicterus. Kernicterus produces cerebral damage and usually causes death **(icterus gravis neonatorum).** Infants who do not die may have mental retardation, cerebral palsy, or high-frequency deafness.

Blood typing in mothers and infants reveals those at risk. Indirect Coombs test reveals antibodies in mothers, and direct Coombs test demonstrates antibodies bound to fetal erythrocytes. In patients with a prior history of HDN, diagnostic tests to determine risk include maternal antibody titers, fetal blood sampling, amniotic fluid spectrophotometry, and fetal ultrasound. Immunoprophylaxis with Rh immunoglobulin (RhoGAM) for at-risk mothers has been very successful.

3. Describe childhood sickle cell disease.

Study pages 539-542; refer to Figures 21-2 through 21-6 and Table 21-2.

Sickle cell disease is an inherited, autosomal recessive disorder most common in the United States among blacks. The disease is characterized by the presence of **hemoglobin S (HbS)** within the erythrocytes. This hemoglobin becomes *elongated and sickle shaped* whenever it is *deoxygenated or dehydrated or the pH decreases*.

Acute complications or crises occur in sickle cell disease and may be provoked by infection, exposure to cold, low Po_2, acidosis, or localized hypoxemia. Infections are frequent in childhood and may generate various levels of other triggers. Triggers may lead to crises.

Vasoocclusive crises result from a logjam effect produced by stiff, sickled erythrocytes in the *microcirculation*. Symptoms include symmetrical swelling of the hands and feet, which may be the first clinical manifestation in infancy. In older children, swollen painful joints, priapism, severe abdominal pain from infarctions of abdominal organs, and strokes may occur. Other complications include sickle cell retinopathy, renal necrosis, and necrosis of the femoral head.

Sequestration crises occur only in the young child. Large amounts of blood may pool in the liver and spleen, which can contain as much as one fifth of the blood volume and, thus, *precipitate shock*. Mortality rates of up to 50% have been reported with these crises. **Hyperhemolytic crises**, although unusual, may occur with some drug use or with infections.

Aplastic crises may occur because of the decreased survival of sickled erythrocytes; fewer erythrocytes peak at 10 to 20 days after initiation of the crisis. This development may lead to *aplastic anemia* if compensatory mechanisms are not intact. Most sickle cell deaths result from overwhelming infection and sepsis.

The parents' medical history and clinical findings may generate an index of suspicion about the child's condition. The sickle solubility test and hemoglobin electrophoresis are used to assist in diagnosis. Prenatal chorionic villus sampling is now available.

The sickle cell trait does not affect life expectancy or markedly interfere with daily activities. Treatment consists of supportive care to prevent consequences of anemia and crises.

4. Describe the thalassemias.

Study pages 542 and 543; refer to Figures 21-7 and 21-8.

The alpha- and beta-thalassemias are inherited *autosomal recessive disorders* that cause an impaired rate of synthesis of one of the two chains—alpha or beta—of adult hemoglobin. Beta-thalassemia is more common than alpha-thalassemia.

Beta-thalassemia involves slowed or defective synthesis of the beta globin chain and is prevalent among Greeks, Italians, some Arabs, and Sephardic Jews. Alpha-thalassemia, wherein the alpha globin chain is affected, is most common among Chinese, Vietnamese, Cambodians, and Laotians. Both thalassemias are common among blacks. The effects range from mild microcytosis to death in utero, and the pathophysiology depends on the number of defective genes and the mode of inheritance.

The fundamental defect in beta-thalassemia is the *uncoupling of alpha and beta chain* synthesis. The free alpha chains are unstable and easily precipitated in the cell. Most erythroblasts that contain precipitates are *destroyed by mononuclear phagocytes* in the marrow, resulting in ineffective erythropoiesis and anemia. Individuals with beta-thalassemia minor, the mild form, are usually asymptomatic. Persons with beta-thalassemia major, the severe form, may become quite ill. Anemia is severe and results in significant cardiovascular overload with high-output congestive heart failure. Today, blood transfusion can increase the life span of patients with beta-thalassemia by a decade or two. Death is usually caused by hemochromatosis.

There are four forms of **alpha-thalassemia**, with each dependent on the number of defective alpha-chain-forming genes. The severity is variable. Individuals who inherit the mildest form of alpha-thalassemia, the alpha trait, usually are symptom free or have mild microcytosis. *Alpha-thalassemia major causes hydrops fetalis and fulminant intrauterine congestive heart failure*. The fetus has a grossly enlarged heart and liver. Diagnosis usually is made postmortem. In children with alpha-thalassemia major that is untreated, cardiovascular compromise causes death by 5 to 6 years of age.

Individuals who are carriers or have alpha-thalassemia minor generally have few symptoms and require no specific treatment. For those with alpha-thalassemia major, therapies to support and prolong life are necessary. *There is no* cure for either condition. Prenatal diagnosis and amniotic fluid genetic counseling are important.

5. Describe childhood hemophilias and their complications.
Study pages 544 and 545; refer to Tables 21-3 and 21-4.

Hemophilia, or spontaneous bleeding, is rare in the first year of life, although significant bleeding may occur during circumcision. However, this is an unusual complication, because hemostasis in these hemophilic infants is achieved through the extrinsic pathway, which does not require factors VIII, IX, and XI, the factors whose absence is responsible for 90% to 95% of cases of bleeding. A deficiency of *factor VIII* (antihemophilic factor) is responsible for *hemophilia A,* and that of *factor IX* (plasma thromboplastin component) *causes hemophilia B.*

Hematoma formation is a more common problem during the first year of life and may be caused by injection or firm holding. These incidents also may precipitate bleeding in the joints. Spontaneous hematuria and epistaxis are bothersome, but rarely serious. Life-threatening intracranial and cervical bleeding may result from normal childhood traumatic injury. The administration of recombinant coagulation factors to replace factors that are deficient or absent has enhanced the physical capabilities of individuals suffering hemophilic defects.

6. Describe the pathophysiology of idiopathic thrombocytopenic purpura and identify its most likely etiology.
Study page 545.

Idiopathic thrombocytopenic purpura (ITP; also called autoimmune acute thrombocytopenia purpura) is the most common thrombocytopenic purpura of childhood. Antiplatelet antibodies attach to platelets that are then sequestered in the spleen, where they are destroyed by mononuclear phagocytes.

Classic symptoms of bruising and petechiae are usually preceded by viral illness occurring 1 to 3 weeks earlier that may cause sensitization of the platelets, which triggers an antibody response; high levels of IgG have been found on the platelets of affected children.

The prognosis is excellent. The acute phase lasts 1 to 2 weeks, although thrombocytopenia may persist longer. Complete recovery occurs in approximately 75% of individuals at 3 months after onset, with 80% of afflicted children recovering by 6 to 9 months. Serious complications are few; severe intracranial bleeding does occur in about 1% of cases.

7. Describe childhood leukemias.
Study pages 546 and 547; refer to Figure 21-9 and Table 21-6.

Leukemia, in its various forms, is the most common childhood malignancy; it accounts for 33% of neoplasms in children. Acute lymphoblastic leukemia (ALL) represents 80% to 85% of all childhood leukemias. Peak incidence of ALL occurs at between 2 and 5 years of age and is twice as common in white children as in nonwhite children. The etiology of leukemia is probably multifactorial, with genetic predisposition, environment, and viruses playing a role. The appearance of the **blast cell** in the bone marrow with a reduction of RBCs and granulocytes is the hallmark of acute leukemia. Manifestations may be rapid or slow, but generally reflect the effects of bone marrow failure. Findings include decreased RBCs and platelets and changes in white blood cells. Pallor, fatigue, petechiae, purpura, and fever are generally present. Fever may be caused by a hypermetabolic state brought on by the rapid production and destruction of leukemic cells or by a secondary infection due to neutropenia. Renal failure may ensue as a result of high uric acid levels that produce precipitates of urates in the renal tubules. Other symptoms, such as bone and joint pain, may be the result of infiltration of leukemic cells into other organs. The CNS is a common site of extramedullary infiltration, although few children have this problem at diagnosis; it occurs later in the course of the disease. Combination chemotherapy with or without radiation therapy to localized sites, such as the CNS, is the treatment of choice for leukemia.

8. Distinguish between non-Hodgkin lymphoma and Hodgkin lymphoma.
Study pages 547-549; refer to Figures 21-10 through 21-10.

Non-Hodgkin lymphoma (NHL) and **Hodgkin lymphoma** make up approximately 11% of all childhood cancers; *NHL is more common.* Either group of diseases is rare before the age of 5 years, and the relative incidence rises throughout childhood. Boys are affected more often than girls. At particular risk are children with inherited or acquired immunodeficiency syndromes. A viral etiology is suggested; a strong correlation between the Epstein-Barr virus and lymphoma exists.

Childhood **NHL** is a *diffuse, rather than nodular, disease*; nodular is less aggressive. Disease sites commonly involve extranodal sites such as the brain, lungs, bone, and skin. Rapidly enlarging lymphoid tissue and painless lymphadenopathy are common with abdominal sites. Symptoms often include abdominal pain and vomiting, but a palpable mass is not always present. An anterior mediastinal mass, with or without pleural effusion, may be present. If the mass is large, respiratory compromise, tracheal compression, and superior vena cava syndrome may arise. CNS involvement is common.

Most children with NHL are cured. Optimal treatment is evolving, but combination chemotherapy, with or without radiation therapy, is successful.

The incidence of **Hodgkin lymphoma** gradually rises through the age of 11 years. There is a marked increase during adolescence that continues into the 30s. Histologically, the tumor consists of neoplastic *Reed-Sternberg cells* typically surrounded by small lymphocytes, macrophages, neutrophils, and plasma cells.

Painless lymphadenopathy in the lower cervical chain, with or without fever, is the most common symptom. Mediastinal involvement can lead to airway obstruction. Extranodal primary involvement is rare in Hodgkin lymphoma.

Treatment for Hodgkin lymphoma includes chemotherapy and radiation therapy. The survival rate for children with Hodgkin lymphoma is high; 70% to 90% is common.

PRACTICE EXAMINATION

True/False

1. During fetal life, the synthesized hemoglobin is composed of two alpha and two beta chains.

2. Although a frequent problem, ABO incompatibility seldom results in significant disease.

3. Sequestration crisis is a serious complication of sickle cell disease that is unique to childhood.

4. Rh incompatibility is a problem only for an Rh-positive woman bearing an Rh-negative fetus during a second pregnancy.

5. Because hemostasis in the newborn is chiefly attained through the extrinsic pathway, serious bleeding in the newborn period usually is not a problem in hemophiliacs.

6. ITP is a genetically transmitted disease.

7. Leukemias are multifactorial diseases, with genetic disposition, environment, and bacterial infections playing a role in their etiologies.

Multiple Choice

Circle the correct answer for each question:

8. Which is the most common blood disorder of infancy and childhood?
   a. iron deficiency anemia
   b. pernicious anemia
   c. folate deficiency anemia
   d. sideroblastic anemia

9. Maternal-fetal blood incompatibility may exist in which condition?
   a. Rh-positive mother, Rh-negative fetus
   b. Rh-negative mother, Rh-positive fetus
   c. Rh-negative father, Rh-positive mother
   d. Rh-negative father, Rh-positive mother

10. Beta-thalassemia is:
    a. common among Italians.
    b. an X-linked recessive disorder.
    c. an autosomal recessive disorder.
    d. Both a and b are correct.
    e. Both a and c are correct.

11. Which statement is correct?
    a. Sickle cell disease is an autosomal dominant disorder.
    b. Sickle cell disease is an X-linked recessive disorder.
    c. Sickle cell disease is an X-linked dominant disorder.
    d. Sickle cell disease is an autosomal recessive disorder.

12. ITP involves antibodies against:
    a. neutrophils.
    b. eosinophils.
    c. platelets.
    d. basophils.

13. Which are factors associated with iron deficiency anemia?
    a. rapid growth
    b. low socioeconomic status
    c. cow's milk for infants
    d. Both a and c are correct.
    e. a, b, and c are correct.

14. What is the most likely cause of ITP?
    a. stress and fatigue
    b. genetic predisposition
    c. prolonged occult bleeding
    d. viral sensitization
    e. Both b and c are correct.

15. Hodgkin lymphoma has:
    a. extensive extranodal involvement.
    b. rare extranodal involvement.
    c. painless cervical lymphadenopathy.
    d. Both a and c are correct.
    e. Both b and c are correct.

16. In sickle cell disease, vasoocclusive crisis is the result of:
    a. damage to platelets caused by IgG.
    b. "plugging" of microcirculation by "stiff" sickled erythrocytes.
    c. ingestion of sulfa drugs.
    d. sequestration of large numbers of erythrocytes in the spleen.

17. Which factor may play a part in the development of childhood leukemia?
    a. genetic predisposition
    b. environmental factors
    c. viral infections
    d. radiation
    e. All of the above are correct.

18. Which statement is true about acute lymphocytic leukemia?
    a. It is the most common childhood leukemia.
    b. It usually occurs between 2 and 6 years of age.
    c. It is uniformly fatal.
    d. It is easily predicted through genetic testing.
    e. Both a and b are correct.

Matching

Match the circumstance with the alteration:

_______ 19. Leukocyte counts approaching 100,000/mm^3

_______ 20. Low platelet counts

_______ 21. Lack of coagulation factors VIII, IX, and XI

_______ 22. May manifest early as symmetric, painful swelling of hands and feet

_______ 23. May cause severe hemolysis in the newborn period

_______ 24. May result in aplastic crises

_______ 25. May result in fetal death

a. leukemia
b. ITP
c. sickle cell disease
d. Rh incompatibility
e. hemophilia

Complete the follow table distinguishing among childhood hemophilias:

Childhood Hemophilias

Type	Cause

CASE REVIEW

Steven D. is a 10-year-old white boy referred for medical attention because of possible physical abuse observed by his gym teacher. The teacher noticed severe bruising over much of his upper body when his shirt rode up during an exercise. Steven emphatically stated, "I have never been abused by anyone." He denied any accidents and did not tell anyone about his bruises because he thought they might "get me into trouble." His mother could not explain the bruises either and did not see them before today because her son does all of his own hygiene and is modest about revealing his body, even to family members. Findings of Steven's physical examination are benign except for multiple, irregular dark purple bruises over most of his torso and lower extremities. His complete blood count is well within normal limits, except for a low platelet count, which is 18,000/mm^3.

What is Steven's diagnosis?

22 Structure and Function of the Cardiovascular and Lymphatic Systems

FOUNDATIONAL OBJECTIVES

After reviewing this chapter, the learner will be able to do the following:

1. **Describe the function of the circulatory system; distinguish between pulmonary and systemic circulation.**
   Review page 551; refer to Figure 22-1.

2. **Describe the heart and its wall, chambers, fibrous skeleton, valves, and great vessels; trace the blood flow through the heart.**
   Review pages 551-555; refer to Figures 22-2 through 22-7 and Table 22-1.

3. **Describe the coronary and lymphatic vessels.**
   Review pages 556 and 557; refer to Figure 22-8.

4. **Describe the initiation and conduction sequence of electrical impulses through the heart; identify the autonomic innervation and its effects on the heart.**
   Review pages 557-560; refer to Figures 22-9 through 22-11 and Table 22-2.

5. **Identify the structure and characteristics of myocardial cells.**
   Review pages 560-562; refer to Figures 22-12 through 22-14.

6. **Describe myocardial contraction and relaxation in relation to the calcium-troponin-tropomyosin complex.**
   Review pages 562 and 563; refer to Figure 22-15.

7. **Use the Frank-Starling law and Laplace law to demonstrate interrelationships that affect cardiac function; indicate the influence of output, preload, afterload, and myocardial contractility.**
   Review pages 563 and 564; refer to Figures 22-16 and 22-17 and Table 22-3.

8. **Describe the determinants of heart rate.**
   Review page 565, refer to Figure 22-18.

9. **Contrast the structure and function of arteries, capillaries, and veins within the systemic circulation.**
   Review pages 567, 569, and 570; refer to Figures 22-19 through 22-25 and Table 22-4.

10. **Describe the determinants of blood flow.**
    Review pages 570, 572, and 573; refer to Figures 22-26 through 22-29.

11. **Identify the factors that regulate arterial and venous blood pressure.**
    Review pages 573, 574, 576, and 578; refer to Figures 22-30 through 22-34.

12. **Describe the autoregulation of coronary circulation.**
    Review pages 578 and 579.

13. **Describe the normal structure and function of the lymphatic system.**
    Review pages 579 and 580; refer to Figures 22-35 through 22-37.

13. **Describe cardiovascular function in the elderly.**
    Review Table 22-3.

PRACTICE EXAMINATION

Multiple Choice

Circle the correct answer for each question:

1. Oxygenated blood flows through the:
   a. superior vena cava.
   b. pulmonary veins.
   c. pulmonary arteries.
   d. coronary veins.
   e. None of the above is correct.

2. The hepatic vein carries blood from the:
   a. vena cava to the liver.
   b. liver to the vena cava.
   c. aorta to the liver.
   d. liver to the aorta.

3. The position of the heart in the mediastinum is:
   a. inferior to the diaphragm and between the lungs.
   b. between the lungs and superior to the diaphragm.
   c. posterior to the trachea and anterior to the esophagus.
   d. posterior to the lungs and anterior to the diaphragm.

4. The pericardial space is found between the:
   a. myocardium and parietal pericardium.
   b. endocardium and visceral pericardium.
   c. visceral pericardium and parietal pericardium.
   d. visceral pericardium and epicardial pericardium.

5. In the normal cardiac cycle, which of the following occurs? (More than one answer may be correct.)
   a. The right atrium and right ventricles contract simultaneously.
   b. The two atria contract simultaneously, whereas the two ventricles relax.
   c. The two ventricles contract simultaneously, whereas the two atria relax.
   d. Both the ventricles and atria contract simultaneously to increase cardiac output.

6. The QRS complex of the ECG represents:
   a. atrial depolarization.
   b. ventricular depolarization.
   c. atrial contraction.
   d. ventricular repolarization.
   e. atrial repolarization.

7. A person having a heart rate of 100 bpm, a systolic blood pressure of 200 mm Hg, and a stroke volume of 40 mL would have an average cardiac output of:
   a. 0.5 mL/min.
   b. 5 L/min.
   c. 4 mL/min.
   d. 8000 mL/min.
   e. None of the above is correct.

8. During atrial systole, the:
   a. atrioventricular valves are open.
   b. atria are filling.
   c. ventricles are emptying.
   d. semilunar valves are open.

9. Which do(es) not significantly affect heart rate?
   a. sympathetic nerves
   b. parasympathetic nerves
   c. atrioventricular valves
   d. acetylcholine

10. One cardiac cycle:
    a. has a duration that changes if the heart rate changes.
    b. usually requires less than 1 second to complete.
    c. is equal to stroke volume × heart rate.
    d. pumps approximately 5 liters of blood.
    e. Both a and b are correct.

11. Compared with arteries, veins:
    a. have a larger diameter.
    b. are thick-coated.
    c. recoil quickly after distension.
    d. Both a and b are correct.

12. Normal systolic pressure within the left ventricle is in the range of:
    a. 90 to 140 mm Hg.
    b. 15 to 30 mm Hg.
    c. 0 to 10 mm Hg.
    d. None of the above is correct.

13. Backflow of blood from the arteries into the relaxing ventricles is prevented by the:
    a. venous valves.
    b. pericardial fluid.
    c. semilunar valves.
    d. atrioventricular valves.

14. Adrenomedullin (ADM):
    a. exhibits powerful vasoconstriction activity.
    b. is present only in cardiovascular tissue.
    c. mediates sodium reabsorption.
    d. exhibits powerful vasodilatory activity.

15. The Frank-Starling law of the heart concerns the relationship between:
    a. the length of the cardiac muscle fiber and the strength of contraction.
    b. stroke volume and arterial resistance.
    c. the rapidity of nerve conduction and stroke volume.
    d. systolic rate and cardiac output.

16. Cardiac muscle differs from skeletal muscle in that cardiac muscle is: (More than one answer may be correct.)
    a. arranged in parallel units.
    b. arranged in branching networks.
    c. multinucleated.
    d. singly nucleated.
    e. more accessible to sodium and potassium ions.

17. Blood pressure is measured as the:
    a. pressure exerted on the ventricular walls during systole.
    b. pressure exerted by the blood on the wall of any blood vessel.
    c. pressure exerted on arteries by the blood.
    d. product of the stroke volume times heart rate.

18. Identify the correct sequence of the portions of the pulmonary circulation.

a. 1, 5, 3, 2, 4	(1) pulmonary veins
b. 4, 2, 3, 1, 5	(2) pulmonary arteries
c. 4, 1, 3, 2, 5	(3) lungs
d. 5, 2, 3, 1, 4	(4) right ventricle
e. 5, 1, 3, 2, 4	(5) left atrium

19. The normal heartbeat is initiated by the:
    a. coronary sinus.
    b. atrioventricular bundle.
    c. right ventricle.
    d. SA node.
    e. AV node.

20. If the sympathetic nervous system stimulation of the heart predominates over parasympathetic nervous system stimulation, the heart will:
    a. increase its rate.
    b. contract with greater force and at a slower rate.
    c. decrease its rate and force of contraction.
    d. contract with less force and at a higher rate.

21. When blood exhibits a turbulent flow:
    a. resistance increases.
    b. greater blood viscosity is present.
    c. the fluids have greater velocity than with laminar flow.
    d. hydrostatic pressure is greater than when the fluids demonstrate laminar flow.

22. Identify the normal sequence of an electrical impulse through the heart's conduction system.

a. 4, 1, 2, 5, 3	(1) atrioventricular bundle
b. 4, 2, 5, 1, 3	(2) AV node
c. 2, 4, 1, 5, 3	(3) Purkinje fibers
d. 4, 2, 1, 5, 3	(4) SA node
	(5) right and left bundle branches

23. Which factor might increase resistance to the flow of blood through the blood vessels?
    a. an increased inner radius of diameter of blood vessels
    b. decreased numbers of capillaries
    c. decreased blood viscosity
    d. decreased numbers of red blood cells

24. Depolarization of cardiac muscle cells occurs because of:
    a. the cell's interior becoming more negatively charged.
    b. the cell's interior becoming less negatively charged.
    c. impermeability of the cell membrane to sodium.
    d. impermeability of the cell membrane to potassium.

25. Which of the following statements is true?
    a. Lymphatic walls consist of multiple layers of flattened endothelial cells.
    b. Lymph from the entire body, except for the upper right quadrant, eventually drains into the thoracic duct.
    c. The thoracic duct has approximately the same diameter as the great veins.
    d. Lymph contains more proteins than does blood plasma.
    e. The lymphatic system, like the circulatory system, is a closed circuit.

Fill in the Blank

Complete the following table describing cardiovascular function in the elderly:

Cardiovascular Function in the Elderly

Determinant	Resting Performance	Exercise Performance
Heart rate		
Cardiac output		
Contraction		

23 Alterations of Cardiovascular Function

FOUNDATIONAL OBJECTIVES

a. Describe blood flow through the heart.
Refer to Figures 22-5, 22-7, and 22-8.

MEMORY CHECK!

- The pumping action of the heart consists of contraction and relaxation of the myocardial layer of the heart wall. During relaxation, termed *diastole,* blood fills the chambers. The contraction that follows, termed *systole,* forces the blood from the chamber into the pulmonary, or systemic, circulation. During diastole, blood from the veins of the systemic circulation enters the thin-walled *right atrium* from the *superior vena cava* and *the inferior vena cava.* Venous blood from the *coronary circulation* enters the right *atrium* through the *coronary sinus.* The right atrium fills, and its fluid pressure pushes open the right atrioventricular (AV), or *tricuspid valve,* to fill the *right ventricle.* Flow and contraction occur a fraction of a second earlier in the left heart. Unoxygenated blood leaves the right ventricle via the *pulmonary semilunar valve* into the *pulmonary artery* to deliver the blood to the lungs, where it is oxygenated. The four *pulmonary veins,* two from the right lung and two from the left lung, carry oxygenated blood from the pulmonary circulation to the *left atrium.* As the left atrium fills, its fluid pressure pushes the cusps of the *mitral valve* open, and blood flows into the *left ventricle.* From the left ventricle, blood flows via the *aortic semilunar valve* into the *aorta* for systemic circulation. Blood circulates from the left ventricle and returns to the right atrium because of a progressive fall in pressure from the left ventricle to the right atrium of approximately 120 mm Hg. Blood always flows from a higher-pressure area toward a lower-pressure area.
- The blood within the heart chambers does not supply oxygen and other nutrients to the cells of the heart. Like all other organs, heart structures are nourished by vessels of the systemic circulation. *The coronary circulation consists of coronary arteries and cardiac veins.* The right and left coronary arteries traverse the epicardium and branch several times. The left coronary artery divides into two branches, the left anterior descending artery and the circumflex artery. The *left anterior descending artery* delivers blood to portions of the left and right ventricles and much of the interventricular septum. The *circumflex artery* supplies blood to the left atrium and the lateral wall of the left ventricle, and it often branches to the posterior surfaces of the left atrium and left ventricle. Three major branches of the *right coronary artery* supply blood to the right atrium, and upper right ventricle.
- Collateral arteries are connections, or anastomoses, between two branches of the same coronary artery or connections of branches of the right coronary artery with branches of the left. They are particularly common within the interventricular and interatrial septa, at the apex of the heart, over the anterior surface of the right ventricle, and around the sinus node. The heart has an extensive capillary network with *about one capillary per muscle cell.* Blood travels from the arteries to the arterioles, then into the capillaries, where exchange of oxygen and other nutrients takes place.
- Blood from the coronary arteries drains into the cardiac veins, which travel alongside the arteries. The cardiac veins feed into the great cardiac vein and then into the coronary sinus located between the atria and ventricles. The coronary sinus empties into the right atrium.

b. Describe the conduction system of the heart.
Review pages 557-560; refer to Figures 22-10 and 22-11.

MEMORY CHECK!

- Continuous, rhythmic repetition of the cardiac cycle, or systole and diastole, depends on the continuous, rhythmic transmission of electrical impulses. As an electrical impulse passes from cell to cell in the myocardium, muscular contraction or systole occurs. After the action potential passes, the fibers relax and return to their resting length; this relaxation is diastole.
- The myocardium differs from other muscle tissues; it contains its *own intrinsic conduction system.* It can generate and transmit action potentials without stimulation from the nervous system. These cells are concentrated at certain sites in the myocardium called nodes. Although the heart is innervated by both sympathetic and parasympathetic fibers, neural impulses are not needed to maintain the cardiac cycle.
- Normally, electrical impulses arise in the *sinoatrial (SA) node,* often called the pacemaker of the heart. Numerous autonomic nerve endings within the node enable it to respond to the nervous system. In the resting adult, the SA node generates about 75 action potentials per minute. Each action potential travels rapidly from cell to cell and through special pathways in the atrial myocardium, causing both atria to contract. Atrial contraction initiates systole. Transmission of the action potential from the atrial to the ventricular myocardium occurs through muscle fibers of the conduction system. The action potential travels first to the *AV node,* then to the *AV bundle,* then to the *common bundle,* and finally through the *bundle branches* of the interventricular septum to *Purkinje fibers* in the heart wall.
- *The extensive network of Purkinje fibers enables the rapid spread of the impulse to the ventricular apices.*
- Electrical activation of the muscle cells, or *depolarization*, is caused by the movement of electrically charged solutes, primarily sodium and potassium, across cardiac cell membranes. Deactivation, or *repolarization,* occurs by ion movement in the opposite direction. Movement of ions into and out of the cell creates an electrical or voltage difference across the cell membrane. This difference or potential of charged ions causes the impulse to flow within cells and from cell to cell.
- *Sympathetic* neural *stimulation* of the myocardium and coronary vessels depends on the presence of *adrenergic receptors* that are able to bind specifically with neurotransmitters of the sympathetic nervous system. Binding of *norepinephrine* to receptors *increases* the rate of impulse generation and conduction and also the *strength of myocardial contraction* during systole. Also, coronary arterioles dilate to supply the heart with more oxygen and nutrients. These effects enable the heart to pump more blood. *Parasympathetic* or vagus nerve activity *decreases the heart rate*. The vagus nerve releases *acetylcholine*.

c. Describe the interrelationships among myocardial stretch and chamber wall dimensions and the contractible force of the heart.
Review pages 563-564; refer to Figures 22-16 and 22-17.

MEMORY CHECK!

- Cardiac muscle, like other muscle, increases its strength of contraction within certain limits when it is stretched. The Frank-Starling law of the heart states that there is a direct relationship between the volume of blood in the heart and stretch or length of cardiac fibers at the end of diastole and the force of contraction during the next systole. *The greater the stretch from preload blood volume, the stronger the contraction.*
- Laplace law describes the relationships among wall thickness, pressure, and wall tension. Wall tension is related directly to the product of intraventricular pressure and internal radius and inversely to the wall thickness. Stated another way, the pressure or contractible force is directly related to wall thickness and wall tension and indirectly related to the radius. *The thicker the wall and greater the wall tension and smaller the radius, the greater the force of contraction.*

d. Establish the determinants of blood flow.
Review pages 570, 572, and 573; refer to Figures 22-26 through 22-29.

MEMORY CHECK!

- Blood flow is determined primarily by two factors: pressure and resistance. Pressure in a liquid system is the force exerted on the liquid per unit area. Fluid moves from the arterial "side" of the capillaries, which is a region of greater pressure, to the venous side, which is a region of lesser pressure. Resistance opposes force. In the cardiovascular system, most opposition to blood flow occurs because of the diameter and length of the blood vessels themselves.
- The relationship between blood flow, pressure, and resistance can be stated as blood *flow equals pressure difference divided by resistance,* or *Q equals P divided by R.*
- Resistance to fluid flow considers the length of the tube or vessel, the viscosity of the fluid, and the radius of the lumen. According to the Poiseuille formula, *resistance equals viscosity of blood times length of vessel divided by the fourth power of the lumen's radius.*
- Because the Poiseuille equation was derived using straight, rigid tubes with steady, streamlined flow, it cannot be applied exactly to the vascular system. Nevertheless, it is a useful model for vascular resistance assessment. *Small changes in the lumen's radius lead to large changes in vascular resistance.* Because vessel length is relatively constant, length is not as important as lumen size in determining flow through a single vessel. However, blood flowing through the distributing arteries encounters more resistance than blood flowing through the capillary bed. In the capillary bed, flow is distributed among many short, tiny branches.
- If the definition of resistance (viscosity times length divided by the fourth power of radius) is substituted into the formula "Q equals P divided by R," a helpful summary of likely factors affecting blood flow rate can be expressed. Now, blood flow equals pressure times radius to the fourth power divided by the viscosity times the length. *The higher the pressure and greater the vessel radius and lesser the viscosity of blood and length of vessel, the greater the flow of blood.*

e. Establish the determinants of blood pressure.
Review pages 573-574, 576, and 578; refer to Figures 22-30 through 22-34.

MEMORY CHECK!

- The mean arterial pressure, which is the average pressure in the arteries throughout the cardiac cycle, depends on the elastic properties of the arterial walls and the mean volume of blood in the arterial system. The main determinants of venous blood pressure are the volume of fluid within the veins and the compliance or distensibility of their vessel walls. The venous system accommodates approximately 60% of the total blood volume at any given moment with a *venous pressure averaging less than 10 mm Hg.* Conversely, the *arteries* accommodate about 15% of the total blood volume with a pressure of *about 100 mm Hg.* Some important relationships are as follows:
  - Mean blood pressure equals cardiac output times peripheral resistance.
  - Cardiac output equals heart rate times stroke volume.
  - Peripheral resistance equals blood viscosity times vessel length divided by vessel radius raised to the fourth power.
  - Blood pressure equals heart rate times stroke volume times viscosity times length divided by the radius to the fourth power. *The higher the heart rate, stroke volume, blood viscosity, and vessel length and the less the vessel radius to the fourth power, the greater the blood pressure.*

LEARNING OBJECTIVES

After studying this chapter, the learner will be able to do the following:

1. Describe venous occlusive diseases.
Study pages 585-587; refer to Figures 23-1 and 23-2.

A **varicose vein** is a vein in which blood has *pooled.* Varicose veins are distended, tortuous, and palpable. Varicose veins in the legs are caused by trauma to the saphenous veins that damages one or more valves or by venous distention from a combination of standing for long periods and the action of gravity on blood within the legs. If a valve is damaged and permits backflow, a section of the vein is subjected to the pressure exerted by a larger volume of blood under the influence of gravity. The *vein swells* as it becomes engorged, and *surrounding tissue becomes edematous* because increased hydrostatic pressure pushes plasma through the stretched vessel wall.

Varicose veins and valvular incompetence can progress to **chronic venous insufficiency (CVI)**. This condition is characterized by chronic pooling of blood in the veins of the lower extremities and leads to *hyperpigmentation* of the skin over the feet and ankles. Edema of the feet and ankles may progress proximally to the knees.

Any trauma or pressure lowers the oxygen supply by further reducing blood flow into the area. Cell death occurs and necrotic tissue evolves into **venous stasis ulcers.** Persistent ulceration develops because the existing compromised circulation cannot meet the high metabolic demands of healing tissue.

Treatment of varicose veins and CVI begins conservative. Wound healing results following noninvasive treatments, such as leg elevation, compressive stockings, and physical therapy. Invasive management consists of sclerotherapy or surgical ligation, vein resection, and vein stripping.

Venous thrombi are more common than arterial thrombi because flow and pressure are lower in the veins than in the arteries. With aging, the deep veins in the lower extremities become especially susceptible to thrombus formation. This development is notable in individuals who experience long-term bed rest or who wear constrictive clothing. Genetic abnormalities increase the risk for venous thrombosis. Persons who have conditions that predispose them to blood flow stasis, endothelial injury, or hypercoagulability are at increased risk for **deep venous thrombosis (DVT).**

The inflammatory response triggered by the clotting cascade causes extreme tenderness, swelling, and redness in the area of thrombus formation. With venous occlusion, the skin is discolored rather than pale, edema is prominent, and pain is most marked at the site of occlusion. Treatment of varicose veins and chronic venous insufficiency begins conservatively with compression stockings and exercise. If conservative treatment is ineffective, saphenous vein stripping may be performed.

Superior vena cava syndrome (SVCS) is a progressive occlusion of the superior vena cava (SVC) that leads to *venous distention in the upper extremities and head.* The leading cause of SVCS is bronchogenic cancer, followed by lymphomas and metastasis of other cancers. The SVC is a relatively low-pressure vessel that lies in the closed thoracic compartment; therefore, tissue expansion within the thoracic compartment can easily compress the SVC.

Clinical manifestations of SVCS include edema and venous distention in the upper extremities and face, including the ocular beds. Cerebral and central nervous system edema may cause headache, visual disturbance, or impaired consciousness. Respiratory distress may be present because of edema of the bronchial structures or compression of the bronchus by a carcinoma.

SVCS is generally not a vascular emergency, but rather *an oncologic problem.* Treatment consists of radiotherapy for the neoplasm and the administration of diuretics, steroids, and anticoagulants.

2. Describe primary, secondary, complicated, and malignant hypertension.
Study pages 587-591; refer to Figures 23-3 through 23-5 and Tables 23-1 and 23-2.

Normal adult blood pressure prevails when the systolic pressure < 120 mm Hg and the diastolic pressure < 80 mm Hg. Adult hypertension begins when the systolic pressure exceeds 140 mm Hg and the diastolic pressure exceeds 90 mm Hg. Increasing pressures in both systolic and diastolic pressures categorize stages of hypertension (HTN): *prehypertension* exists when systolic pressure is 120 mm to 139 mm Hg and diastolic pressure is 80 mm to 89 mm Hg; *stage 1 HTN* exists when systolic pressure is 140 mm to 159 mm Hg and diastolic pressure is 90 mm to 99 mm Hg; and *stage 2 HTN* is present when systolic pressure ≥ 160 mm Hg and diastolic pressure ≥ 100 mm Hg.

HTN is caused by increases in cardiac output, total peripheral resistance, or both. Cardiac output is increased by any condition that increases heart rate or stroke volume, whereas peripheral resistance is increased by any factor that increases blood viscosity or reduces vessel diameter.

Isolated systolic hypertension (ISH) is defined as systolic pressure ≥140 mm Hg and diastolic pressure < 90 mm Hg. ISH is substantial in all age groups and is strongly associated with cardiovascular and cerebrovascular events. An increased pulse pressure (the *difference between systolic and diastolic pressures,* normally 30 mm to 40 mm Hg) indicates reduced vascular compliance of the large arteries and is always present in ISH. Rigidity of the aorta is the chief vascular cause of ISH

Primary HTN *affects 92% to 95% of hypertensive individuals.* The exact cause of primary HTN is *unknown,* although several factors are proposed, including: (1) a family history of HTN, (2) advancing age, (3) gender (men younger than women), (4) black race, (5) high sodium intake, (6) glucose intolerance, (7) cigarette smoking, (8) obesity, 9) heavy alcohol consumption, and (10) low dietary intake of potassium, calcium, and magnesium. Multiple pathophysiologic mechanisms mediate primary HTN, including the SNS, the renin-angiotensin-aldosterone system, and the natriuretic peptides. Inflammation, endothelial dysfunction, obesity-related hormones, and insulin resistance also increase peripheral resistance and blood volume and decrease renal excretion of salt into the urine.

Secondary HTN is caused by any systemic disease process that *raises peripheral vascular resistance or cardiac output*. Causes include renal disease, adrenal disorders, vascular disease, and drugs (corticosteroids, oral contraceptives, and antihistamines). Fortunately, if the cause is identified and removed before permanent structural changes occur, blood pressure can return to normal.

Complicated HTN is *sustained primary HTN that has pathologic effects in addition to causing hemodynamic alterations and fluid and electrolyte imbalances.* Complicated HTN compromises the structure and function of vessels, the heart, kidneys, eyes, and the brain. Cardiovascular complications include left ventricular hypertrophy, angina pectoris, congestive heart failure or left side heart failure, coronary artery disease, myocardial infarction, and sudden death.

Malignant HTN is a rapidly progressive HTN in which *diastolic pressure usually exceeds 140 mm Hg.* It can cause profound cerebral edema, which disrupts cerebral function and causes loss of consciousness. High hydrostatic pressures in the capillaries cause vascular fluid to move into the interstitial space. If blood pressure is not reduced, cerebral edema and dysfunction increase until death occurs.

Generally, the early stages of HTN have no specific clinical manifestations; thus, HTN is called a *"silent disease."* Consequently, some HTN individuals never have signs, symptoms, or complications; others become very ill and their HTN can cause death. Anatomic and physiologic damage could have been caused by past hypertensive disease even if current blood pressure is within normal ranges. *Most of the clinical manifestations of hypertensive disease are caused by complications that damage organs and tissues other than the vascular system.* Besides elevated blood pressure, the signs and symptoms are specific for the organs or tissues affected. Heart disease, renal insufficiency, central nervous system dysfunction, impaired vision, impaired mobility, vascular occlusion, or edema can be caused by sustained HTN.

HTN is usually managed with both pharmacologic and nonpharmacologic methods. Treatment begins with reducing or eliminating risk factors. The usual recommendations are to restrict sodium intake, increase physical training, and discontinue cigarette smoking.

Groups of drugs are used to manage HTN: thiazide diuretics, angiotensin-converting enzyme inhibitors, angiotensin receptor blockers, calcium channel blockers, and adrenergic blockers. Diuretics and beta-blockers are initially used because they reduce morbidity and mortality. If the response is inadequate, other agents are added.

3. Define and identify the causes of orthostatic or postural hypotension.
Study page 591.

Orthostatic or **postural hypotension** is a *drop in both systolic and diastolic arterial blood pressure upon standing from a reclining position.* The normal or compensatory vasoconstrictor response to standing is replaced by a marked vasodilation and blood pooling in the muscle vasculature and in the splanchnic and renal beds. Acute orthostatic hypotension may be the result of: (1) anatomic variation, (2) altered body chemistry, (3) antihypertensive and antidepressant therapy, (4) prolonged immobility caused by illness, (5) starvation, (6) physical exhaustion, (7) fluid volume depletion (dehydration), and (8) venous pooling.

Chronic orthostatic hypotension may be secondary to a specific disease. The diseases that may cause secondary orthostatic hypotension are adrenal insufficiency, diabetes mellitus, intracranial tumors, cerebral infarcts, and peripheral neuropathies.

Orthostatic hypotension is often accompanied by dizziness, blurring or loss of vision, or syncope or fainting caused by insufficient vasomotor compensation and reduced brain blood flow. No curative treatment is available; however, increased fluid and salt intake, thigh-high stockings, mineralocorticoids, and vasoconstrictors can manage the symptoms.

4. Define aneurysm and list the types.
Study pages 591-592; refer to Figures 23-5 and 23-6.

An **aneurysm** is a localized dilation or outpouching of a vessel wall or cardiac chamber. The tension on the wall increases as the vessel becomes thinner, *so the possibility of rupture increases.* This is an example of the law of Laplace. The stretching produces infarct expansion, a weak and thin layer of necrotic muscle, and fibrous tissue that bulges with each systole. With time, the aneurysm can leak, cause pressure on surrounding organs, impair blood flow, or rupture.

The aorta is particularly susceptible to aneurysm formation because of the constant stress on its vessel wall and the absence of penetrating vasa vasorum in its adventitial layer. Three fourths of all aneurysms occur in the abdominal aorta.

True aneurysms are fusiform and circumferential in nature and involve all three layers of the arterial wall; there is weakening of the vessel wall. **False aneurysms or saccular aneurysms** are usually the result of trauma. These aneurysms are caused by a break in the wall or a dissection of the layers of the arterial wall; blood is contained at the point of aneurysm by the adventitial layer.

Treatment of aneurysms is nearly always surgical. Leaking cerebral aneurysms are treated with clot-stabilizing drugs and a number of clinical measures designed to reduce intracranial pressure and promote hemodynamic stability before surgical intervention.

5. Distinguish between a thrombus and an embolus.
Study pages 592-593; refer to Table 23-3.

A **thrombus** is a blood clot that *remains attached to a vessel wall.* Thrombi tend to develop wherever intravascular conditions promote activation of the coagulation cascade or there is stasis of blood flow.

In the arteries, *activation of the coagulation cascade* is usually caused by roughening of the tunica intima by atherosclerosis. Infectious agents also roughen the normally smooth lining of the artery, which causes platelets to adhere readily. Pooling of arterial blood within an aneurysm can stimulate thrombus formation. In the veins, thrombus formation is more often associated with *inflammation.* Thrombi also form on heart valves if there is inflammation of the endocardium or rheumatic heart disease.

A thrombus poses two threats to the circulation. *First,* the thrombus may be large enough to occlude the artery and cause ischemia in the tissue supplied by the artery. *Second,* the thrombus may become dislodged and may travel through the vascular system until it occludes flow into a distal systemic or pulmonic vascular bed.

Diagnosis is made with Doppler ultrasonography and angiography. Pharmacologic treatment includes the administration of heparin, warfarin, and streptokinase. A balloon-tipped catheter can be used to remove or compress a thrombus.

Embolism is the obstruction of a vessel by an **embolus,** or a bolus of matter that *circulates* in the bloodstream. The embolus may be a dislodged thrombus, an air bubble, or an aggregate of fat, bacteria, or cancer cells. An embolus travels in the bloodstream until it reaches a vessel through which it cannot pass; an embolus eventually lodges in a systemic or pulmonary vessel. *Pulmonary emboli* originate mostly from the *deep veins of the legs* or in the *right heart. Systemic emboli* most commonly originate in the *left heart* and are associated with thrombi after myocardial infarction, valvular disease, left heart failure, endocarditis, and dysrhythmias.

Embolism of a coronary or cerebral artery is an immediate threat to life if the embolus severely obstructs these important vessels. Occlusion of a coronary artery causes myocardial infarction, whereas occlusion of a cerebral artery causes a stroke, or cerebral vascular accident (CVA).

6. Describe arterial occlusive disease.
Study pages 593-594.

Thromboangiitis obliterans, or **Buerger disease,** tends to occur in young men who are heavy cigarette smokers. It is an inflammatory disease of the *peripheral arteries.* Inflammation, thrombus formation, and vasospasm can eventually occlude and obliterate portions of small- and medium-sized arteries in the feet and sometimes in the hands. The pathogenesis of the disease is unknown.

The chief symptom of thromboangiitis obliterans is pain and tenderness of the affected part. Clinical manifestations are caused by sluggish blood flow and include rubor, caused by dilated capillaries under the skin, and cyanosis, caused by blood that remains in the capillaries after its oxygen has diffused into the interstitium.

The most important part of treatment is cessation of cigarette smoking. Vasodilators may alleviate vasospasm. If vasospasm persists, sympathectomy may be performed, and gangrene necessitates amputation.

Raynaud phenomenon and **Raynaud disease** are characterized by attacks of *vasospasm* in the small arteries and arterioles of the fingers and, less commonly, the toes. Raynaud phenomenon is secondary to systemic diseases such as collagen vascular disease, pulmonary hypertension, thoracic outlet syndrome, myxedema trauma, and serum sickness and to long-term exposure to environmental conditions, such as cold and vibrating machinery in the workplace. Raynaud disease is a primary vasospastic disorder of unknown origin tending to affect young women. It consists of vasospastic attacks triggered by brief exposure to cold or by emotional stress. Genetic predisposition may play a role in its development.

The vasospastic attacks of either disorder cause changes in skin color and sensation because of ischemia. Vasospasm occurs with varying frequency and severity and causes pallor, numbness, and the sensation of cold in the digits. Also, sluggish blood flow resulting from ischemia may cause the skin to appear cyanotic. Rubor follows as vasospasm ends and the capillaries become engorged with oxygenated blood.

Treatment for Raynaud phenomenon consists of removing the stimulus or treating the primary disease process. Treatment of Raynaud disease is limited to prevention or alleviation of vasospasm itself. Exposure to cold temperatures, emotional stress, and cigarette smoking are avoided. Exercises that build centrifugal force in the extremities are also helpful in the early stages of vasospasm for either entity.

7. Describe the development of atheromatous plaque and its manifestations. (See atherogenesis flow chart on next page.)
Study pages 594-595 and 597; refer to Figures 23-7 through 23-10.

Atherosclerosis is the common form of arteriosclerosis (arterial hardening) in which the *thickening* of vessel walls is caused by hardening *of soft deposits of intra-arterial fat and fibrin that reduce lumen size.* Atherosclerosis can take several forms, depending on the anatomic location of the affected vessel, the individual's age and genetic and physiologic status, and the risk factors to which the individual may have been exposed. It is the leading contributor to coronary artery and cerebrovascular disease.

8. Describe peripheral artery disease.
Study page 597.

Peripheral artery disease (PAD) refers to atherosclerotic disease of arteries perfusing the limbs, particularly the lower legs. It is prevalent in individuals with diabetes. In most individuals, atherosclerotic obstruction results in pain during ambulation, which is called *intermittent claudication.* When a thrombus overlies the lesion, acute blood flow obstruction can be acute, with severe pain, pulse loss, and altered skin color.

Atherosclerosis

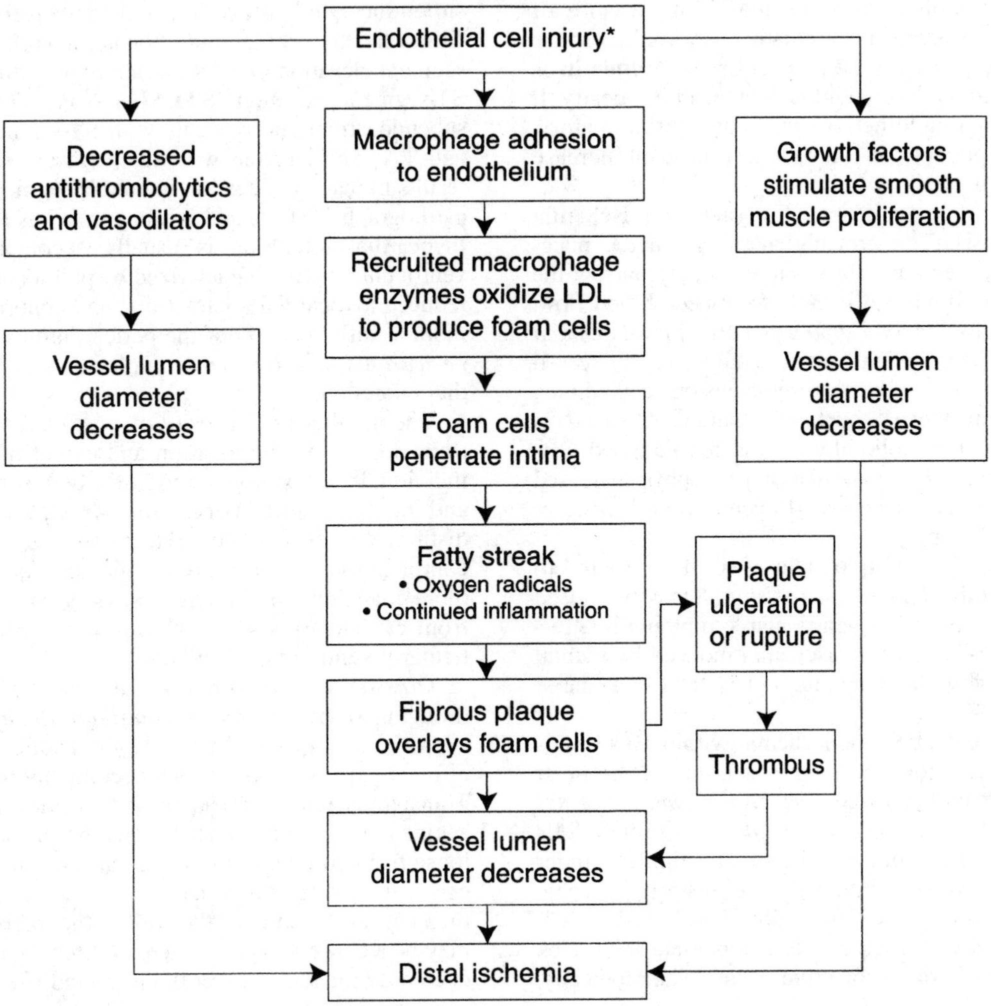

*There is increasing evidence that inflammation and infection may be causes of endotheliel injury.

9. **Characterize coronary artery disease (CAD); distinguish between myocardial ischemia and myocardial infarction, and list complications of each.**
Study pages 597-607 and 609; refer to Figures 23-10 through 23-25 and Tables 23-4 and 23-5. (See the table on page 164 comparing myocardial ischemia with myocardial infarction and the flow chart illustrating the consequences of each on page 165.)

CAD, myocardial ischemia, and **myocardial infarction** all impair the pumping ability of the heart by *depriving the heart muscle of oxygen and nutrients.* CAD diminishes the myocardial blood supply until deprivation impairs myocardial metabolism. The myocardial cells remain alive, but they are unable to function normally. Persistent ischemia or the complete occlusion of a coronary artery causes infarction or death of the deprived myocardial cells and tissues.

In the United States, CAD is the single largest killer of individuals. The risk factors for CAD are classified as either *modifiable or nonmodifiable.* The nonmodifiable risk factors for CAD are variables that cannot be altered by people who wish to decrease their risk of cardiovascular disease. These include advanced age, being male, being a postmenopausal female, and family history. The modifiable risk factors include *dyslipidemia, hyperhomocysteinemia,* HTN, cigarette smoking, diabetes and insulin resistance, obesity, sedentary lifestyle, and atherogenic diet. *High levels* of low-density lipoprotein (LDL) cholesterol and lipoprotein(a) [Lp(a)], which are genetically determined, and *low levels* of high-density lipoprotein (HDL) cholesterol have been shown to be high-risk factors for CAD. *High levels of HDL cholesterol* may be more protective for the development of atherosclerosis than low levels of LDL cholesterol. The postmenopausal state is characterized by an increase in LDL and total cholesterol. Newly identified risk factors for atherogenesis and CAD include high levels of fibrinogen, serum amyloid, *C-reactive protein,* uric acid, and infectious agents, notably, *Chlamydia pneumoniae* and *Helicobacter pylori*. C-reactive protein is an acute-phase reactant that is a measure of atherosclerosis-related inflammation. Adipokines are hormones released from adipose cells. **Adiponectin** is normally *antiatherogenic* and is decreased in obesity. It protects vascular endothelium and is anti-inflammatory. Decreased adiponectin is linked to a significant increase in cardiovascular risk.

The most common cause of **myocardial ischemia** is atherosclerosis. The growing mass of plaque, platelets, fibrin, and cellular debris can eventually narrow the coronary artery lumen sufficiently to impede blood flow. *Imbalances between blood supply and myocardial demand* cause myocardial ischemia. Supply is reduced by increased resistance in coronary vessels, hypotension, arrhythmia, valvular incompetence, shock, or anemia. Demand is increased by high systolic blood pressure, increased ventricular volume, left ventricular hypertrophy, increased heart rate, and valvular disease. Ischemia occurs whether demand exceeds supply.

Ischemia can be asymptomatic; if so, it is referred to as **silent ischemia.** The absence of angina may be caused by an abnormality in left ventricular symptomatic afferent innervation. Myocardial ischemia induced by mental stress can exist without angina and is thus considered silent.

Myocardial cells become ischemic within 10 seconds of coronary occlusion. After several minutes, the heart cells lose their ability to contract. *Anaerobic processes* take over, and *lactic acid accumulates*. Cardiac cells remain viable for approximately 20 minutes under ischemic conditions. If blood flow is restored, aerobic metabolism resumes, and contractility is restored.

If the coronary arteries cannot compensate for a lack of oxygen, **myocardial infarction** occurs. Pathologically, there are two major types of myocardial infarction: **subendocardial infarction** and **transmural infarction.** Clinically, myocardial infarction is categorized as non–ST-segment elevation myocardial infarction **(non-STEMI)** or ST-segment elevation **(STEMI).** Non-STEMI is usually subendocardial and presents with ST-segment depression and T wave inversion without Q waves. *Transmural MI* results in marked elevation in the ST segments on electrocardiography (ECG) and is categorized as STEMI. Acute myocardial infarction is usually accompanied by left ventricular failure characterized by pulmonary congestion, reduced myocardial contractility, and abnormal heart wall motion. Inflammation of the pericardium, which is called *pericarditis*, is a frequent complication of acute myocardial infarction.

The number and severity of *postinfarction complications* depend on the location and extent of necrosis, the individual's physiologic condition before the infarction, and the therapeutic intervention. *Arrhythmias*, which are disturbances of cardiac rhythm, are the most common complication of acute myocardial infarction and affect more than 90% of individuals. Sudden death resulting from cardiac arrest is often caused by arrhythmias, particularly ventricular fibrillation.

Dressler's postinfarction pericarditis syndrome is thought to be an *antigen-antibody response to the necrotic myocardium*. Pain, fever, friction rub, pleural effusion, and arthralgias may accompany this syndrome. Transient ischemic attacks or an outright cerebrovascular accident may result from thromboemboli that have broken loose from coronary arteries or cardiac valves to occlude cerebral vessels. Pulmonary emboli are especially common causes. Rupture of the wall of the infarcted ventricle may be a consequence of aneurysm formation because of decreased muscle mass at the infarcted site.

Myocardial Ischemia/Infarction

		Acute Coronary Syndromes (Thrombus Formation)	
Stable Angina	**Prinzmetal Angina**	**Unstable Angina**	**Infarction**
Cause			
Temporary ischemia, exertion; vessels cannot dilate in response to increased demand	Vasospasm, with or without atherosclerosis; occurs at night and at rest	Advanced reversible ischemia; occurs at rest	Prolonged and irreversible ischemia, cellular necrosis with repair or scarring
Electrocardiographic Findings			
Normal, possible transient ST-segment depression and T wave inversion	Transient ST-segment elevation	Transient ST-segment depression and T wave inversion	Elevated ST segments; later, pronounced Q waves
Plasma Enzyme Levels			
Normal	Normal	Normal	Elevations of CPK-MB fraction, LDH, SGOT, and troponins I and T indicate severity

Myocardial Ischemia/Infarction—Cont'd

Stable Angina	Prinzmetal Angina	Acute Coronary Syndromes (Thrombus Formation) Unstable Angina	Acute Coronary Syndromes (Thrombus Formation) Infarction
Pain Relief and Treatment*			
Rest and nitroglycerin, beta-blockers, calcium antagonists	Nitroglycerin, beta-blockers, calcium antagonists	Rest and nitroglycerin ineffective, beta-blockers, calcium antagonists, anticoagulant therapy	Narcotics, anti coagulant therapy (aspirin), thrombolytic agents, ACE inhibitors, beta-blockers, statins, surgery

*When medical therapy fails to relieve angina, percutaneous transluminal intervention (PTCI) or coronary artery bypass grafting (CABG) may be required.

Note: The first symptom of myocardial ischemia or infarction is usually sudden, severe chest pain. The pain of infarction is more severe and persistent than the pain of ischemia; it may be heavy and crushing and may radiate to neck, jaw, back, shoulder, or left arm. Exercise stress testing is useful in differentiating angina from other types of chest pain. Radioisotope imaging with thallium-201 is another diagnostic test to detect CAD. Single-photon emission computed tomography (SPECT) is able to identify ischemia and coronary risk.

Consequences/Complications of Myocardial Ischemia/Infarction

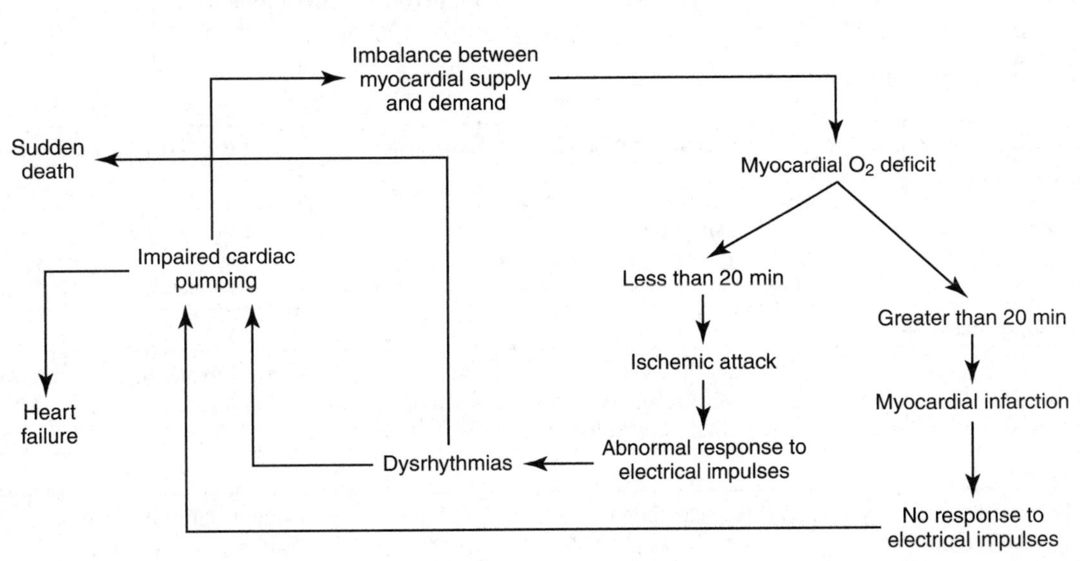

10. Characterize the terms associated with pericardial disease.
Study pages 609-611; refer to Figures 23-22 through 23-24.

Pericardial disease is often a localized manifestation of another disorder. Infection, trauma or surgery, neoplasms, or metabolic, immunologic, or vascular disorders can elicit a pericardial response. Pericarditis, pericardial effusion, and constrictive pericarditis are the consequences of the elicited response. **Acute pericarditis**, although idiopathic, is commonly caused by infection, connective tissue disease, or radiation therapy. It is also the most common cardiovascular complication of HIV infection.

Symptoms include sudden onset of severe chest pain that *worsens with respiratory movements.* Individuals with acute pericarditis also may report dysphagia, restlessness, irritability, anxiety, weakness, and malaise. Friction rub or a short, scratchy, grating sensation similar to the sound of sandpaper may be heard at the cardiac apex and left sternal border; this finding is pathognomonic for pericarditis. Treatment for uncomplicated acute pericarditis consists of relieving symptoms with anti-inflammatory agents.

Pericardial effusion is the accumulation of *fluid in the pericardial cavity* and is possible with all forms of pericarditis. The fluid may be a transudate or an exudate. Pericardial effusion indicates an underlying disorder. If the fluid creates *sufficient pressure to cause cardiac compression*, it becomes a serious condition known as **tamponade**. The danger of tamponade is that pressure exerted by the pericardial fluid eventually *equals diastolic pressure* within the heart chambers. The first structures to be affected by tamponade are the *right atrium and ventricle* because diastolic pressures are normally lowest therein. Subsequent decreased atrial filling leads to *decreased ventricular filling*, decreased stroke volume, and reduced cardiac output. Life-threatening circulatory collapse may develop.

The most significant clinical finding in tamponade is **pulsus paradoxus**. In this circumstance, arterial blood pressure during expiration exceeds arterial pressure during inspiration by more than 10 mm Hg. There is impairment of diastolic filling of the left ventricle, plus *reduction of blood volume within all cardiac chambers*.

Treatment of pericardial effusion or tamponade generally consists of aspiration of the excessive pericardial fluid. Persistent pain is treated with analgesics, anti-inflammatory agents, or steroids. Surgery may be required if the tamponade cause is trauma or aneurysm.

Constrictive pericarditis is either idiopathic or associated with radiation exposure, rheumatoid arthritis, uremia, or coronary artery bypass grafting. In constrictive pericarditis, fibrous scarring with occasional calcification of the pericardium causes the visceral and parietal pericardial layers to adhere; thus, the pericardial cavity is obliterated. Like tamponade, *constrictive pericarditis compresses* the heart and eventually reduces cardiac output. Unlike tamponade, however, constrictive pericarditis always develops gradually.

Symptoms are exercise intolerance, dyspnea on exertion, fatigue, anorexia, weight loss, edema, distention of the jugular vein, and hepatic congestion. Chest radiographs often show prominent pulmonary vessels and calcification of the pericardium.

Initial treatment for constrictive pericarditis involves digitalis glycosides, diuretics, and sodium restriction. Surgical removal of the pericardium may be indicated because its removal does not compromise cardiac function.

11. Compare the cardiomyopathies.

Study pages 611-612; refer to Figure 23-25 through 23-27.

The **cardiomyopathies** are a diverse group of diseases that primarily *affect the myocardium* itself and are not secondary to the usual cardiovascular disorders, such as CAD, hypertension, and valvular dysfunction. Cardiomyopathy may be secondary to infectious disease, exposure to toxins, systemic connective tissue disease, infiltrative and proliferative disorders, or nutritional deficiencies; most cases of cardiomyopathy are idiopathic.

Characteristics of Cardiomyopathies

Dilated Cardiomyopathy	Hypertrophic Cardiomyopathy	Restrictive Cardiomyopathy
Associated Conditions		
Alcoholism, pregnancy, infection, nutritional deficiency, toxin exposure	Possible inherited defect of muscle growth and development	Infiltrative disease
Structural Changes		
Globular shape, largest circumference of left ventricle is midway between base and apex	Thick left ventricular wall, left ventricular V chamber is small, dilated left atrium	Normal left ventricular chamber, dilated left atrium
Manifestations		
Eventual left heart failure, dyspnea, fatigue, pedal edema	Dyspnea, fatigue, dizziness, angina, syncope, palpitations, ventricular arrhythmias, eventual left heart failure,	Dyspnea, fatigue, eventual right heart failure

Valvular Stenosis and Regurgitation

Valvular Disorders	Causes	Manifestations
Aortic stenosis	Rheumatic heart disease, congenital malformation, calcification degeneration	Decreased stroke volume, left ventricular failure, dyspnea, angina, systolic murmur
Mitral stenosis	Acute rheumatic heart fever, bacterial endocarditis	Decreased stroke volume, right ventricular failure, chest pain, orthopnea, pulmonary hypertension, dysrhythmia, palpitations, induced thrombi, ascites, diastolic murmurs
Aortic regurgitation	Bacterial endocarditis, hypertension, connective disease disorders	Congestive left heart failure, dyspnea, throbbing peripheral pulse, palpitations, chest pain, diastolic and systolic murmurs

Valvular Stenosis and Regurgitation—Cont'd

Valvular Disorders	Causes	Manifestations
Mitral regurgitation	Rheumatic heart disease, mitral valve prolapse, CAD, infective endocarditis, connective tissue disorders	Left heart failure, pulmonary hypertension, dyspnea, hemoptysis, palpitations, murmur throughout systole
Tricuspid regurgitation	Congenital, high blood pressure in pulmonary circulation or right ventricle	Right heart failure, peripheral edema, ascites, hepatomegaly, murmur throughout systole
Mitral valve prolapse	Autosomal dominant pattern, hyperthyroidism related	Regurgitant murmur, fatigue and lethargy, greater risk for infective endocarditis

12. Identify the causes and manifestations of valvular dysfunction.
Study pages 612-616; refer to Figures 23-28 through 23-31 and Table 23-6. (See previous table on valvular stenosis disorders.)

In **valvular stenosis**, the valve orifice is constricted or narrowed. This narrowing impedes the forward flow of blood and increases the workload of the cardiac chamber *"in front" of or before the diseased valve*. Increased volume and pressure cause the myocardium to work harder, and myocardial hypertrophy develops.

In **valvular regurgitation**, known also as insufficiency or incompetence, the valve leaflets or cusps fail to close completely, permitting blood flow to continue even when the valve should be closed. During systole, some blood *leaks back into the atrial "upstream" chamber*. This condition increases the workload of *both atrium and ventricle*. Increased volume leads to chamber dilation; increased workload leads to hypertrophy. Although all four heart valves may be affected, those of the left heart are more commonly affected than those of the right heart.

13. Distinguish between rheumatic heart disease (RHD) and infective endocarditis.
Study pages 616-619; refer to Figures 23-32 through 23-34 and Table 23-7.

Rheumatic Heart Disease and Infective Endocarditis

Cause	Pathophysiology	Manifestations	Treatment
Rheumatic Heart Disease			
Sequel to pharyngeal infection with group A beta-hemolytic streptococci, immune response to streptococcal cell membrane antigens (M proteins)	Carditis of all three layers of heart wall, endocardial inflammation and vegetative growth on valves, valvular stenosis, Aschoff bodies	Fever, lymphadenopathy, acute migratory polyarthritis, chorea, erythema marginatum or truncal rash, history of streptococcal pharyngeal infection, high anti–streptolysin O titer, ECG abnormalities	10 days of oral penicillin or erythromycin, salicylates or nonsteroidal anti-inflammatory drugs, surgical repair of damaged valves for chronic disease; to prevent recurrence: continuous prophylactic antibiotic therapy for as long as 5 years
Infective Endocarditis			
Staphylococcus aureus followed by viridans streptococci, viruses, fungi, rickettsiae	Prior endothelial damage to valves leads to thrombotic endocarditis; blood-borne microbes colonize damaged valve; adhered microbes multiply and form endocardial vegetations	Fever, cardiac murmur, petechial lesions of skin and mucosa, bacteremia, Osler nodes, Janeway lesions	Long-term (4 to 6 weeks) antimicrobial therapy: penicillin and streptomycin; prophylactic antibiotics for procedures that increase the risk of transient bacteremia

14. Generalize dysrhythmias of the heart.
Study page 619; refer to Tables 23-8 and 23-9.

Dysrhythmias or *arrhythmias* can be caused by either an abnormal rate of impulse generation or an abnormal conduction of impulses. Dysrhythmias can impair the pumping of the heart and cause heart failure. One kind of dysrhythmia is a heart block. In AV node block, impulses are prevented from reaching the ventricular myocardium; the ventricles contract at a slower rate than normal.

Bradycardia is a *slow* heart rhythm, less than 60 beats per minute. Bradycardia can result from vagal hyperactivity, hyperkalemia, and digoxin toxicity. Pacemakers can assist in blocks and bradycardia if rhythmic medication is inadequate.

Tachycardia is a *rapid* heart rhythm of more than 100 beats per minute. Tachycardia results because of improper autonomic control mechanisms, heart disorders, lung disease, shock, and fever.

Sinus dysrhythmia is a *variation* in heart rate during breathing. The causes of sinus dysrhythmia are unknown. This phenomenon is common in young people and infrequently requires treatment.

Premature contractions or *extrasystoles* are contractions that occur before the next expected contraction. Premature contractions may occur with hyperkalemia or hypercalcemia. Frequent premature contractions can lead to fibrillation, during which cardiac muscle fibers contract out of sequence one another. In fibrillation, the affected heart chambers do not effectively pump blood, so tissue and organ perfusion is impaired. **Ventricular fibrillation** is a life-threatening condition, as the *ventricle cannot fill* or eject blood to vital tissues because contractions are so rapid. If fibrillation is not corrected immediately by defibrillation or some other method, death may occur within minutes.

15. Discuss contractility, preload, and afterload as mechanisms for left heart failure.
Study pages 624-626; refer to Figures 23-37 through 23-30.

According to the Frank-Starling law of the heart, contractility is optimal within a certain range of myocardial cell lengths; *the more the myocardium is stretched, the harder it contracts.* Normally, an increase of diastolic stretch results in a larger systolic ejection force and a larger stroke volume. Increases of **preload** or left ventricular end-diastolic volume (LVEDV) increase myocardial oxygen consumption by requiring a greater force of contraction to accomplish systole. The increased force of cardiac contraction is accompanied by greater metabolic demand in the myocardium, and more oxygen is required to support myocardial metabolism. Unfortunately, increased myocardial stretch *decreases myocardial capillary perfusion by mechanically narrowing coronary capillary lumina.* Also, if preload increases beyond the ventricle's ability to empty, the coronary artery blood supply drops as *the ejection fraction decreases.* These two factors cause the overworked and overstretched myocardium to become hypoxic. Myocardial ischemia results in **ventricular remodeling**. This remodeling alters ventricular wall structure in the noninfarcted myocardium even after the infarction area has healed. *The process causes progression of myocyte contractile dysfunction.*

Afterload is the force or pressure against which a cardiac chamber must eject blood during systole. Increased afterload is associated with increased *systemic vascular resistance (SVR) or pulmonary vascular resistance,* such as occurs in systemic or pulmonary hypertension. The ventricle responds to the resistance by becoming hypertrophic. The hypertrophied ventricular myocardium must use greater force during ejection and must consume more oxygen with each contraction. Thickened myocardium changes the myocytes; ventricular remodeling and the hypertrophy deposits collagen between the myocytes. The deposits decrease contractility, leading to dilation and heart failure.

16. Differentiate between left and right heart failure; describe high-output heart failure.
Study page 626; refer to Figure 23-39 and 23-40. (See left side and right side heart failure charts on following pages.)

High-output heart failure is the inability of the heart to adequately supply the body with blood-borne nutrients despite adequate blood volume and normal or elevated myocardial contractility. In high-output failure, the heart increases its output, *but the body's metabolic needs are still not met.* Common causes of high-output failure are anemia, septicemia, hyperthyroidism, and beriberi.

Anemia decreases the oxygen-carrying capacity of the blood. *Metabolic acidosis* occurs as the body's cells switch to anaerobic metabolism (see Chapter 4). In response to metabolic acidosis, heart rate and stroke volume increase in an attempt to circulate blood faster. If anemia is severe, however, even maximum cardiac output does not supply the cells with enough oxygen for metabolism.

In septicemia, disturbed metabolism, bacterial toxins, and the inflammatory process cause systemic vasodilation and fever. Faced with a lowered SVR and an elevated metabolic rate, cardiac output increases to maintain blood pressure and prevent metabolic acidosis. In overwhelming septicemia, however, the heart may not be able to raise its output enough *to compensate for vasodilation.* Body tissues show signs of inadequate blood supply despite high cardiac output.

Hyperthyroidism accelerates cellular metabolism through the actions of elevations of thyroxine from the thyroid gland. This elevation may occur chronically (thyrotoxicosis) or acutely (thyroid storm). Because the body's demand for oxygen threatens to cause *metabolic acidosis*, cardiac output increases. *If blood levels of thyroxine are high* and the metabolic response to thyroxine is vigorous, even an abnormally elevated cardiac output may be inadequate.

Left Side Failure (Congestive Heart Failure*)

Pathology sequence

Systolic or diastolic ventricular dysfunction

↓

Decreased left ventricular emptying (end-diastolic volume and preload increases)

↓

Increased volume and pressure in left ventricle

↓

Increased volume and pressure in left atrium (increased preload)

↓

Increased volume in pulmonary veins

↓

Increased volume in pulmonary capillary bed

↓

Fluid transudation from capillaries to alveoli

↓

Aleveolar space fluid

↓

Pulmonary edema

↓

Increased pulmonary vascular resistance

↓

Right ventricular failure

Manifestations of the left side heart failure

- Exertional and nocturnal dyspnea
- Blood-tinged sputum
- Orthopnea
- Cough
- Cyanosis
- Decreased urinary output
- Rales
- Fatigue
- S_3 gallop

NOTE: Treatment for left heart failure is to correct the underlying cause. Valvular dysfunction may require surgery. Vasodilators can improve coronary artery perfusion.
The hypotension associated with left ventricular failure is usually treated with a cardiotonic antihypotensive. Oxygen is administered continuously to increase the supply of oxygen to the myocardium. Diuretics are given to decrease pulmonary edema and blood volume, and sodium and fluid intake are restricted. ACE inhibitors reduce preload and afterload by decreasing aldosterone levels and peripheral vascular resistance. Morphine sulfate dilates the pulmonary and systemic vessels, which decreases pulmonary and systemic capillary hydrostatic pressure. Also, morphine sulfate is an analgesic and an opiate, which improves the emotional state of the individual and may limit the cerebrally mediated release of epinephrine. Surgery or heart transplant may be necessary.

* CHF can be categorized as (a) systolic or (b) diastolic heart failure.
Systolic dysfunction is an increase in left ventricular end-diastolic pressure that results in pulmonary edema.
Diastolic dysfunction is increased left ventricular end-diastolic pressure increase, even if volume and cardiac out are normal.

Right Side Failure (Cor Pulmonale)

Pathology sequence

Left heart failure
↓
Increased pulmonary vascular resistance
↓
Decreased right ventricular emptying
↓
Increased volume and pressure in right ventricle (end-diastolic volume and preload increases)
↓
Increased volume and pressure in right atrium
↓
Increased volume and pressure in the great veins
↓
Increased volume in the systemic venous circulation
↓
Increased volume in distensible organs
↓
Increased capillary pressure
↓
Peripheral edema and serous effusion

Manifestations of the right side heart failure

- Fatigue
- Ascites
- Gastrointestinal disorders
- Liver and spleen engorgement
- Cyanosis
- Distended jugular veins
- Elevated venous pressure
- Dependent edema

NOTE: Treatment for right heart failure begins with treatment of the underlying left heart failure or pulmonary disease. Diuretics and restricted water and sodium intake are used to reduce venous blood volume or preload. Myocardial contractility is enhanced with digoxin or other cardiotonic medications.

17. Characterize impaired cellular metabolism due to shock.
Study pages 627 and 629; refer to Figure 23-41.
The final outcome of any type of shock is impaired cellular metabolism and cellular lysis. (The diagram on the previous page illustrates these events.)

18. Classify the different types of shock by etiology; note the consequences of shock.
Study pages 629 and 631-634; refer to Figures 23-44 through 23-48 and Table 23-10. (See table on the following page.)

Shock is a condition in which the cardiovascular system fails *to perfuse the tissues* adequately. This failure results in widespread impairment of cellular metabolism. Any factor that alters heart function, blood volume, or blood pressure can cause shock.

Ultimately, shock, irrespective of its cause, *progresses to organ failure and death* unless compensatory mechanisms or clinical intervention reverse the process. Shock causes many diverse signs and symptoms. The individual in shock may feel sick, weak, cold, hot, nauseated, dizzy, confused, afraid, thirsty, and short of breath. Blood pressure, cardiac output, and urinary output usually decrease. Respiratory rate usually increases.

Shock's Impairment of Cellular Metabolism

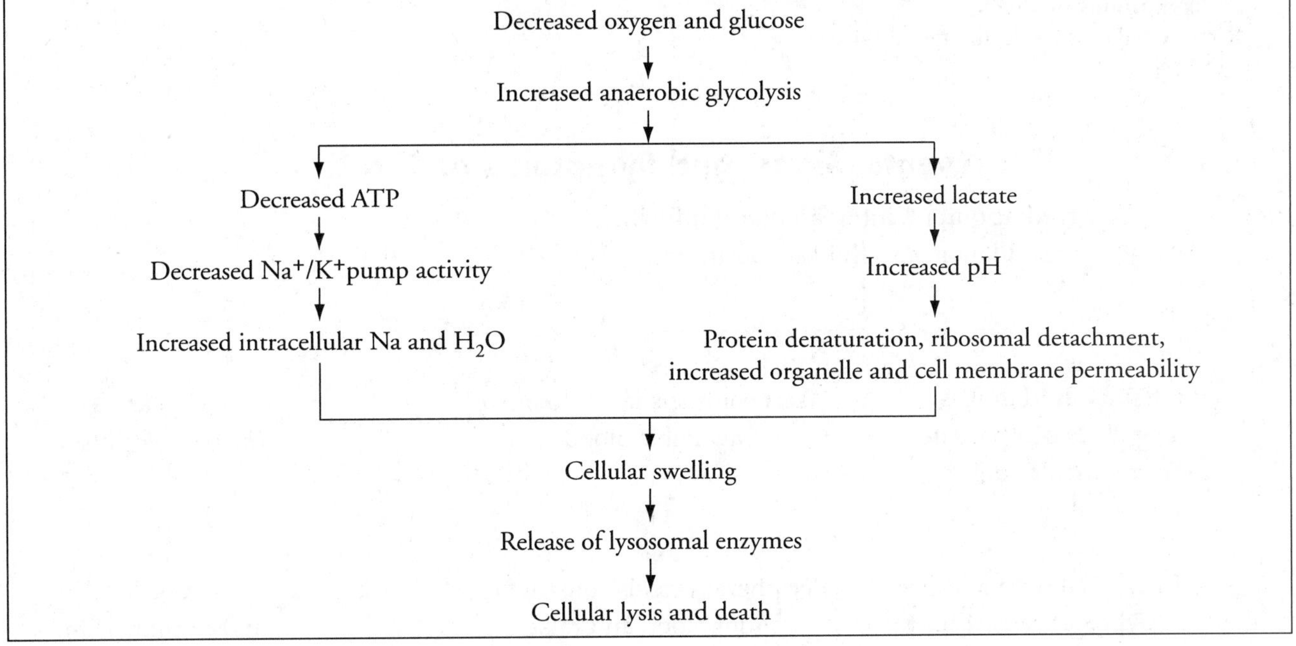

Types of Shock

Type	Etiology
Cardiogenic (heart failure)	Myocardial ischemia, myocardial infarction, congestive heart failure, myocardial or pericardial infections, dysrhythmias, excessive right ventricular afterload, drug toxicity
Hypovolemic (insufficient intravascular fluid volume; begins when loss is 15%)	Loss of whole blood plasma or interstitial fluid, fluid sequestration
Neurogenic (neural alterations of vascular muscle smooth muscle tone)	Sympathetic understimulation or parasympathetic overstimulation of vascular muscle causes ensuing vasodilation, decreased systemic vascular resistance
Anaphylactic (immunologic alterations)	Hypersensitivity leads to vasodilation, increased vascular permeability, and peripheral blood pooling
Septic* (infectious processes)	Bacteremia and triggering substances released by the bacteria, including endotoxins from gram-negative organisms, lipoteichoic acids and peptidoglycans from gram-positive organisms, and superantigens, cause the host to initiate a proinflammatory response; vasodilation; then a compensatory host anti-inflammatory response; next, a mixed antagonistic response between inflammatory and anti-inflammatory mediators leads the host into multiple organ dysfunction syndrome (MODS)

*Septic shock is one component of a continuum of progressive dysfunction called **systemic inflammatory response syndrome (SIRS)**. The syndrome begins with an infection that progresses to bacteremia, sepsis, septic shock, and finally MODS.

Note: The consequence of all types of shock is reduced tissue perfusion and impaired cellular metabolism. Treatment of shock requires removing the underlying cause. After correction of the cause, supplemental oxygen, vasopressors, and intravenous fluid are given to expand the intravascular volume. Depending on the type of shock, corticosteroids, anti-inflammatory drugs, antibacterials, and nitric oxide synthetase inhibitors may be indicated.

19. Briefly diagram the common events found in all types of shock, and relate the events to the signs and symptoms of shock.
Refer to Figures 23-42 through 23-46.

Events, Signs, and Symptoms of Shock

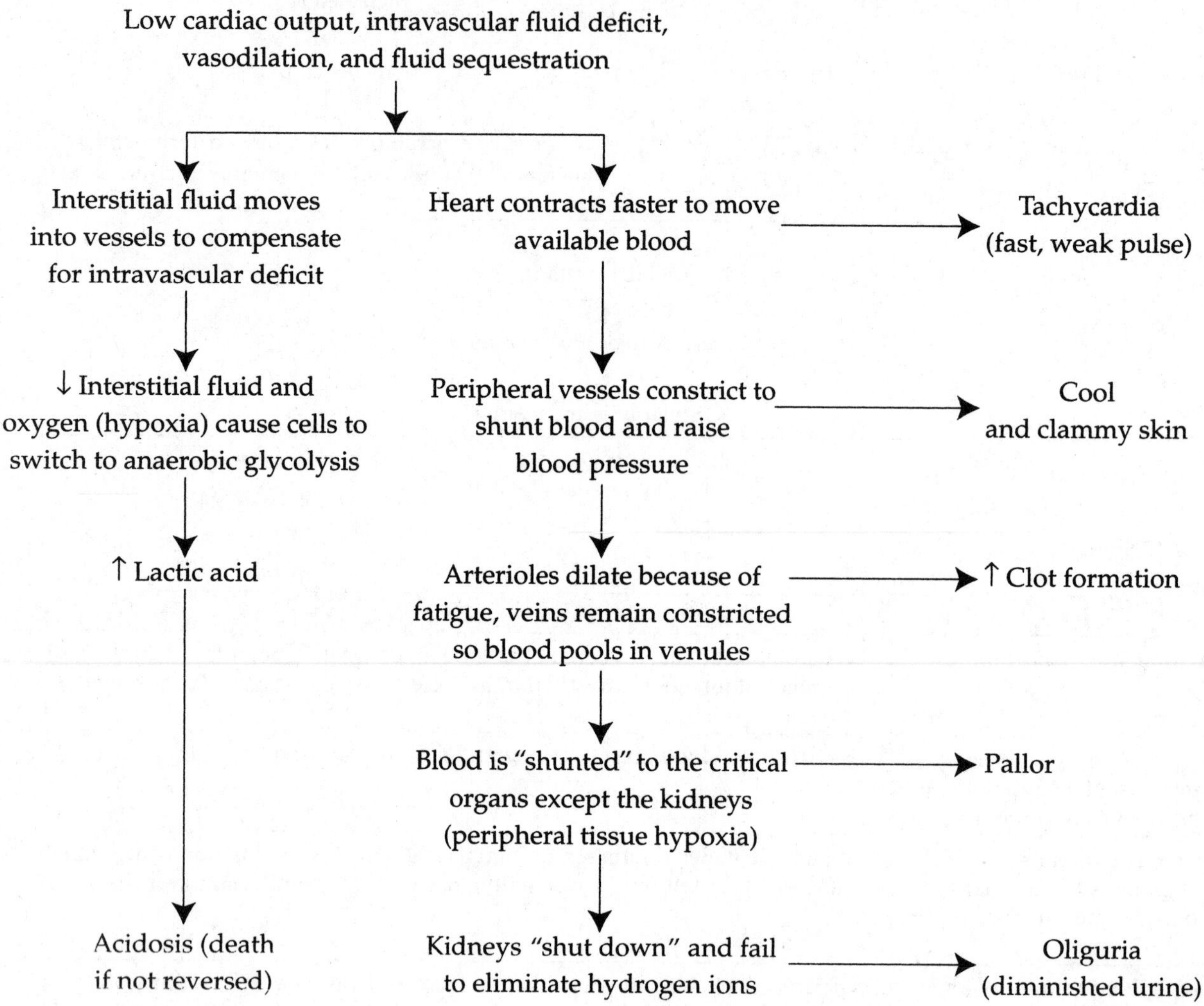

20. Illustrate the pathogenic sequence of MODS due to shock.
Study pages 634-637; refer to Figure 23-47 and Table 23-11.

Sepsis and septic shock are the most common causes of ***MODS***. Severe trauma, burns, and respiratory or renal failure also contribute to MODS. The following diagram illustrates the pathogenesis of MODS:

Pathogenesis of Multiple Organ Dysfunction Syndrome (MODS)

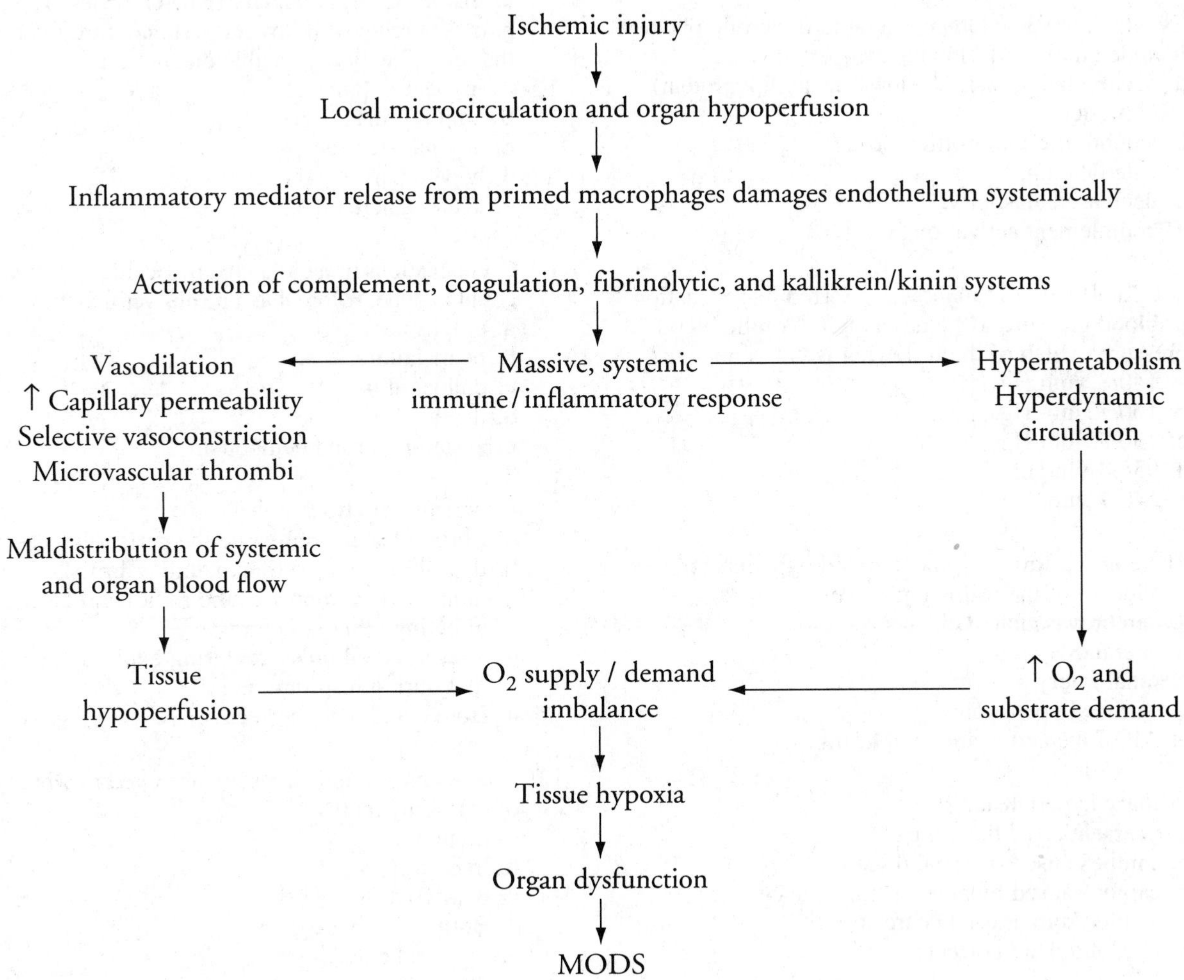

PRACTICE EXAMINATION

Multiple Choice

Circle the correct answer for each question:

1. Adiponectin is:
   a. an enzyme.
   b. increased in obesity.
   c. inflammatory.
   d. antiatherogenic.

2. Events in the development of atherosclerotic plaque include all of the following *except:*
   a. accumulation of LDL (low-density lipoprotein) cholesterol.
   b. smooth muscle proliferation.
   c. calcification.
   d. decreased elasticity.
   e. complement activation.

3. G.P., a 50-year-old man, was referred for evaluation of blood pressure. If he has a high diastolic blood pressure, which of the following is G.P.'s reading?
   a. 140/82 mm Hg
   b. 160/72 mm Hg
   c. 130/95 mm Hg
   d. 95/68 mm Hg
   e. 140/72 mm Hg

4. The complications of uncontrolled hypertension include all of the following *except:*
   a. cerebrovascular accidents.
   b. anemia.
   c. renal injury.
   d. cardiac hypertrophy.
   e. All of the above are complications.

5. Primary hypertension:
   a. is essentially idiopathic.
   b. can be caused by renal disease.
   c. can be caused by hormone imbalance.
   d. results from arterial coarctation.
   e. b, c, and d are correct.

6. Orthostatic hypotension is caused by all of the following *except:*
   a. increased age.
   b. increased blood volume.
   c. autonomic nervous system dysfunction.
   d. bed rest.
   e. severe varicose veins.

7. Localized outpouching of a vessel wall or heart chamber is:
   a. a thrombus.
   b. an embolus.
   c. a thromboembolus.
   d. an aneurysm.
   e. a vegetation.

8. Which is a possible cause of varicose veins?
   a. gravitational forces on blood
   b. long periods of standing
   c. trauma to the saphenous veins
   d. Both b and c are correct.
   e. a, b, and c are correct.

9. A 76-year-old man came to the emergency room after experiencing chest pain while shoveling snow. Laboratory tests revealed essentially normal blood levels of SGOT, CPK, and LDH enzymes. The chest pain was relieved following rest and nitroglycerin therapy. The most probable diagnosis is:
   a. myocardial infarct.
   b. emphysema.
   c. angina pectoris.
   d. hepatic cirrhosis.
   e. acute pancreatitis.

10. Complications of an infarcted myocardium likely could include: (More than one answer may be correct.)
    a. emphysema.
    b. heart failure.
    c. endocarditis.
    d. death.
    e. systemic thromboembolism.

11. In pericardial effusion:
    a. fibrotic lesions obliterate the pericardial cavity.
    b. there is associated rheumatoid arthritis.
    c. tamponade compresses the right heart before affecting other structures.
    d. arterial blood pressure during expiration exceeds that during inspiration.
    e. Both c and d are correct.

12. Chamber volume increase is observed in what type of cardiomyopathy?
    a. dilated
    b. hypertrophic
    c. restrictive
    d. Both a and b are correct.
    e. a, b, and c are correct.

13. Which statement is true regarding rheumatic heart disease? (More than one answer may be correct.)
    a. It is caused by staphylococcal infections.
    b. It is caused by hypersensitivity/immunity to streptococci.
    c. It damages the tricuspid valve most often.
    d. It usually damages the mitral valve.

14. Transmural myocardial infarction:
    a. displays non-STEMI.
    b. occurs when infarction is limited to part of the heart wall.
    c. is categorized as STEMI.
    d. displays I-wave inversion.

15. Bacterial infective endocarditis differs from rheumatic heart disease because of which of the following? (More than one answer may be correct.)
    a. Bacterial endocarditis is an infection of the heart, endocardium, and valves.
    b. It always follows rheumatic fever.
    c. It may occur following dental or bladder catheterization procedures.
    d. It commonly involves the vena cava valve.
    e. It is caused by a type III hypersensitivity.

16. Individuals with only left heart failure would exhibit which of the following? (More than one answer may be correct.)
    a. hepatomegaly
    b. dyspnea
    c. ankle swelling
    d. pulmonary edema
    e. peripheral edema

17. In congestive heart failure, the pump or myocardium itself fails because of which of the following? (More than one answer may be correct.)
    a. loss of contractile force of the heart
    b. hypertension
    c. cardiac dysrhythmias
    d. intermittent claudication from occlusive vascular disease

18. Shock is a complex pathophysiologic process involving all of the following *except:*
    a. decreased blood perfusion to kidneys.
    b. acidosis.
    c. rapid heart rate.
    d. hypertension.
    e. anaerobic glycolysis.

19. SIRS begins with an infection that progresses to:
    a. bacteremia.
    b. sepsis.
    c. septic shock.
    d. MODS.
    e. All of the above are correct.

20. Which statement is *incorrect* concerning hypertension?
    a. Malignant hypertension is characterized by a diastolic pressure higher than140 mm Hg.
    b. More than 90% of cases are of the essential or primary type.
    c. Headache is the most reliable symptom.
    d. When it is left untreated, the major risks include CVAs and cardiac hypertrophy.

21. A 53-year-old man was admitted to the emergency room after experiencing shortness of breath, weakness, cardiac dysrhythmias, and chest pain that did not subside after nitroglycerin therapy. Laboratory tests showed that the patient had an elevations of serum CPK, troponin, and SCOT or AST. ECG tracings revealed a prominent Q wave and an elevated ST segment. The most probable diagnosis is:
    a. a transient ischemic attack.
    b. an acute myocardial infarct.
    c. an attack of unstable angina pectoris.
    d. Prinzmetal angina.
    e. coronary artery vasospasm.

Matching

Match the valvular dysfunction with its consequence:

_______ 22. Aortic stenosis

_______ 23. Tricuspid regurgitation

_______ 24. Mitral stenosis

_______ 25. Mitral regurgitation

a. right ventricular hypertrophy
b. left ventricular hypertrophy
c. right atrial hypertrophy
d. left atrial hypertrophy
e. left atrial/right ventricular hypertrophy
f. right and left ventricular/left atrial hypertrophy
g. hypertrophy of all chambers

Fill in the Blank

Complete the following table describing the effects of sustained primary HTN:

Effects of Sustained Primary Hypertension

Injury Site	Injurious Mechanism	Pathology
Heart	Myocardial overload, coronary artery atherosclerosis	Left ventricular hypertrophy, myocardial ischemia
Kidneys		
Brain	Reduced blood flow and O_2, weakened vessel walls	TIAs, thrombosis, aneurysm, hemorrhage, infarction
Retina		
Aorta		
Lower extremity arteries		

CASE REVIEW 1

Mr. T., a 45-year-old black man employed as a midlevel corporate manager, came to the doctor's office seeking a physical examination. He appeared somewhat overweight. He denied taking any medications or smoking, but admitted drinking alcohol. His father and older brother have hypertension (HTN) and his paternal grandfather experienced a myocardial infarction (MI) and a CVA at a young age. Mr. T. stated, "A year ago at a health fair my cholesterol was tested. I was told later by mail that my cholesterol was 250 and I had to recheck my blood pressure."

What presumptive diagnosis seems likely? What other questions should the practitioner ask this patient? What laboratory tests are indicated?

CASE REVIEW 2

W.S., a 51-year-old white man, was assisting in the launching of his best friend's water-ski boat from a faulty boat trailer when he began to experience chest discomfort. At first, he believed his discomfort was caused by the extreme July heat. Gradually, the discomfort became a crushing pain in his sternal area that radiated into his left arm and lower jaw. His friend suspected an ensuing heart attack and persuaded W.S. to check into a nearby emergency department.

On arrival at the emergency department, W.S.'s skin was cool, clammy, and pale. His blood pressure was low, and his pulse was weak and irregular. An electrocardiogram showed evidence of myocardial injury, and blood was drawn to check enzyme and electrolyte levels. While reporting his history, W.S. stated, "I am under a lot of executive pressure at work and am being treated for hypertension." He later acknowledged smoking three packs of cigarettes a day for 30 years and that his father died of a heart attack at the age of 47. Serum levels of CPK, troponin, LDH, and SGOT verified anterior MI.

Knowing the diagnosis, identify W.S.'s risk factors and the early causes and precipitating events of his infarction, and suggest possible treatment for his condition.

24 Alterations of Cardiovascular Function in Children

FOUNDATIONAL OBJECTIVES

Review Foundational Objectives a, b, c, and d from Chapter 23.

MEMORY CHECK!

- The heart arises from the *mesenchyme* and begins its development as an enlarged blood vessel with a large lumen and muscular wall. The midsection of this tube begins to grow faster than its ends, so the tube bulges and twists until both ends of the tube come together and fuse. The superior part of the tube is the *truncus arteriosus*, which divides longitudinally into the *pulmonary artery and aorta;* the lower part of the tube becomes the *superior and inferior venae cavae*. The development of the cardiac septa eventually divides the heart into the four chambers. If development of the septa proceeds normally, the four-chambered heart will be present by the sixth or seventh week of gestation.
- Blood for the fetus is oxygenated in the *placenta* and returns to the fetus through the umbilical vein. Part of this blood passes through the *liver*, but about half the flow is diverted from the liver through the *ductus venosus* (a connection between the hepatic vessels and the inferior vena cava) and into the inferior vena cava. This blood flows into the heart and passes through the *foramen ovale* (an opening between the right and left atria), through the left ventricle, and into the aorta. From there, it flows to the head and upper extremities. Blood returning from the upper body collects in the superior vena cava. A small portion of this blood enters the lungs; the largest amount, however, flows through the *ductus arteriosus* (a connection between the pulmonary artery and the aorta), into the descending aorta, to the body, and then back to the placental vein through two umbilical arteries.
- After birth, *systemic resistance rises, and pulmonary resistance falls*. Pulmonary vascular resistance drops suddenly at birth because the lungs expand and the pulmonary vessels dilate; it continues to decrease gradually over the first 6 to 8 weeks after birth. Decreased resistance causes the right myocardium to thin. Systemic vascular resistance increases markedly at birth because severance of the umbilical cord removes the low-resistance placenta from the systemic circulation. Greater systemic resistance causes the right myocardium to thicken. *Changes in resistance cause the fetal connections between the pulmonary and systemic circulatory systems to disappear.* The *foramen ovale closes* functionally at birth and anatomically several months later. The *ductus arteriosus closes* functionally 15 to 18 hours after birth and anatomically within 10 to 21 days. The *ductus venosus* closes within 1 week after birth.

LEARNING OBJECTIVES

After studying this chapter, the learner will be able to do the following:

1. Characterize congenital heart disease.
Study pages 643 and 644; refer to Figures 24-1 and 24-2 and Tables 24-1 and 24-2.

Most **congenital heart diseases** have both environmental and genetic causes. Most environmental risk factors are associated with maternal conditions, such as viral infections, diabetes, drug intake, and advanced maternal age. Genetic factors include, but are not limited to, trisomy 13 or 18, cri du chat syndrome, and Turner syndrome.

Classification of congenital heart defects is based on whether they: (1) cause blood flow to the lungs to increase, decrease, or remain normal; (2) cause cyanosis; or (3) obstruct blood flow. Cyanosis, a bluish discoloration of the skin, can be caused by defects that restrict blood flow into the pulmonary circulation, overload the pulmonary circulation, lead to pulmonary edema, or cause unoxygenated blood to shunt from the pulmonary to the systemic circulation. Shunting of blood flow from the left heart to the right heart is *left-to-right* shunting and causes *no cyanosis. Cyanosis* develops when blood is shunted from the right heart into the left heart, a condition known as a *right-to-left shunt.*

2. Identify the most common congenital defects that obstruct ventricular outflow and describe their pathophysiology and treatment.
Study pages 644, 646 and 647; refer to Figures 24-3 through 24-5.

Coarctation of the aorta (COA) is caused by a *narrowing of the aorta* anywhere between the origin of the aortic arch and the abdominal bifurcation. This defect may be considered in terms of its proximity to the ductus arteriosus. A narrowing near the ductus arteriosus results in *increased blood flow to the head and upper extremities* and decreased blood flow to the lower extremities. *Disparities* between the blood pressures *in the upper and lower extremities* are often diagnostic. Surgical correction includes resection of the affected site on the aorta with various grafts and closure of the ductus.

Aortic stenosis (AS) is a *narrowing or stricture of the aortic valve* that causes *resistance* to blood flow from the left ventricle, decreased cardiac output, left ventricular hypertrophy, and pulmonary *vascular* congestion.

Children with AS show signs of exercise intolerance, chest pain, and dizziness. There is a characteristic systolic *ejection murmur*. Individuals are at risk for bacterial endocarditis, coronary insufficiency, and ventricular dysfunction.

Aortic valvotomy is an early palliative procedure. A valve replacement may be required as a subsequent procedure.

Pulmonic stenosis (PS) is caused by the *restriction or thickening of the leaflets of the pulmonary valve.* Outflow is restricted from the right ventricle, resulting in *increased afterload;* if the restriction is severe, right ventricular hypertrophy and dilation may result. If pressures are high enough, the foramen ovale may reopen, resulting in a *right-to-left* shunt; cyanosis is usually not present. Mild cases cause little or no symptomatology, whereas severe cases may require surgical correction.

3. Describe the congenital defects with increased pulmonary blood flow and their pathophysiology and treatment.

Study pages 647-649; refer to Figures 24-6 and 24-7.

Patent ductus arteriosus (PDA) results from the *failure of the ductus arteriosus to close* within the first weeks of life. Continued patency of the ductus permits blood to flow from the higher-pressure aorta to the lower-pressure pulmonary artery, causing a left-to-right shunt to develop. Clinical manifestations are usually without cyanosis and include a *"machinery" murmur* and pulmonary vascular obstructive disease in later life. Treatment usually consists of placement of an occlusive device or surgical ligation.

Atrial septal defects (ASDs) are *abnormal communications across the interatrial septum.* The size of the ASD determines the direction of flow. If the ASD is small, the shunt direction is left to right; if it is large, the pressures in the atria are equal, and resistance determines the shunt direction of the ventricles. At birth, atrial size and resistance are generally equal; as the infant grows, the left ventricle thickens, and systemic pressure rises, causing a left-to-right shunt. These defects may be so mild that they go undetected until preschool age. A *soft murmur* is often audible at the second intracostal space, and the examiner may also hear a fixed splitting of the second heart sound; this finding indicates right ventricular *overload.* Treatment involves placement of a closure device or surgical correction.

Ventricular septal defect (VSD) is essentially a *defect in the intraventricular septum* that leads to blood flow between the ventricles of the heart. Small defects have very little associated pathology and often close on their own, with the shunt usually flowing left to right. Large defects are a different matter. In a large VSD, pressures may become equal in the two chambers, with blood flow again being *left to right* because of higher systemic pressures. In this case, large amounts of blood flow into the lungs through the pulmonary artery and back to the left heart and cause a great deal of *left ventricular stress;* heart failure may eventually result. Treatment ranges from observation in mild cases to correction involving open-heart surgery in more serious cases.

Atrioventricular canal (AVC) defect consists of a low *atrial septal defect* that is continuous with a high *ventricular septal defect* and clefts of the *mitral and tricuspid valves.* A large central atrioventricular defect allows blood to flow between all four chambers of the heart. The directions of flow are determined by pulmonary and systemic resistance, left and right ventricular pressures, and the compliance of each chamber. Flow is generally from *left to right.* There is usually moderate to severe left heart failure and a characteristic *systolic murmur and a middiastolic rumble.* There may be little to mild cyanosis; the cyanosis increases with crying. Complete surgical repair of AVC defects can be performed in infants. If the mitral valve defect is severe, a valve replacement may be necessary.

4. Describe the congenital defects with decreased pulmonary blood flow and their pathophysiology and treatment.

Study pages 649 and 651; refer to Figures 24-8 and 24-9.

Tetralogy of Fallot is a syndrome of four defects. The associated defects that make up tetralogy are: (1) a ventricular septal defect (VSD), (2) an overriding aorta that straddles the VSD, (3) PS, and (4) right ventricular hypertrophy. The pathophysiology associated with tetralogy of Fallot may be varied and depends on the degree of pulmonary stenosis, as well as the size of the VSD and pulmonary and systemic pressures. The shunt direction may be *either left to right or right to left* (blue spells). In any event, these defects result in hypoxia in the systemic circulation while the body attempts to compensate by increasing red blood cell production and increasing blood flow to the lungs through collateral bronchial vessels. Cyanotic episodes may also be accompanied by syncope or seizures because of *hypoxia.* Treatment is usually accomplished by various surgical procedures that increase blood flow to the pulmonary arteries.

Tricuspid atresia is the *failure of the tricuspid valve to develop.* Thus, there is no communication from right atrium to right ventricle. Blood flows through an ASD or a patent foramen ovale to the left heart and through a VSD to the right ventricle and then to the lungs. It is often associated with PS and transposition of the great arteries. *The unoxygenated blood and oxygenated blood completely mix in the left heart.*

Cyanosis is usually observed during the newborn period in a patient with tricuspid atresia. There may be tachycardia, dyspnea, and a murmur. Older children exhibit chronic hypoxemia with clubbing. Individuals are at risk for bacterial endocarditis, brain abscess, and stroke.

Palliative treatment involves the placement of a shunt to increase blood flow to the lungs. Staged repair consists of several surgical procedures that eventually connect the inferior vena cava and the pulmonary artery.

5. Describe defects that permit mixing of pulmonary blood and systemic blood.

Study pages 651-653; refer to Figures 24-10 through 24-13.

Complete transposition of the great vessels results in the effective switching of the aorta and pulmonary arteries so *the pulmonary artery leaves the left ventricle and the aorta leaves the right ventricle.* This switch creates two separate circulatory systems with *no communication between them.* Children with minimum communication are severely cyanotic. If large septal defects exist, cyanosis may be less but symptoms of left heart failure occur. Cardiomegaly develops a few weeks after birth. Switching procedures to make the left ventricle the systemic pump may be the best of the various available surgical corrections.

Total anomalous pulmonary venous connection (TAPVC) is a disorder in which *the pulmonary circulation enters the right atrium instead of the left.* TAPVC has variations with the same resultant pathophysiology, all of which are associated with ASDs. TAPVC in any form results in the pumping of a mixture of oxygenated and unoxygenated blood to the systemic circulation. The shunt direction is usually right to left. The amount of cyanosis generated by this anomaly depends on the mixture of unoxygenated and oxygenated blood. Thus, the greater the pulmonary blood flow, the less the cyanosis. Congestive heart failure (CHF) is a common complication. The surgical approach varies with the defect; generally, attachments are made to enable proper directional blood flow through the heart.

Truncus arteriosus is *failure of normal septation and division of the embryonic vessel* trunk into the pulmonary artery and the aorta; the resulting single vessel overrides both ventricles. Blood from both ventricles *mixes* in the common great artery and causes *desaturation and hypoxemia.* Blood ejected from the heart flows to the lower-pressure pulmonary arteries and causes increased pulmonary blood flow and reduced systemic blood flow.

Most infants have moderate to severe left heart failure and variable cyanosis, poor growth, and activity intolerance. Children are at risk for brain abscess and bacterial endocarditis.

Corrective surgery involves closing the defect so that the truncus arteriosus receives the outflow from the left ventricle, excising the pulmonary arteries from the aorta, and attaching them to the right ventricle with a homograft.

Hypoplastic left heart syndrome is *underdevelopment of the left heart,* which results in a hypoplastic left ventricle and aortic atresia. Most blood from the left atrium flows across the patent foramen ovale to the right atrium, to the right ventricle, and out the pulmonary artery.

Mild cyanosis and signs of left heart failure are present until the patent ductus arteriosus closes. Then there is progressive deterioration with cyanosis and decreased cardiac output, which leads to cardiovascular collapse. Without intervention, this condition is usually fatal in the first months of life.

A several-stage surgical repair approach is used to correct this condition. Some authorities believe that heart transplantation in the newborn period is the best option for infants with hypoplastic left heart syndrome.

6. Summarize the causes and consequences of blood flow defects in congenital heart disease (see following diagram).

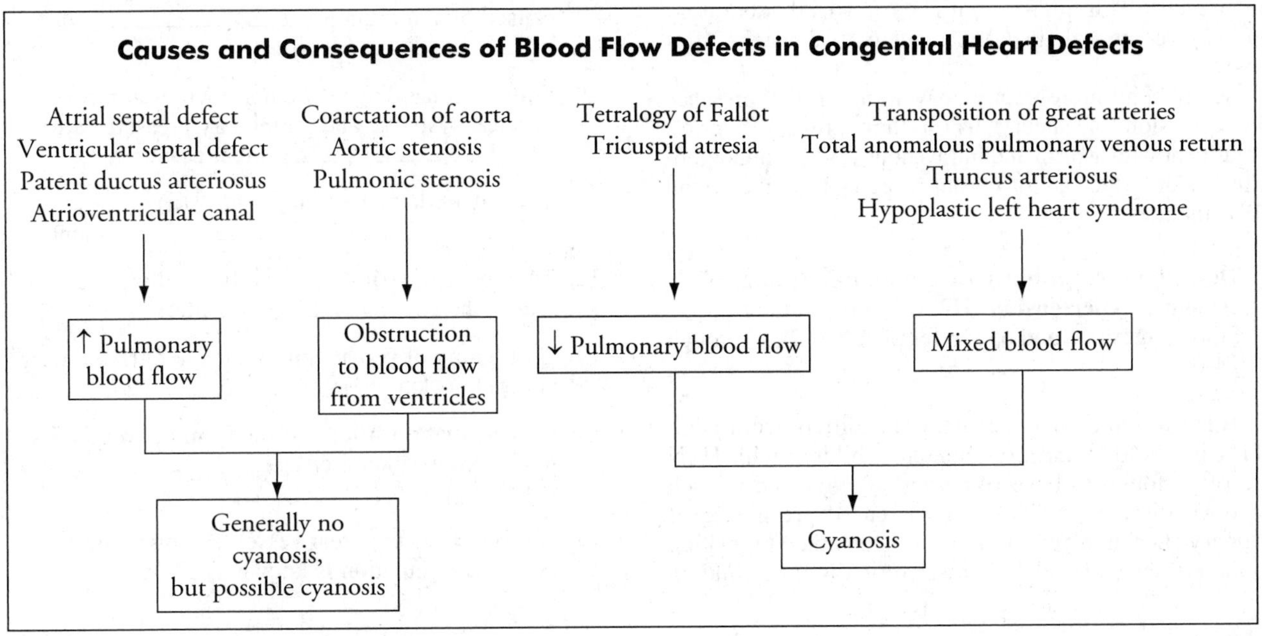

7. Describe childhood CHF and its manifestations.
Study pages 686 and 687; refer to Table 24-3.

CHF is a common complication of many congenital heart defects. It results from heart defects that *increase blood volume and pressure* in the pulmonary circulation.

Dyspnea on exertion often manifests in infants with CHF, as does difficulty with feeding. When the infant tries to suck and swallow, breathing is interrupted and the child easily becomes exhausted. Poor feeding and failure to thrive are primary indicators of left CHF in infants. In severe left heart failure, tachypnea may be accompanied by retractions, grunting, nasal flaring, coughing, and rales. Hepatomegaly is usually caused by right ventricular failure.

8. Describe the pathophysiology related to Kawasaki disease.
Study pages 654 and 655.

Kawasaki disease is an acute, *acquired self-limiting vasculitis* that may have cardiac sequelae. Eighty percent of cases occur in children younger than 5 years; incidence peaks in toddlers. This disease tends to cluster in mini-epidemics and may be related to an *infectious process with an autoimmune component.* The disease process progresses through distinct clinical phases: acute, subacute, and convalescent.

In the *acute phase*, the child has fever, conjunctivitis, "strawberry" tongue, rash, and lymphadenopathy, and is often irritable. Myocarditis may develop. The *subacute phase* begins when the fever ends and continues until the clinical signs have resolved. This is the time of the greatest risk for coronary artery aneurysm development and thrombosis. The *convalescent phase* is marked by continued elevation of the erythrocyte sedimentation rate and platelet count. Arthritis may be present. This phase continues until all laboratory values are normal, usually about 6 to 8 weeks after onset.

Serial echocardiography may monitor the presence or regression of aneurysms in the coronary arteries. Treatment with aspirin and intravenous (IV) immunoglobulins reduces the risk of coronary artery thrombosis and abnormalities.

9. Describe susceptibility to and manifestations of systemic hypertension (HTN) in children.
Study pages 655 and 656; refer to Tables 24-4 through 24-6.

HTN in children is acquired and differs from adult HTN in etiology and presentation. Children with HTN are often found to have some *underlying disease*, such as renal disease or COA. An increased prevalence of primary HTN in older children has been noted in relation to the presence of early atherosclerotic disease. Children who are overweight *(the obesity epidemic)* and who smoke are often hypertensive.

To treat most children with secondary HTN (known cause), the cause must be identified. Drug therapy is controversial in children with primary HTN. However, when nonpharmacologic therapy fails, the approach is similar to the treatment of adult HTN.

PRACTICE EXAMINATION

True/False

1. Shunts are usually independent of systemic or pulmonary pressures and are solely the result of heart defects.
2. A patent ductus arteriosus or VSD is sometimes helpful when it is associated with other cardiac defects.
3. VSDs always require surgical closure.
4. In ASDs or VSDs, murmurs indicate defects.
5. Cyanosis is *not* a major finding in transposition of the great vessels because the blood is free to travel normally to the lungs.

Fill in the Blanks

6. Abnormal blood flow within the heart is usually referred to as a(n) ______________.
7. In VSD, the shunt direction is generally ______________ to ______________.
8. Cyanotic defects usually shunt to ______________ to ______________.
9. Cyanosis that results from cardiac defects is usually caused by a mixture of ______________ and ______________ blood.
10. Some cardiac defects are not obvious at birth because systemic and pulmonary pressures are nearly ______________ at that point.
11. The patent ductus arteriosus has a(n) ______________ -to- ______________ shunt.
12. The ductus arteriosus should be totally closed within the ______________ of life.
13. Thickening or restriction of the valve from the right ventricle is known as ______________.
14. Defects that obstruct outflow from the ventricles tend to cause increased ______________, which may lead to ______________.
15. Narrowing of the great vessel leading to the systemic circulation is known as ______________.

Matching

Match the description with the alteration:

_______ 16. Associated with dyspnea when feeding

_______ 17. Likely associated with an infectious etiology and an autoimmune response

_______ 18. Vasculitis associated with aneurysm

_______ 19. If mild, often self-correcting

_______ 20. Blue spells

_______ 21. ASD, overriding aorta, PS, right ventricular hypertrophy

_______ 22. Common complication of congenital heart defects

_______ 23. Immediate cyanosis and distress after birth

_______ 24. Two separate circulatory systems

_______ 25. May be associated with coronary thrombosis

a. Kawasaki disease
b. VSD
c. tetralogy of Fallot
d. transposition of the great vessels
e. left heart failure

Complete the following table identifying causes of childhood sustained HTN by age group:

Common Causes of Childhood Sustained Hypertension

Age Group	Causes
Newborn	
> 6 yr	Renal parenchymal disease (RPD), COA, renal artery stenosis
6-10 yr	
> 10 yr	

CASE STUDY

David M. is a 7-year-old boy being presented for a routine physical examination. His past medical and family history is not unusual. His activity level is normal, and his mother stated, "David is quite healthy." David's physical findings are normal until the cardiovascular system is evaluated. He is noted to have a systolic murmur. David also has bounding pulses in his arms and severely decreased pulses in his legs. The practitioner requests a pediatric cardiology consultation.

Which cardiac defect causes such a striking discrepancy in blood flow to the upper and lower extremities?

25 Structure and Function of the Pulmonary System

FOUNDATIONAL OBJECTIVES

After reviewing this chapter, the learner will be able to do the following:

1. **Identify the sequence of structures of the pulmonary system as air moves into and out of the lungs; list the defense mechanisms of the pulmonary system.**
   Review pages 660, 661, and 664-666; refer to Figures 25-1 through 25-7 and Table 25-1.

2. **Describe lung volumes and capacities.**
   Refer to Table 25-2.

3. **Describe the neurochemical control of ventilation; characterize types of lung receptors.**
   Review pages 666 and 667; refer to Figure 25-9.

4. **Relate changes in the thoracic volume to muscular contractions, alveolar surface tension, elastic properties of the lungs and chest wall, and conducting airway resistance.**
   Review pages 668-670; refer to Figures 25-10 through 25-12.

5. **Identify the factors in oxygen transport to the cells of the body, and describe oxyhemoglobin association and disassociation; identify the factors in carbon dioxide transport from the cells.**
   Review pages 670-675; refer to Figures 25-13 through 25-15 and 25-17.

6. **Identify the normal values for arterial and venous blood gases.**
   Refer to Figure 25-16.

7. **Describe the factors controlling pulmonary vasodilation and vasoconstriction.**
   Review page 676.

8. **Note the pulmonary changes that occur with normal aging.**
   Review page 676.

PRACTICE EXAMINATION

Multiple Choice

Circle the correct answer for each question:

1. Considering the sequence of structures through which air enters the pulmonary system, the pharynx is to the trachea as the:
   a. bronchioles are to the segmental bronchi.
   b. alveoli are to the alveolar ducts.
   c. alveolar ducts are to the respiratory bronchioles.
   d. respiratory bronchioles are to the alveolar ducts.
   e. All of the above are correct.

2. The cilia of the bronchial wall:
   a. ingest bacteria.
   b. trigger the sneeze reflex.
   c. trap and remove bacteria.
   d. propel mucus and trapped bacteria toward the oropharynx.
   e. Both a and c are correct.

3. As the terminal bronchioles are approached:
   a. the epithelium becomes thicker.
   b. mucus-producing glands increase.
   c. the epithelium becomes thinner.
   d. cartilaginous support increases.
   e. the smooth muscle layer thickens.

4. The left bronchus:
   a. is shorter and wider than the right.
   b. is symmetrical with the right.
   c. has a course more vertical than that on the right.
   d. is more angled than the right.
   e. has more bronchial wall layers than the right.

5. The respiratory unit consists of:
   a. cilia.
   b. bronchiolar arteries and veins.
   c. goblet cells and alveoli.
   d. respiratory bronchioles and alveoli.
   e. All of the above are correct.

6. Alveoli are excellent gas exchange units because of:
   a. their large surface area.
   b. a very thin epithelial layer.
   c. extensive vascularization.
   d. Both b and c are correct.
   e. a, b, and c are correct.

7. Surfactant:
   a. facilitates O_2 exchange.
   b. produces nutrients for the alveoli.
   c. permits air exchange between alveolar ducts.
   d. facilitates alveolar expansion during inspiration.
   e. All of the above are correct.

8. During expiration, which relationship is true?
   a. As the lung volume decreases, the number of gas molecules increases.
   b. As the lung pressure increases, the number of gas molecules increases.
   c. As the lung volume decreases, the pressure increases.
   d. As the partial pressure increases, less gas will dissolve in a liquid.

9. When the diaphragm and external intercostal contract:
   a. the intrathoracic volume increases.
   b. the intrathoracic pressure increases.
   c. the intrathoracic volume decreases.
   d. None of the above is correct.

10. Oxygen diffusion from the alveolus to the alveolar capillary occurs because:
   a. the Pao_2 is less in the capillary than in the alveolus.
   b. the Pao_2 is greater in the atmosphere than in the arterial blood.
   c. oxygen diffuses faster than CO_2.
   d. the Pao_2 is higher in the capillary than in the alveolus.

11. A shift to the right in the oxyhemoglobin dissociation curve:
   a. prevents oxygen release at the cellular level.
   b. causes oxygen to bind more tightly to hemoglobin.
   c. improves oxygen release and increases oxygen movement into the cells.
   d. Both a and b are correct.
   e. None of the above is correct.

12. In which sequence does Pao_2 progressively decrease?
   a. blood in aorta, atmospheric air, body tissues
   b. body tissues, arterial blood, alveolar air
   c. body tissues, alveolar air, arterial blood
   d. atmospheric air, aortic blood, body tissues

13. Most O_2 is carried in the blood ____________; most CO_2 is carried in the blood ____________.
   a. dissolved in plasma; associated with salt or an acid
   b. bound to hemoglobin; associated with bicarbonate/carbonic acid
   c. combined with albumin; associated with carbonic acid and hemoglobin
   d. bound to hemoglobin; bound to albumin

14. Alveoli are well-suited for diffusion of respiratory gases because:
   a. they are small and, thus, have a small total surface area.
   b. vascularization is minimal, allowing greater air circulation.
   c. they contain four thick layers, preventing air leakage.
   d. they contain surfactant, which helps prevent alveolar collapse.

15. Which ordinarily brings about the greatest increase in the rate of respiration?
   a. excess carbon dioxide
   b. increased O_2
   c. increased arterial pH
   d. a sudden rise in blood pressure

16. Given that the oxygen content of blood equals 1.34 mL of O_2 per gram of hemoglobin times the arterial oxygen saturation percentage, if hemoglobin concentration is 15 g/dL and arterial saturation is 98%, what is the arterial oxygen content?
   a. 13.2 mL per dL of blood
   b. 19.7 mL per dL of blood
   c. 14.7 mL per dL of blood
   d. None of the above is correct.

17. The major muscle(s) of inspiration is/are the:
   a. diaphragm.
   b. sternocleidomastoid.
   c. external intercostals.
   d. internal intercostals.
   e. Both a and c are correct.

18. Stretch receptors:
   a. are sensitive to volume changes in the lung.
   b. are located in airway smooth muscles.
   c. decrease ventilatory rate when stimulated.
   d. prevent lung overinflation when stimulated.
   e. All of the above are correct.

19. Which of the following increases the respiratory rate?
   a. increased $Paco_2$, decreased pH, decreased Pao_2
   b. increased $Paco_2$, increased pH, decreased Pao_2
   c. decreased $Paco_2$, decreased pH, increased Pao_{22}
   d. decreased $Paco_2$, decreased pH, decreased Pao_{22}

20. The dorsal respiratory group (DRG) of neurons:
   a. sets the automatic rhythm of respiration.
   b. modifies the rhythm of respiration.
   c. is active when increased ventilation is required.
   d. None of the above is correct.

Matching

Match each term with its description or example:

_______ 21. Inspiratory reserve volume

_______ 22. Vital capacity

a. amount of air remaining in lungs after a forced expiration
b. taking an extra-deep breath of air just before diving
c. includes sum of tidal, expiratory reserve, and inspiratory reserve volumes
d. the extra air pushed out during a forced exhalation

Match the normal range of blood gases with its arterial or venous state:

_______ 23. $Paco_2$ of 40 mm Hg

_______ 24. Oxygen saturation of 70%

_______ 25. Oxygen content of blood of 19 to 20 mL/dL

a. arterial blood
b. mixed venous blood

Fill in the Blank

Complete the following table identifying pulmonary defense mechanisms:

Pulmonary Defensive Mechanisms

Effector	Mechanism of Defense
Upper tract mucosa, nasal hairs, and turbinates	
Mucus blanket	
Cilia	
Alveolar macrophages	Phagocytosis ingests and removes particles and bacteria from the alveoli
Irritant receptors in nares	
Irritant receptors in trachea and large airways	

26 Alterations of Pulmonary Function

FOUNDATIONAL OBJECTIVES

a. Compare the structures of the lower airway as generations of division move toward the alveoli.
Refer to Figures 25-1 and 25-3 through 25-6.

MEMORY CHECK!
• The trachea and mainstem bronchi are composed mainly of cartilage with a lining of mucous membrane. When the bronchi enter the lungs, they branch further. Instead of cartilaginous rings, smooth muscle encircles the bronchi with cartilage interspersed among the muscle bundles. By the time they reach the bronchioles, supportive cartilage is no longer present. The bronchioles are *capable of constriction* because of their layer of smooth muscle. Smooth muscle becomes thinner in the terminal bronchioles. The epithelium changes from pseudostratified and ciliated columnar in the bronchi to nonciliated cuboidal in the terminal bronchioles and, finally, to squamous in the alveoli. *Macrophages* must remove any debris that reaches the respiratory bronchioles and alveoli because of the *absence of cilia*.

b. Identify the measurements of lung volume.
Refer to Table 25-2.

MEMORY CHECK!
• *Tidal volume* (TV) is the amount of gas inspired and expired during normal breathing. *Inspiratory reserve volume* (IRV) is the amount of gas that can be inspired in addition to the tidal volume. *Expiratory reserve volume* (ERV) is the amount of gas that can be expired after a passive or relaxed expiration. *Residual volume* (RV) is the volume of gas that cannot be expired and is always present in the lungs. • *Total lung capacity* (TLC) is the total gas volume in the lung when the lung is maximally inflated. It consists of RV, ERV, TV, and IRV. *Vital capacity* (VC) is the maximum amount of gas that can be expired from the lung after maximal inspiration. It consists of IRV, TV, and ERV. *Functional residual capacity* (FRC) is the amount of gas remaining in the lung at the end of a passive expiration or RV and ERV. Inspiratory capacity (IC) is the amount of gas that can be inspired after a passive expiration from FRC. It consists of TV and IRV. The lung capacities are always the sum of two or more volumes. Normal values for volumes and capacities are based on age, sex, and height. • With each breath, a portion of the tidal volume remains in the conducting airways. This is the anatomic dead space. In certain disease conditions, some of the respiratory bronchioles and alveoli receive adequate ventilation, but do not participate in gas exchange because they are not perfused by the pulmonary circulation. The volume of gas in unperfused alveoli is known as alveolar dead space.

c. Describe the diaphragmatic movements in inspiration and expiration; indicate other factors involved in the mechanism of breathing.
Review pages 668-670; refer to Figures 25-10 and 25-11.

MEMORY CHECK!

Equilibrium between lungs and thorax
↓
Stimulation of respiratory centers
↓
Contraction of the diaphragm
↓
Increased size of the thorax
↓

Increased intrathoracic volume → Increased alveolar size → Lungs inflate–Inspiration

Decreased intrapleural pressure → Intra-alveolar pressure becomes less than atmospheric pressure → Lungs inflate–Inspiration

Lungs inflate–Inspiration
(Because of the higher concentration of oxygen in the atmosphere than in the alveoli, oxygen moves into the alveoli for gaseous exchange. Oxygen is loaded onto hemoglobin by the driving pressure of PaO_2 in the plasma. As pressure decreases at the tissue level, oxygen dissociates from hemoglobin and enters tissue cells by diffusion.)
↓
Relaxation of the diaphragm to a passive position
↓
Thorax and lungs return to equilibrium
↓

Decreased intrathoracic volume → Decreased alveolar size → Lungs empty–Expiration

Increased intrapleural pressure → Intra-alveolar pressure becomes greater than atmospheric pressure → Lungs empty–Expiration

Lungs empty–Expiration
(Carbon dioxide diffuses readily from tissue cells into plasma. Carbon dioxide returns to the lungs dissolved in plasma and bound to hemoglobin. Carbon dioxide is expelled because of its higher concentration in the alveoli than in the atmosphere.)

*Gases move from high concentrations or high pressures to low concentrations or low pressures.

MEMORY CHECK—Cont'd

- Other factors involved in the mechanics of breathing include alveolar *surface tension*, elasticity of the lungs and chest wall, and resistance to airflow through the conducting airways. Surface tension occurs at any gas-liquid interface and is the tendency for liquid molecules exposed to air to adhere to one another. This phenomenon decreases the surface area exposed to the air. According to the law of Laplace, the pressure (P) required to inflate a sphere is equal to 2 times the surface tension (T) divided by the radius (r) of the sphere, or $P = 2T/r$. *As the surface tension increases and the radius of the sphere or alveolus becomes smaller, more pressure is required to inflate it.*
- *Surfactant* in the alveoli has a detergent-like effect that separates the liquid molecules, thus *decreasing alveolar surface tension.* Surfactant reverses the law of Laplace. The alveoli are much easier to inflate at low lung volumes after expiration than at high volumes after inspiration. The decrease in the surface tension caused by surfactant also is responsible for keeping the alveoli free of fluid. *In the absence of surfactant, the surface tension tends to attract fluid into the alveoli.*
- The lung and chest wall have elastic properties that permit expansion during inspiration and relaxation to original dimension during expiration. *During inspiration*, the diaphragm and intercostal muscles contract, air flows into the lungs, and the *chest wall expands*. Muscular effort is needed to overcome the resistance of the lungs to expansion. *During expiration*, the muscles relax, and the elastic recoil of the lungs causes the *thorax to decrease in volume* until the chest wall and lung recoil forces are balanced.
- Compliance is the measure of lung and chest wall *distensibility*. It represents the relative ease with which these structures can be stretched. Compliance is, therefore, the reciprocal of elasticity. An *increase in compliance* indicates that the lungs or chest wall is abnormally *easy to inflate* and has lost some elastic recoil. A *decrease* indicates that the lungs or chest wall is abnormally stiff or *difficult to inflate.*
- Airway resistance is determined by the length, radius, and cross-sectional area of the airways and density, viscosity, and velocity of the gas. Resistance (R) is computed by dividing change in pressure (P) by rate of flow (F), or $R = P/E$. Resistance is inversely proportional to the fourth power of the radius; thus, *anything that decreases the radius of the airways increases airway resistance.*

LEARNING OBJECTIVES

After studying this chapter, the learner will be able to do the following:

1. Define the terms used in describing the signs and symptoms of pulmonary disease.
Study pages 679-681; refer to Figure 26-1.

Dyspnea is the subjective sensation of uncomfortable breathing. It is often described as breathlessness, air hunger, shortness of breath, or *labored breathing*. Dyspnea occurs if increased airway resistance or decreased compliance causes respiratory effort greater than appropriate for the ventilation achieved. The signs of dyspnea include flaring of the nostrils, use of accessory muscles of respiration, and retraction of the intercostal spaces. *Paroxysmal nocturnal dyspnea* occurs in individuals with left ventricular failure who wake up at night gasping for air and have to sit up or stand to relieve the dyspnea. This dyspnea results from redistribution of body water into the lungs while the individual is recumbent. *Orthopnea* is experienced in the horizontal position.

Coughing is a protective reflex that cleanses the lower airways by an *explosive expiration* that removes inhaled particles, accumulated mucus, or foreign bodies. Stimulation of the irritant receptors in the airway initiates the cough.

Hemoptysis is *coughing up blood* or bloody secretions. It indicates that a localized infection or inflammation has damaged the bronchi or the lung parenchyma.

An **abnormal sputum** occurs with different pulmonary disorders. Changes in the amount and consistency of sputum provide information about the progression of disease and the effectiveness of therapy.

Hypoventilation is inadequate alveolar ventilation in relation to metabolic demands. It is caused by alterations in pulmonary mechanics or in the neurologic control of breathing. With hypoventilation, CO_2 removal does not keep up with production, and CO_2 rises in the blood, causing ***hypercapnia***.

Hyperventilation is alveolar ventilation that exceeds metabolic demands. The lungs remove CO_2 at a faster rate than it is produced, resulting in *hypocapnia* or low levels of CO_2 in the blood.

Strenuous exercise or metabolic acidosis induces **Kussmaul respiration** or **hyperpnea.** Kussmaul respiration is characterized by a slightly increased ventilatory rate, effortless tidal volumes, and no *expiratory pause*.

Cheyne-Stokes respirations are characterized by *alternating periods of deep and shallow breathing.* Apnea, cessation of breathing lasting from 15 seconds to 60 seconds, is followed by increased ventilation, after which ventilation decreases again to apnea. Cheyne-Stokes respirations occur in any condition that slows either the blood flow to the brain stem or impulses to the respiratory centers of the brain stem.

Cyanosis is a *bluish discoloration* of the skin and mucous membranes caused by increasing amounts of desaturated or reduced hemoglobin in the blood. Cyanosis can result from decreased arterial oxygenation or decreased cardiac output.

Clubbing is the selective *bulbous enlargement of the end of a finger or toe*. Its pathogenesis is unknown, but it is associated with diseases that interfere with oxygenation and cause long-term *hypoxia*.

Pain is caused by pulmonary disorders that originate in the *pleurae, airways, or chest wall.* Infection and inflammation of the parietal pleura cause pain when the pleura stretches during inspiration. Pain that is pronounced after coughing occurs in individuals with infection and inflammation of the trachea or bronchi. Pain in the chest wall occurs with excessive coughing, which makes the muscles sore.

2. Characterize lung conditions caused by pulmonary disease or injury.

Study pages 681-687; refer to Figures 26-2 through 26-6 and Table 26-1.

Conditions Caused by Pulmonary Disease or Injury

Condition	Pathology	Cause
Oxygen and Carbon Dioxide Tension		
Hypercapnia	Increased carbon dioxide in arterial blood	Drug depression of respiratory center, infections of CNS, or trauma to the medulla; spinal cord disruption or poliomyelitis; neuromuscular junction disease, as in myasthenia gravis or muscular dystrophy affecting respiratory muscles; thorax cage abnormalities; airway obstruction; emphysema due to physiologic dead space
Hypoxemia	Reduced oxygenation of arterial blood	Decreased oxygen content of inspired gas, hypoventilation diffusion abnormalities in emphysema, abnormal ventilation/perfusion ratios in bronchitis, right-to-left shunts in RDS or atelectasis
Disorders of the Chest Wall and Pleura		
Chest wall restriction	Compromised ventilation, decreased tidal volume	Gross obesity, lateral bending and rotation of spine, arthritis of spine, depression of the sternum, neuromuscular disease
Flail chest	Compromised ventilation	Fracture of ribs or sternum
Pneumothorax	Air or gas in pleural space collapses the lung partially or totally	Rupture of pleura or chest wall or spontaneous rupture of pleura blebs
Pleural effusion	Transudative or exudative fluid in the pleural space collapses the lung partially or totally	Fluid from blood or lymphatic vessels from CHF, hypoproteinemia, infections or malignancies causing mast cell release of capillary permeability mediators, trauma that damages blood vessels
Empyema	Pus in pleural space	Bacterial pneumonia, surgical complications, tumor obstruction

Conditions Caused by Pulmonary Disease or Injury—Cont'd

Condition	Pathology	Cause
Restrictive Lung Disorders		
Aspiration	Passage of fluid and solids into lungs, obstruction of airway, localized inflammation, noncompliant lungs, disrupted surfactant production, edema, collapse	Decreased levels of consciousness, CNS abnormalities
Atelectasis	Collapse of lung tissue	External pressure from tumor, fluid, or air in the pleural space; abdominal distention; bronchi obstruction; inhalation of concentrated oxygen or anesthetics
Bronchiectasis	Persistent abnormal dilation of bronchi	Obstruction of airway, atelectasis, infection, cystic fibrosis, tuberculosis, weakness of bronchial wall
Bronchiolitis	Inflammatory obstruction of bronchioles	Chronic bronchitis, infection, inhalation of toxic gases
Bronchiolitis obliterans	Fibrotic process occludes airways and scars lungs	Same as for bronchiolitis; common after lung transplantation
Fibrosis	Fibrous or connective tissue in lung	Scar tissue following ARDS, tuberculosis, or inhalation of dust or asbestos
Toxic gas exposure	Inflammation of airways, alveolar and capillary damage, pulmonary edema	Inhalation of smoke, ammonia, hydrogen chloride, sulfur dioxide, chlorine, phosgene, or nitrogen dioxide; prolonged high concentrations of oxygen
Pneumoconiosis	Fibrous tissue or nodules in lungs	Silicosis (inhalation of silica), anthracosis (inhalation of coal dust), asbestosis (inhalation of asbestos)
Allergic alveolitis	Lung inflammation or hypersensitivity pneumonitis	Inhalation of allergens—grains, silage, bird droppings, feathers, cork dust, animal pelts, molds, mushroom compost
Pulmonary edema	Excess water in lungs	Heart disease increases pulmonary capillary hydrostatic pressure, so fluid moves into interstitium; ARDS or inhalation of toxic gases injures capillaries and increases permeability; blockage of lymphatic vessels by CHF, edema, or tumors

ARDS, acute respiratory distress syndrome; CHF, congestive failure; CNS, central nervous system; RDS, respiratory distress syndrome.

3. In a diagrammatic scheme, interrelate the pathogenic factors in acute respiratory distress syndrome (ARDS).
Study pages 689 and 690; refer to Figure 26-7. (See diagram on next page.)

4. Compare and contrast the obstructive pulmonary diseases. (See table on page 193.)
Study pages 691, 692, 694, and 695; refer to Figures 26-8 through 26-12 and Table 26-2.

Obstructive pulmonary disease is characterized by *difficult expiration*. More force or the use of accessory muscles of expiration is required to expire a given volume of air. The most common obstructive diseases are asthma, chronic bronchitis, and emphysema. Because many individuals have both chronic bronchitis and emphysema, these diseases are grouped together and are called chronic obstructive pulmonary disease (COPD). Asthma is more acute and intermittent than COPD, but it also can be chronic and is included as a type of COPD.

Symptoms develop progressively: Dyspnea and hypoxemia → hyperventilation and respiratory alkalosis → decreased tissue perfusion → organ dysfunction → metabolic acidosis → increased breathing work → decreased tidal volume → hypoventilation → respiratory acidosis and worsening hypoxia → hypotension → decreased cardiac output → death.

ARDS Pathophysiology

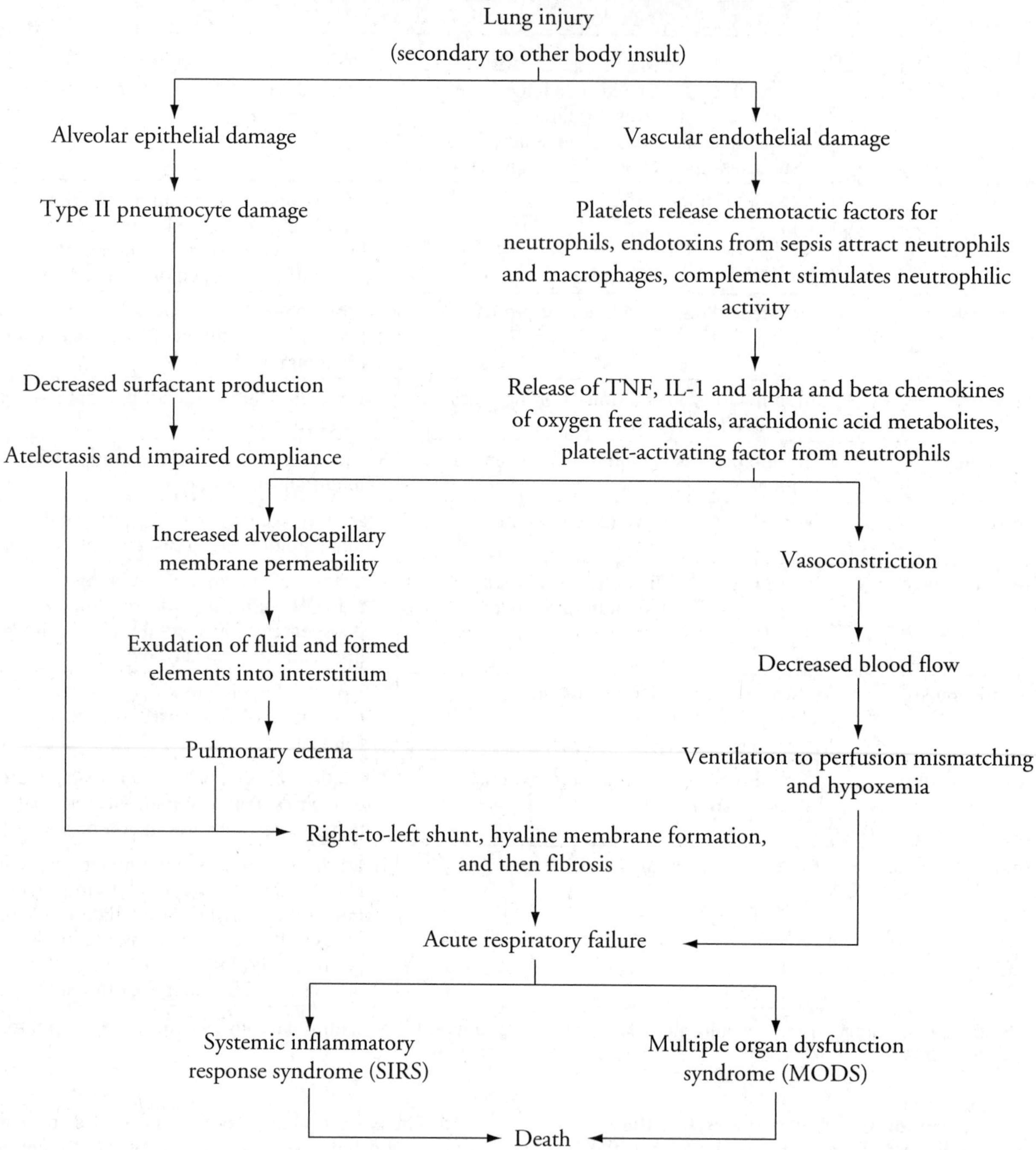

Obstructive Pulmonary Diseases

	Asthma	Emphysema	Chronic Bronchitis
Cause of airway obstruction	Bronchial inflammation, smooth muscle spasm mucosal edema, and increased production of thick mucus	Enlargement and destruction of alveoli, loss of elasticity, trapping of air during expiration	Inflammation and thickened mucous membrane, production of thick, tenacious mucus with pus
Precipitating causes and risk factors	Familial hyperresponsiveness to inflammatory mediators—allergens, histamine, interleukins, IgE, prostaglandins, and leukotrienes—leads to mucus and bronchoconstriction	α_1-antitrypsin deficiency, tobacco smoke	Tobacco smoke, air pollutants, infections
Manifestations	Dyspnea; wheezing; nonproductive cough early but later mucoid, prolonged expiration; tachycardia; tachypnea; acidosis	Marked dyspnea; no productive cough early but cough later with infection; tachypnea with prolonged expiration; accessory muscles used for ventilation; barrel chest; normal or elevated hematocrit; late cor pulmonale	Exercise intolerance, late dyspnea, wheezing, productive cough, chronic hypoventilation, polycythemia and cyanosis, cor pulmonale, CHF
Treatment	Inhaled antiinflammatory agents, inhaled corticosteroids, immune therapies for allergic individuals	Prophylactic antibiotics for acute infections, inhaled corticosteroids, cautious oxygen administration	Bronchodilators, expectorants, postural drainage, percussion, anti-inflammatory agents

Note: Acute bronchitis is an acute infection or inflammation of the bronchi following a viral infection and is usually self-limiting.

5. Describe pneumonia and describe its causes, manifestations, and treatment.
Study pages 695-698; refer to Figure 26-13.

Pneumonia is an acute infection of the lower respiratory tract or the lung caused by bacteria, bacteria-like microbes, fungi, viruses, protozoa, or parasites. Common infectious agents in **community-acquired pneumonia** include *Streptococcus pneumoniae, Mycoplasma pneumoniae, Haemophilus influenzae,* and *Legionella* species. *Pseudomonas aeruginosa, Staphylococcus aureus, Klebsiella pneumoniae, and Escherichia coli* are the most common etiologic agents in **nosocomial pneumonia**. **Immunocompromised individuals** are susceptible to *Pneumocystis jiroveci, Mycobacterium tuberculosis,* and fungal infections.

Pathogenic microorganisms can reach the lung by inspiration and through aspiration of oropharyngeal secretions. The lungs' defense mechanisms—namely, the cough reflex, mucociliary clearance, and phagocytosis by alveolar macrophages—normally prevent infection by pathogens. The body's immune system and various components of the inflammatory response further aid healthy individuals to prevent disease. In susceptible individuals, the invading pathogen is not contained. Instead, it multiplies, releases damaging *toxins,* and stimulates full-scale inflammatory and immune responses. Inflammation and edema cause the acinus and terminal bronchioles to fill with infectious debris and exudate; *ventilation-perfusion* abnormalities follow. If the pneumonia is caused by staphylococci or gram-negative bacteria, necrosis of lung parenchyma also may occur.

Most cases of bacterial pneumonia are preceded by an *upper respiratory viral infection.* Individuals then demonstrate fever, chills, productive or dry cough, malaise, pleural pain, and sometimes dyspnea and hemoptysis. The white blood cell count is usually elevated, but it may be low if the individual is debilitated. Chest radiographs reveal infiltrates that may involve a single lobe of the lung *(lobar pneumonia)* or may be more diffuse *(bronchopneumonia).*

Antibiotics are used to treat bacterial and mycoplasmal pneumonias. Viral pneumonia is treated with supportive therapy unless secondary bacterial infection is present. Adequate hydration, deep breathing, coughing, and chest physical therapy are important in treating all types of pneumonia.

6. Describe the pathogenesis of tuberculosis (TB).
Study page 698.

Tuberculosis is an infection caused by *Mycobacterium tuberculosis,* an acid-fast bacillus that usually affects the lungs but may invade other body systems. Individuals with AIDS are highly susceptible to respiratory infections, including tuberculosis. Tuberculosis is transmitted from person to person in airborne droplets. Once the bacilli are inspired into the lung, they multiply and cause nonspecific lung inflammation. Some bacilli migrate through the lymphatics and become lodged in the lymph nodes, where they encounter lymphocytes and initiate an immune response.

Neutrophils and alveolar macrophages wall off the colonies of bacilli and form a *granulomatous lesion* called a *tubercle*. Infected tissues within the tubercle die and form a cheeselike material; this is called *caseation necrosis*. Collagenous scar tissue then grows around the tubercle, which prevents further multiplication of bacilli.

Once the live bacilli are isolated in tubercles and immunity develops, tuberculosis may *remain dormant for life*. However, *if the immune system is impaired or if live bacilli escape* into the bronchi, active disease occurs and may spread through the blood and lymphatics to other organs. Endogenous reactivation of dormant bacilli in the elderly may be caused by poor nutritional status, insulin-dependent diabetes, long-term corticosteroid therapy, and renal failure.

In many infected individuals, tuberculosis is *asymptomatic.* In others, symptoms develop so gradually that they are not noticed until the disease is well advanced. Common clinical manifestations include fatigue, weight loss, lethargy, loss of appetite, and a low-grade fever that usually occurs in the afternoon. A cough with purulent sputum develops slowly and becomes more frequent after weeks or months. "Night sweats" and general anxiety are often present.

A *positive tuberculin skin response* indicates that an individual has been infected and has produced antibodies against the bacillus. Chest radiographs and culturing of the bacillus from the sputum aid in diagnosing tuberculosis.

Treatment consists of antibiotic therapy to control active tuberculosis or prevent reactivation of dormant tuberculosis and transmission of the disease. Today, with drug-resistant bacilli, the recommended treatment for persons at high risk is a combination of four drugs to which the organism is susceptible. Treatment continues until sputum cultures show that the active bacilli have been eliminated.

7. Compare and contrast pulmonary embolism, pulmonary hypertension, and cor pulmonale.
Study pages 699-701; refer to Figures 26-14 and 26-15.

Blood flow through the lungs can be disrupted by a number of disorders that occlude the vessels, increase pulmonary vascular resistance, or destroy the vascular bed. Major disruptive disorders include pulmonary embolism, pulmonary hypertension, and cor pulmonale. (See the following table on pulmonary vascular disease.)

Pulmonary Vascular Disease

	Embolism	Hypertension	Cor Pulmonale
Cause	Blood-borne substances or emboli from venous stasis, pulmonary vessel injury, or hypercoagulation lodge in a branch of pulmonary artery and obstruct blood flow	Pulmonary arterial pressure is elevated (> 25 mm Hg) by increased blood flow in pulmonary circulation, obstruction or constriction of vascular bed, or left heart failure	Right ventricular enlargement because of primary pulmonary disease and long-standing hypertension
Manifestations	Earlier evidence of deep venous thrombosis of legs or pelvis; tachypnea, tachycardia, dyspnea, chest pain, anxiety, hypoxemia, respiratory alkalosis	Fatigue, chest discomfort, tachypnea, dyspnea with exercise, jugular venous distention, accentuated second heart sound, a radiograph or electro-cardiogram that shows right ventricular hypertrophy	Chest pain; second heart sound or closure of pulmonic valve is accentuated; tricuspid valve murmur; radiograph and electrocardiogram show right ventricle enlargement
Treatment	Avoidance of venous stasis; anticoagulant therapy; fibrinolytic agent if life threatening; possible surgical thrombectomy; and warfarin or heparin for several months after stabilization	Supplemental oxygen, digitalis, and diuretics are supportive; prostacyclin analogs and endothelin-receptor antagonists; lung transplantation is therapeutic	Same as for pulmonary hypertension; success depends on reversal of underlying lung disease

8. Describe laryngeal cancer.
Study pages 701 and 702; refer to Figure 26-17.

The risk for **laryngeal cancer** is increased by, and related to, the amount of *tobacco* smoked; the risk heightens when smoking is combined with *alcohol* consumption. Carcinoma of the glottis is more common than that of the epiglottis, aryepiglottic folds, arytenoids, and false cords. Squamous cell carcinoma is the most common cell type.

Progressive hoarseness is the most significant symptom and can result in voice loss. Dyspnea is rare with supraglottic tumors, but can be severe in subglottic tumors. Laryngeal pain, or a sore throat, is likely with supraglottic lesions. Cough may occur after swallowing.

Combined chemotherapy and radiation have shown good results. Partial laryngectomy is used for glottis malignancies. Total laryngectomy is required when lesions are extensive and involve the cartilage.

9. Describe the major histologic types of lung cancer.
Review pages 702-704; refer to Figure 26-18 and Table 26-3.

Lung cancers or **bronchogenic carcinomas** arise from the bronchial epithelium. Lung cancer is divided into two categories: non–small cell lung carcinomas (NSCLCs), which constitute 75% to 85% of all lung cancers, and small cell lung cancers (SCLCs) or neuroendocrine tumors, which account for the other 15% to 20%.

The most common cause of lung cancer is tobacco smoking. Smokers with obstructive lung disease are at a greater risk. Other risk factors are *secondhand smoke,* occupational exposures to certain workplace toxins, radiation, and air pollution. Genetic risks include polymorphisms of the genes responsible for growth factor receptors, DNA repair.

Characteristics of Lung Cancer

Type; Frequency	Growth Rate	Speed of Metastasis and Site	Manifestations	Treatment
Non–small Cell Lung Carcinomas (NSCLCs)				
Adenocarcinoma; 35%-40%	Moderate	Early; to lymph nodes, pleura, bone, brain, and adrenal glands	Pleural effusion	Surgical treatment/ adjunctive chemotherapy
Squamous cell; 30%	Slow	Late; to hilar lymph nodes	Cough, sputum production, hemoptysis, airway obstruction	Surgical treatment/ adjunctive chemotherapy and irradiation
Large cell; 10%-15%	Rapid	Early and widespread	Pain, pleural effusion, cough, sputum production, hemoptysis; airway obstruction results in pneumonia	Surgical treatment
Small Cell Lung Cancers (SCLCs) or Neuroendocrine Tumors				
Small cell carcinoma; 20%-25%	Very rapid	Very early; to mediastinum, lymph nodes, brain, bone marrow	Airway obstruction, cough, chest pain, hemoptysis, wheezing, excessive adrenocorticotropic hormone (ACTH) secretion with its signs and symptoms	Chemotherapy and irradiation to lungs, central nervous system, and thorax

Note: The currently accepted system for the staging of lung cancer is the TNM classification. In this system, *T* denotes the extent of the primary tumor, *N* indicates the nodal involvement, and *M* describes the extent of metastasis.

PRACTICE EXAMINATION

Multiple Choice

Circle the correct answer for each question:

1. High altitudes may produce hypoxemia by:
   a. right-to-left shunts.
   b. hypoventilation.
   c. decreased oxygen inspiration.
   d. diffusion abnormalities.
   e. All of the above are correct.

2. In ARDS, increased alveolocapillary membrane permeability is caused by:
   a. platelet-activating factor (PAF).
   b. oxygen-free radicals.
   c. tumor necrosis factor (TNF).
   d. Both a and c are correct.
   e. a, b, and c are correct.

3. Type II pneumocyte damage causes:
   a. increased alveolocapillary permeability.
   b. chemotaxis for neutrophils.
   c. exudation of fluid from capillaries into interstitium.
   d. decreased surfactant production.
   e. All of the above are correct.

4. Pulmonary edema may be caused by abnormal:
   a. capillary hydrostatic pressure.
   b. capillary oncotic pressure.
   c. capillary permeability.
   d. Both a and c are correct.
   e. a, b, and c are correct.

5. In bronchial asthma:
   a. bronchial muscles contract.
   b. bronchial muscles relax.
   c. mucous secretions decrease.
   d. imbalances within the CNS develop.

6. Asthma is precipitated by which of the following inflammatory mediators? (More than one answer may be correct.)
   a. histamine
   b. prostaglandins
   c. leukotrienes
   d. neutrophilic infiltration

7. In emphysema:
   a. there is increased area for gaseous exchange.
   b. there are prolonged inspirations.
   c. the bronchioles are primarily involved.
   d. diaphragm movement is increased.
   e. None of the above is correct.

8. Chronic bronchitis: (More than one answer may be correct.)
   a. is caused by lack of surfactant.
   b. is caused by air pollutants.
   c. exhibits a productive cough.
   d. causes collapsed alveoli.

9. Which is *inconsistent* with pneumonia?
   a. chest pain, cough, and rales
   b. involves only interstitial lung tissue
   c. may be caused by mycoplasmas
   d. can be lobar pneumonia or bronchopneumonia

10. Tuberculosis: (More than one answer may be correct.)
    a. is caused by an aerobic bacillus.
    b. may affect other organs.
    c. involves a type III hypersensitivity.
    d. antibodies may be detected by a skin test.

11. Pulmonary emboli usually: (More than one answer may be correct.)
    a. obstruct blood supply to lung parenchyma.
    b. originate from thrombi in the legs.
    c. occlude pulmonary vein branches.
    d. occlude pulmonary artery branches.

12. Pulmonary hypertension:
    a. occurs when left arterial pressure is elevated.
    b. involves deep vein thrombosis.
    c. shows right ventricular hypertrophy on an electrocardiogram.
    d. Both a and c are correct.
    e. a, b, and c are correct.

13. Cor pulmonale:
    a. occurs in response to long-standing pulmonary hypertension.
    b. is right heart failure.
    c. is manifested by altered tricuspid and pulmonic valve sounds.
    d. Both b and c are correct.
    e. a, b, and c are correct.

14. A lung cancer characterized by many anaplastic figures and the production of hormones is most likely:
    a. squamous cell carcinoma.
    b. small cell carcinoma.
    c. large cell carcinoma.
    d. adenocarcinoma.
    e. bronchial adenoma.

15. The metastasis of lung squamous cell carcinoma is:
    a. late.
    b. very early and widespread.
    c. early.
    d. early and widespread.
    e. never seen.

Matching

Match the pulmonary condition with the characteristic or definition:

_______ 16. Kussmaul respiration
_______ 17. Hemoptysis
_______ 18. Cyanosis
_______ 19. Cheyne-Stokes respiration
_______ 20. Atelectasis
_______ 21. Bronchiectasis
_______ 22. Pneumoconiosis
_______ 23. Flail chest
_______ 24. Pneumothorax
_______ 25. Abscess

a. inadequate alveolar ventilation
b. ventilation exceeding metabolic demand
c. coughing blood or bloody secretions
d. abnormal dilation of bronchi
e. fibrous tissue or nodules in lungs
f. fractured ribs or sternum
g. increased ventilatory rate, effortless tidal volume, and no expiratory pause
h. decreased arterial oxygenation
i. alveolar collapse
j. pleural space air
k. pleural space pus
l. apnea, increased ventilations, then apnea again
m. circumscribed area of suppuration

Fill in the Blank

Complete the following table identifying the causes and pathogenic mechanisms leading to pulmonary edema:

Pathogenesis of Pulmonary Edema

Causes	Pathogenic Mechanism
Heart disease:	
Valvular dysfunction	
Left ventricular dysfunction	
Coronary artery disease	
Capillary endothelium injury	Increased capillary permeability and alveolar surfactant disruption, movement of fluid and plasma proteins from capillary to interstitial space and alveoli
Lymphatic vessel blockage	

CASE STUDY 1

A 19-year-old female college student presents to the emergency department complaining of chest tightness and dyspnea. She was cutting and trimming the lawn when these symptoms developed. Rhinorrhea and tearing began soon after she went outside and preceded the chest discomfort. Going inside did not relieve her symptoms.

During the physical examination, she said, "I have had asthma since childhood, and my mother and brother also have asthma." Her respiratory rate was 30 breaths per minute, and she exhibited the use of accessory muscles of respiration. Breath sounds were decreased, except for expiratory wheezes. Heart sounds were distant with tachycardia, but regular.

Identify appropriate laboratory tests. Indicate what therapies might be initiated. What worsening signs and symptoms may manifest?

CASE STUDY 2

Mr. S. is a retired 69-year-old county attorney who was on a buying trip with his wife looking for old, classic cars in the high, mountainous country of Colorado when he became extremely short of breath, much more than usual. His alarmed wife took him to a multispecialty medical clinic for evaluation.

Upon admission, Mr. S. was restless and dyspneic. His past history revealed a habit of smoking two packs of cigarettes a day for 45 years (90 pack years). During the past few years, Mr. S. noticed a cough each morning on arising. Recently, while working in his flower garden, he had to stop at times to catch his breath. He stated, "Even while I'm watching television, it is sometimes hard to breathe."

On examination, the anteroposterior diameter of his chest was enlarged, and upon percussion, his chest exhibited a hyperresonant sound. A chest radiograph was taken, and pulmonary function tests were done. The chest radiograph revealed a flat, low diaphragm with lung hyperinflation, but clear fields. Pulmonary function tests showed decreased tidal volume and vital capacity, increased total lung capacity, and prolonged forced expiratory volume.

Which pulmonary disease is exhibited by Mr. S.'s symptoms? Justify your answer.

27 Alterations of Pulmonary Function in Children

FOUNDATIONAL OBJECTIVES

a. Review Foundational Objectives a, b, and c of Chapter 26 and the following MEMORY CHECK! box.

> **MEMORY CHECK!**
>
> - Infants and young children have *fewer alveoli* than adults; their alveoli *are much smaller* and *less complex* than those of adults. The *small-diameter airways* of infants and children produce *increased resistance to airflow* and are *easily obstructed* by mucosal edema or secretions. The airways and chest walls of the infant are much less rigid than those of the adult. The flexible and compliant infant chest wall may actually flex inward, and the airways may collapse somewhat during times of respiratory stress, thereby limiting functional residual capacity. The premature infant may not have attained adequate *surfactant* production by the time of birth and will be unable to maintain *alveolar surface tension*. Children have greater metabolic rates and oxygen consumption than adults; respiratory distress, acidosis, and dehydration develop more easily in children than in adults. By virtue of their immature immune systems, children have many more respiratory infections than do adults.

LEARNING OBJECTIVES

After studying this chapter, the learner will be able to do the following:

1. Describe different forms of croup and epiglottis, and differentiate among upper airway infections.
Study pages 707-709; refer to Figures 27-1 through 27-4 and Table 27-1.

Croup or laryngotracheobronchitis is an acute upper airway infection generally caused by parainfluenza virus, but also by influenza A and respiratory syncytial virus (RSV). The affected age range is usually 6 months to 5 years, and recurrences are common. Airway obstruction occurs in the narrow subglottic region of the trachea, just below the vocal cords.

Spasmodic croup is characterized by barking cough and *stridor* (hoarse sound), but usually occurs in older children. It is of sudden onset and usually occurs at night without prodromal symptoms. Inflammatory edema of the upper trachea develops. The etiology is unknown, and croup usually resolves quickly. It has been associated with viruses, allergies, asthma, and *gastroesophageal reflux disease (GERD)*.

Bacterial laryngotracheitis is the most common potentially life-threatening upper airway infection in children. It is most often caused by *Staphylococcus aureus,* including methicillin-resistant strains, *Haemophilus influenzae*, and group A beta-hemolytic *Streptococcus*.

Classic symptoms of croup are rhinorrhea, sore throat, and low-grade fever that progress to a high-pitched seal-like barking cough and inspiratory *stridor* that is variable in intensity. Swelling of the subglottic tissues causes obstruction, and spasm of the vocal cords occurs as the inflammation extends. Treatment, when resolution does not occur within 24 to 48 hours, is with oral or injected glucocorticoids and inhaled epinephrine to temporarily decrease airway edema. The presence of stridor at rest requires hospital observation and treatment.

Acute epiglottitis is an acutely life-threatening emergency. The etiologic agent is usually *group A beta-hemolytic streptococcus*, because vaccination has decreased the incidence of *H. influenzae* infections. Children aged 2 to 7 years are affected. The affected swollen structures are the epiglottis and the very small glottic space.

Onset is rapid, and the child with epiglottitis is quite anxious and has a muffled voice. Severe respiratory stridor develops, and *the child is unable to swallow,* causing copious drooling. Treatment consists of establishing an emergency airway by intubation. Appropriate antibiotics are necessary to treat the underlying bacterial infection. Administering oxygen, aerosolized epinephrine, and nebulized glucocorticoids will relieve inflammation and obstruction, when required.

Tonsillar infections are occasionally severe enough to cause upper airway obstruction. *Tonsillitis is secondary to group A streptococcal infections.* Tonsillitis is a complication of infectious mononucleosis and may be complicated by abscess, which further obstructs the airway. Management of severe tonsillitis may require corticosteroids, antibiotics, or tonsillectomy.

2. Describe foreign body aspiration in infants and children.
Study pages 709 and 710.

Foreign body aspiration is common and often life threatening in children. Cough, hoarseness, stridor or wheezing, and dyspnea are common with any foreign body aspiration. Blockage of the larynx or trachea can be fatal. Lodged objects require endoscopic removal.

3. Describe obstructive sleep apnea (OSAS).
Study page 710.

OSAS is partial or complete upper airway obstruction during sleep, with disruption of normal ventilation and sleep patterns. Childhood OSAS is common, with an estimated prevalence of 2% to 13%. OSAS usually occurs in children with adenotonsillar hypertrophy, but also may occur in children who are obese or in whom craniofacial anomalies or neurologic disorders affect the airways. Allergies and asthma may contribute to OSAS.

There is usually a history of *snoring and labored breathing during sleep*, which may be continuous or intermittent. There may be episodes of increased respiratory effort but no audible airflow, often terminated by snorting, gasping, repositioning, or arousal. Daytime sleepiness is occasionally reported. Children are most often referred for tonsillectomy and adenoidectomy (T & A) on the basis of described symptoms and physical findings, such as enlarged tonsils, adenoidal facies, and mouth breathing.

4. Describe respiratory distress syndrome (RDS) of the newborn.
Study pages 710-712; refer to Figure 27-5.

RDS of the newborn consists of *inadequate surfactant* to reduce alveolar surface tension and *inadequate alveolar surface area* for gas exchange due to prematurity. The small, underdeveloped alveoli of the premature infant require high pressures to inflate the lungs. Absence of surfactant compounds this problem, and each breath the infant takes requires as much pressure as the first. Without surfactant, alveoli collapse at the end of each exhalation. Increased pulmonary vascular resistance causes shunting of the blood away from the lungs and results in a *right-to-left shunt*, further compounding the *hypoxia* and *hypercapnia*. Hypoxia and hypercapnia trigger *vasoconstriction* of the pulmonary vascular bed and exacerbate shunting. *Prolonged anaerobic metabolism produces metabolic acidosis.*

Tachypnea, expiratory grunting, intercostal and subcostal retractions, nasal flaring, and cyanosis are clinical manifestations. Treatment is supportive with cautious mechanical ventilation. Exogenous surfactant administration for low-birth weight infants has contributed significantly to the treatment of RDS. Antenatal treatment with glucocorticoids for women in preterm labor induces a significant acceleration of lung maturation and reduces the incidence of RDS.

5. Describe bronchopulmonary dysplasia (BPD).
Study pages 752 and 753; refer to Figure 27-6.

BPD is a severe form of lung damage associated with neonatal *chronic lung injury;* chronic, persistent lung disease follows the initial injury. *"New" BPD* results in poor alveolar architecture. The alveoli are *large and fewer in number*; thus, there is decreased surface area for gas exchange. Also, reduced growth of pulmonary capillaries to form alveolar units leads to *impaired gas exchange.* Risk factors include premature birth with immature lungs, mechanical ventilation toxicity, positive-pressure ventilation, respiratory infection, and ductus arteriosus. Clinically, the infants have hypoxemia and hypercapnia, intermittent bronchospasms, mucus plugging, and pulmonary hypertension.

BPD can cause death within a few weeks, or the child can live for months or years. Death occurs because of infection or respiratory failure. Treatment requires prolonged assisted gentle ventilation. Diuretics can control pulmonary edema.

6. Identify the most common etiologic agent in bronchiolitis; describe the pathophysiology and the usual clinical course of the disease.
Study pages 714 and 716.

Bronchiolitis is a lower respiratory tract infection caused most commonly by *respiratory syncytial virus* in infants, followed by adenoviruses, influenza, parainfluenza, and *Mycoplasma*. Rhinovirus appears to correlate with increased likelihood of asthma after children have experienced bronchiolitis. Viral infection causes necrosis of the bronchial epithelium and *destruction of ciliated epithelial cells.* The submucosa of the *bronchi becomes edematous and plugged* with mucus and cellular debris, and bronchospasm further narrows airways. *Atelectasis* occurs in some areas of the lungs and hyperinflation in others.

The usual manifestations in an infant are rhinorrhea, a tight cough, wheezing, chest retraction, and poor appetite or feeding. Treatment is primarily supportive; supplemental oxygen and increased hydration are used. Bronchodilators and steroids may benefit if underlying lung disease is present.

Bronchiolitis obliterans is *fibrotic obstruction of the respiratory bronchioles* and *alveolar ducts* secondary to inflammation. Most cases are associated with severe viral pulmonary infections; progression of disease is reflected by symptoms of severe airway obstruction. There is no specific treatment; anti-inflammatory agents can reduce airway inflammation and improve function. Some children deteriorate rapidly and die within weeks, whereas others have a chronic course.

7. Describe the most common etiologic agents of pneumonias in children.
Study pages 714-716; refer to Table 27-2.

Pneumonia involves inflammation and infection in the *terminal airways and alveoli.* The most common etiologic agents are viruses, followed by bacteria and *Mycoplasma*.

The *viral pneumonias* tend to occur in infancy and early childhood and are characterized by cough, fever, rhinorrhea, rales, wheezing, apnea, and *mild systemic symptoms*. RSV causes most viral pneumonias in infants. Treatment for viral pneumonia is palliative.

Bacterial pneumonias—due to *Streptococcus pneumoniae* (1 to 4 yr), *S. aureus* (1 wk to 2 yr), and group A beta-hemolytic streptococci (all ages)—tend to have *more dramatic systemic features,* causing high fever, productive cough, shaking, chills, pleuritic pain, and malaise. They are more lobar in nature than those caused by other infectious agents. *Mycoplasma* (an organism much like the one that causes pleuropneumonia in animals) and *Chlamydia* (specialized bacteria) cause *atypical pneumonia* in school-age children and adolescents and exhibit only upper respiratory tract involvement with low-grade fever and cough and require antibiotics therapy for resolution.

Aspiration pneumonitis is caused by inhalation of foreign substances, such as food, secretions, and environmental compounds, into the lungs. The severity of lung injury after an aspiration incident is determined by the *pH of the aspirated material,* the presence of pathogenic bacteria, and the volatility and viscosity of the substance. Very low or very high pH and low viscosity cause significant inflammatory response, whereas high-viscosity substances are less likely to cause a pneumonitis. Treatment generally includes antibiotics.

8. Describe the pathophysiologic processes, manifestations, and treatment of asthma.
Study pages 716 and 718; refer to Figure 27-7.

Asthma is a chronic illness of highly variable severity that tends to be punctuated with more or less frequent episodes of acute exacerbation. In children, asthma reflects a complex interaction between genetic susceptibility and environmental factors or triggers. In infants and toddlers younger than 2 years, the most common of these is RSV. In older children, the major viral trigger is rhinovirus. The pathophysiologic basis of asthma involves *hyperresponsive lower airways* responding in an obstructive manner to *various triggers*. The triggers include allergens, exercise, viruses, and other infectious agents. Responses include spasm of the respiratory smooth muscle that encircles the airways, edema of the airway mucosa, mucus plugging of the airways, and cellular infiltration into the airways. Asthma attacks have two phases. The early phase of the attack is caused by immunoglobulin E (IgE) mediation resulting from mast cell degranulation and histamine, leukotrienes, prostaglandins, platelet-activating factor, and certain cytokines released in response to the triggering factors. The late phase, which follows in 4 to 8 hours, is caused by inflammatory mediators released from the cells attracted to the airways. Epithelial and sensory damage occurs, causing bronchoconstriction. The typical abnormalities in acute asthma are hypoxemia, hypercapnia, and respiratory alkalosis; with severe airway obstruction and respiratory failure with acute CO_2 retention and respiratory acidosis occurs.

Clinical manifestations may include persistent cough, expiratory wheeze, and signs of respiratory distress. On physical examination, there is expiratory wheezing, which is described as high pitched and musical; the expiratory phase of the respiratory cycle is prolonged. The child may speak in clipped sentences or not at all because of dyspnea. Sometimes, hyperinflation (barrel chest) is visible.

Treatment involves the administration of adrenergic and bronchodilator aerosols and inhaled corticosteroids. For allergic asthma, hypersensitivity immune therapy may be appropriate.

9. Describe the pathogenesis of acute respiratory distress syndrome (ARDS) in children.
Study page 718; refer to Figure 27-5.

ARDS is the descriptor for the condition in children that results from a direct pulmonary insult or systemic insult that activates an inflammatory response causing alveolocapillary injury. Its pathogenesis is detailed in the flowchart presented in Chapter 26 for Learning Objective 3.

10. Describe the pulmonary pathophysiology associated with cystic fibrosis (CF), and identify general modes of diagnostic testing and therapy.
Study pages 718-720; refer to Figures 27-8 and 27-9.

CF is an *autosomal recessive*, genetically transmitted, *multisystem disease* in which exocrine or mucus-producing glands secrete abnormally thick mucus that obstructs the lungs and the gastrointestinal system. The CF gene has been located on chromosome 7. Its mutation results in the abnormal expression of the protein **cystic fibrosis transmembrane conductance regulator (CFTR)**, which is a chloride channel present on the surface of many types of epithelial cells. CF results from *defective epithelial chlorine ion transport,* whereby mucus is dehydrated and viscous because of defective chloride secretion and excess sodium absorption.

Although CF is a multiorgan disease, *respiratory failure* is almost always the cause of *death. Thick secretions obstruct the bronchioles* in the lungs and predispose the lungs to recurrent or chronic infection. Chronic inflammation, subsequent to the actions of interleukin-8 (IL-8), neutrophil attraction, and protease activity, leads to destruction of the airway walls and hyperplasia of goblet cells. Bronchiectasis, pneumonia, and widespread pulmonary fibrosis follow in response to bacterial colonization with *S. aureus* and *Pseudomonas aeruginosa*. End-stage disease is characterized by: (1) pulmonary hypertension, (2) chronic hypoxia, and (3) cor pulmonale. An obstructed gastrointestinal system leads to *malabsorption of nutrients* related to pancreatic insufficiency.

Chronic cough, wheeze, sputum production, and purulent mucus, as well as recurrent pneumonia, are common.

Labored ventilation results in hypoxia, finger clubbing, cyanosis, and barrel chest. Less frequent manifestations include chronic sinusitis, nasal polyps, and rectal prolapse.

Genetic testing is available to detect carriers. Sweat chloride testing is a definitive diagnostic test because it measures defective epithelial chloride ion transport. Treatment includes aggressive chest physiotherapy, bronchodilators, mucus liquefiers, and the judicious use of macrolide antibiotics to control infection.

11. Describe sudden infant death syndrome (SIDS).
Study pages 720 and 721.

SIDS refers to the *sudden, unexpected death of any infant or young child* in whom a postmortem examination fails to demonstrate a cause for death. The highest incidence is between 3 and 4 months of age; it mostly occurs during sleep, occurs more frequently during winter months, and is more common in males than females.

The cause of SIDS is unknown. A leading hypothesis is that a *developmental immaturity of ventilation and arousal responses to hypoxemia or hypercapnia is the etiologic basis* for this disorder. It has been associated with low birth weight, prone sleeping, and other environmental factors.

SIDS has no treatment because the death is sudden and unexplained. There is evidence that infants *should not be placed in the prone position* during the first 6 months of life and should not be laid down to sleep on top of any soft surface.

PRACTICE EXAMINATION

True/False

1. Inflammation above the epiglottis causes a barking cough.
2. Laryngotracheobronchitis is more severe than epiglottis.
3. Surfactant production accelerates airway luminal growth.
4. Failure to produce surfactant at birth results in severe atelectasis and RDS.
5. CF is a disease process caused primarily by hyperresponsive airways that are sensitive to certain environmental triggers.
6. Bronchiolitis and asthma produce similar symptoms.

Multiple Choice

Circle the correct answer for each question:

7. Epiglottitis is characterized by:
   a. gradual onset.
   b. severe stridor.
   c. drooling.
   d. All of the above are correct.
   e. Both b and c are correct.

8. Croup (laryngotracheobronchitis) is characterized by:
   a. mild to moderate stridor, which is often worse at night.
   b. antecedent "cold" symptoms.
   c. swelling of subglottic tissues.
   d. a barking cough.
   e. All of the above are correct.

9. The most common cause of bronchiolitis is:
   a. *H. influenzae.*
   b. exposure to allergens.
   c. parainfluenza virus.
   d. RSV.

10. Streptococcal pneumonia in children is acute and tends to occur in:
    a. the winter.
    b. the early spring.
    c. the fall months.
    d. the summer.
    e. any season.

11. Staphylococcal pneumonia in children has its highest incidence at age:
    a. 2 to 3 years.
    b. 1 to 4 years.
    c. 1 week to 2 years.
    d. 1 to 12 years.

12. Bronchiolitis:
    a. causes destruction of ciliated cells.
    b. can cause atelectasis.
    c. can cause hyperinflation.
    d. All of the above are correct.

13. All of the following statements about foreign body aspiration are true *except*:
    a. it is a relatively common occurrence in childhood.
    b. the offending objects include food and toys.
    c. it can cause pneumonia and atelectasis.
    d. it may cause pneumonias and lung abscess.
    e. Both b and c are correct.

14. Which statement is true concerning CF?
    a. It is a multisystem disease.
    b. A cloride secretion defect results in overproduction of viscous mucus.
    c. It is difficult to detect carriers through genetic testing.
    d. Infectious complications are common.
    e. a, b, and d are correct.

15. Which statement is true concerning asthma?
    a. Its triggers include allergy, viruses, and exercise.
    b. Once asymptomatic for a number of years, affected individuals may be assumed to be cured.
    c. It is characterized by hyperresponsive airways.
    d. Both a and c are correct.
    e. a, b, and c are correct.

16. Which statement is true concerning RDS of the newborn? There is:
    a. a right-to-left shunt.
    b. absence of surfactant.
    c. hypoxic vasoconstriction.
    d. All of the above are correct.

Matching

Match the characteristic or cause with the alteration:

_______ 17. Expiratory wheezing

_______ 18. Autosomal recessive disease

_______ 19. A right-to-left shunt

_______ 20. Adenotonsillar hypertrophy

_______ 21. Acute, life-threatening infection

_______ 22. Parainfluenza virus

_______ 23. Prone position increases incidence

_______ 24. Spasm of vocal cords occurs as inflammation intensifies

_______ 25. Inflammatory basis with hyperresponsive airways

a. asthma
b. CF
c. laryngotracheobronchitis
d. SIDS
e. epiglottitis
f. RDS
g. OSAS

Fill in the Blank

Complete the following table identifying common types of pneumonia in children:

Common Types of Childhood Pneumonia

Type	Causal Agent	Age
Viral pneumonia	RSV, influenza, adenovirus, others	Infants for RSV, all ages for others
Pneumococcal pneumonia	*Streptococcus pneumonia*	Usually 1-4 yr
Staphylococcal pneumonia		
Streptococcal pneumonia		
Mycoplasma and *Chlamydia* pneumonia		

CASE STUDY

Styler C., a 2-month-old boy, saw his physician 3 days earlier with a history of mild nasal congestion without fever, cough, vomiting, or other complaints. His parents stated, "We are just getting over terrible winter colds and hope we have not given them to Tyler."

Tyler has returned today because his mother is concerned that he is coughing severely, not feeding well at all, and "breathes funny." He still has no significant fever but is somewhat lethargic, with a high respiratory rate, moderate intercostal retractions, nasal flaring, and light expiratory wheeze. Tyler is admitted to the hospital for further treatment.

What do Tyler's signs and symptoms suggest, and what is causing his signs? Why is hospitalization necessary?

28 Structure and Function of the Renal and Urologic Systems

FOUNDATIONAL OBJECTIVES

After reviewing this chapter, the learner will be able to do the following:

1. **Identify the anatomic features of the kidneys.**
Review pages 724 and 726; refer to Figure 28-2.

2. **Describe the structure of the nephron.**
Review pages 726-728; refer to Figures 28-3 through 28-6.

3. **Identify the kidney's blood vessels; characterize the nephron's blood vessels.**
Review page 728; refer to Figures 28-5 and 28-8.

4. **Describe the ureters, bladder, and urethra.**
Review page 729; Refer to Figures 28-2 and 28-7.

5. **Describe the process of tubular reabsorption and tubular secretion; note the substances reabsorbed and secreted.**
Review pages 774 and 776; refer to Figure 28-10.

6. **Describe the process of glomerular filtration.**
Review pages 774-776; refer to Figures 28-10 and 28-11 and Table 28-1.

7. **Describe the purposes of the countercurrent exchange system; note the actions of diuretics.**
Review pages 776-778; refer to Figures 28-12 and 28-13 and Table 28-2.

8. **Identify the effects of hormones activated or synthesized by the kidney.**
Review pages 778-780.

9. **Distinguish between pediatric and adult renal function.**
Review page 738.

PRACTICE EXAMINATION

Multiple Choice

Circle the correct answer for each question:

1. Which sequence of structures does urine pass through as it leaves the body?

a. 2, 4, 6, 1, 3, 5	(1) ureter
b. 4, 2, 6, 1, 3, 5	(2) renal pelvis
c. 6, 4, 2, 1, 3, 5	(3) urinary bladder
d. 2, 6, 4, 5, 3, 1	(4) major calyx
e. 6, 4, 2, 5, 3, 1	(5) urethra
	(6) minor calyx

2. The functional unit of the human kidney is the:
a. nephron.
b. collecting tubule (duct).
c. major calyx.
d. minor calyx.
e. pyramid.

3. One unique feature of the renal blood circulation is that:
a. blood flows from arterioles into venules.
b. blood flows from venules into arterioles.
c. there is a double set of venules.
d. there are two sets of capillaries.

4. Which has the opposite effect on urine production from the others?
a. decreased solutes in blood
b. decreased blood pressure
c. increased ambient temperature
d. dehydration
e. reduced water consumption

5. The glomerular filtration rate is regulated by:
a. the autonomic nervous system.
b. the renin-angiotensin system.
c. atrial natriuretic factor.
d. All of the above are correct.
e. Both a and b are correct.

6. If the following hypothetical conditions exist in the nephron, what would be the net (effective) filtration pressure?
   Glomerular blood hydrostatic = 80 mm Hg
   Glomerular blood osmotic = 20 mm Hg
   Capsular hydrostatic = 30 mm Hg
   a. 40 mm Hg
   b. 30 mm Hg
   c. 20 mm Hg
   d. 10 mm Hg

7. The capillaries of the glomerulus differ from other capillary networks in the body because they:
   a. have a larger area of anastomosis.
   b. branch from and drain into arterioles.
   c. lack endothelium.
   d. force filtrate from the blood.

8. Which is *not* a function of the kidney?
   a. water volume control
   b. blood pressure control
   c. urine storage
   d. conversion of vitamin D to an active form

9. Potassium is secreted by the _____ and reabsorbed by the _____.
   a. Bowman capsule; loop of Henle
   b. proximal convoluted tubule; distal convoluted tubule
   c. loop of Henle; collecting ducts
   d. distal convoluted tubule; proximal convoluted tubule
   e. collecting ducts; loop of Henle

10. Antidiuretic hormone (ADH) causes water to:
    a. diffuse into the ascending limb of the vasa recta.
    b. return to the systemic circulation.
    c. be reabsorbed at the proximal tubule.
    d. Both a and b are correct.
    e. a, b, and c are correct.

11. Water reabsorbed from the glomerular filtrate initially enters (the):
    a. afferent arterioles.
    b. efferent arterioles.
    c. Bowman' capsule.
    d. glomerulus.
    e. vasa recta.

12. Plasma contains a much greater concentration of _____ than the glomerular filtrate.
    a. sodium
    b. protein
    c. urea
    d. creatinine

13. An increase in water permeability of the distal convoluted tubules and collection duct is the result of:
    a. a decrease in the production of ADH.
    b. an increase in production of ADH.
    c. a decrease in blood plasma osmolality.
    d. an increase in water content within tubular cells.
    e. None of the above is correct.

14. The descending loop of the nephron allows:
    a. sodium secretion.
    b. potassium secretion.
    c. hydrogen ion secretion.
    d. water reabsorption.

15. Which most accurately describes the pressures affecting net glomerular filtration?
    a. Blood osmotic pressure opposes capsular hydrostatic and blood hydrostatic pressures.
    b. Blood hydrostatic pressure opposes capsular hydrostatic and blood oncotic pressures.
    c. Capsular hydrostatic pressure opposes blood osmotic and blood hydrostatic pressures.
    d. None of the above is correct.

16. Tubular secretion of urea is accomplished in the:
    a. glomerulus.
    b. urethra.
    c. renal pelvis.
    d. distal convoluted tubule.
    e. None of the above is correct.

17. Tubular reabsorption and tubular secretion differ in that:
    a. secretion adds material to the filtrate; reabsorption removes materials from the filtrate.
    b. secretion is a passive process; reabsorption is an active transport process.
    c. reabsorption tends to increase urine volume; secretion tends to decrease urine volume.
    d. secretion adds materials to the blood; reabsorption removes materials from the blood.

18. The kidneys: (More than one answer may be correct.)
    a. conserve H^+.
    b. conserve NH_4^+.
    c. eliminate H^+.
    d. eliminate NH_4^+.
    e. conserve HCO_3^-.

19. If a small person excretes about 1 liter of urine during a 24-hour period, estimate the total amount of glomerular filtrate formed.
    a. 4 liters
    b. 10 liters
    c. 18 liters
    d. 100 liters

20. Which should *not* appear in the glomerular filtrate (in any significant quantity) just after the process of glomerular filtration has been accomplished?
   a. protein
   b. urea
   c. glucose
   d. Both a and b are correct.

21. The loop of Henle is to vasa recta as convoluted tubules are to:
   a. afferent arterioles.
   b. peritubular capillaries.
   c. efferent arterioles.
   d. renal arteries.

22. The two "currents" used in the countercurrent exchange system are the:
   a. afferent and efferent arterioles.
   b. glomerulus and glomerular (Bowman) capsule.
   c. ascending and descending limbs.
   d. proximal and distal tubules.
   e. All of the above are correct.

23. The countercurrent exchange system:
   a. prevents reabsorption of water from the collecting duct.
   b. concentrates sodium in the renal cortex.
   c. facilitates osmosis.
   d. concentrates chloride in the renal cortex.
   e. None of the above is correct.

24. Atrial natriuretic factor (ANF):
   a. increases ADH secretion.
   b. is produced by the kidney.
   c. increases urine output.
   d. decreases urine output.

25. A waste product of protein metabolism is:
   a. pepsinogen.
   b. trypsin.
   c. amino acid.
   d. urea.
   e. urine.

Fill in the Blank

Complete the following table identifying glomerular filtration pressures:

Glomerular Filtration Pressures

		Pressures (mm Hg)
Forces	Afferent arteriole	Efferent arteriole
Promoting filtration:		
Glomerular capillary hydrostatic pressure		45
Bowman capsule oncotic pressure		
Total	47	45
Opposing filtration:		
Bowman capsule hydrostatic pressure		
Glomerular capillary oncotic pressure		
Total	35	45
Net filtration pressure	12	0

29 Alterations of Renal and Urinary Tract Function

FOUNDATIONAL OBJECTIVES

a. Define the renal processes of filtration, reabsorption, and secretion.
Review pages 731-733; refer to Figure 28-10.

MEMORY CHECK!

- *Glomerular filtration* is the first step in urine formation in which permeable substances from the blood are filtered at the endothelial-capsular membrane into the Bowman capsule; the filtrate there enters the proximal convoluted tubule.
- *Tubular reabsorption* retains substances needed by the body, including water, glucose, sodium, potassium, and bicarbonate. This process removes materials from the filtrate and returns them to the blood.
- *Tubular secretion* excretes chemicals not needed by the body, including hydrogen and some amino acids, urea, creatinine, and some drugs. Secretion adds material to the filtrate from the blood.

b. Describe the effects of the renin-angiotensin system on renal blood pressure, blood volume, and blood flow.
Refer to Figure 28-9.

MEMORY CHECK!

EFFECTS OF RENIN-ANGIOTENSIN SYSTEM

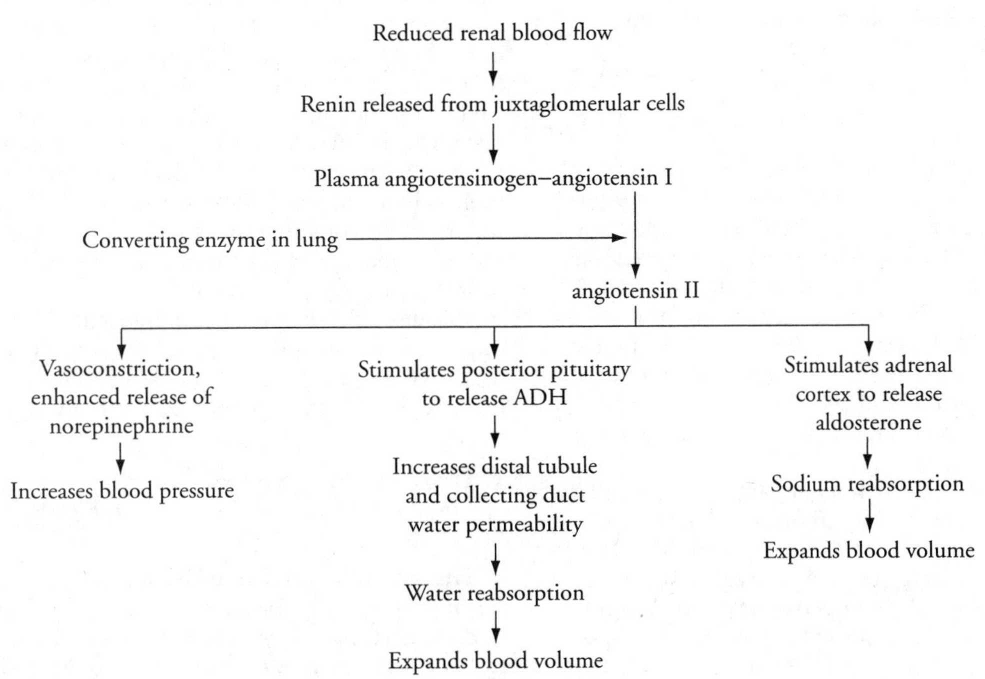

Atrial natriuretic peptide inhibits renin secretion; thus, decreasing blood volume and blood pressure.

c. **Explain the basis of serum and urinalysis examinations to evaluate renal function.**
Review pages 736 and 737; refer to Tables 28-3 and 28-4.

MEMORY CHECK!

LABORATORY TESTS FOR KIDNEY FUNCTION

- *Blood urea nitrogen (BUN)* measures the concentration of urea in the blood. Urea is formed from protein metabolism and is elevated in reduced glomerular filtration. Normal BUN is 10 mg/dL to 20 mg/dL. The BUN rises in states of dehydration and acute and chronic renal failure because passage of fluid through the tubules is slowed.
- The *serum creatinine* level should have a stable value because creatinine is a by-product of muscle metabolism and its levels of production are constant and are proportional to muscle mass. Normally, creatinine is not reabsorbed. A normal serum level, 0.7 mg/dL to 1.2 mg/dL indicates normal renal function. A rise in serum creatinine and its accumulation in the plasma represent decreasing glomerular filtration rate (GFR). If the serum creatinine value is doubled, renal function is probably 50% of normal; if the value is tripled, about 75% of renal function is lost.
- *Creatinine clearance* is the amount of blood theoretically "cleared" of creatinine by the kidney in 1 minute of filtration; 90 mL/min to 130 mL/min is normal. Creatinine clearance provides a good measure of renal blood flow and GFR because serum levels are related to a 24-hour urine volume. Inulin, a substance with a stable plasma concentration, can be used to assess clearance. The amount of inulin filtered is equal to the volume of plasma filtered multiplied by the plasma concentration of insulin.
- The *urinalysis* is an essential part of the examination of all individuals who may have renal disease because materials in the urine can be diagnostic for many disorders. It is normal to have inorganic material such as Na^+, Cl^-, and K^+ and organic materials such as urea and creatinine in the urine. It is abnormal to find red blood cells (RBCs), more than a few white blood cells (WBCs), bacteria, protein, glucose, and ketones in the urine.

LEARNING OBJECTIVES

After studying this chapter, the learner will be able to do the following:

1. **Describe the general anatomic and functional features of urinary tract obstruction.**
Study pages 741-744; refer to Figures 29-1 and 29-3 and Tables 29-1 and 29-2.

Urinary tract obstruction is defined as blockage of urine flow within the urinary tract. **Obstructive uropathy** is any anatomic or functional blockage that leads to urinary stasis, dilates the urinary system, increases the risk of infection, and generally compromises function.

Complete obstruction of the *upper urinary tract* causes dilation of the ureter *(hydroureter)* and of the renal pelvis and calyces *(hydronephrosis)*. Within days, tubulointerstitial fibrosis and apoptosis develop, and if these conditions are not relieved, irreversible renal damage occurs.

Persistent partial obstruction impairs the ability to concentrate urine, reabsorb bicarbonate, excrete ammonia, and regulate metabolic acid-base balance. The body is able to partially counteract the negative consequences of unilateral obstruction by **compensatory hypertrophy**. This hypertrophy results from obligatory growth under the influence of growth hormone and compensatory growth under the influence of yet unidentified hormones. The contralateral, unobstructed kidney consequently increases the size of individual glomeruli and tubules, but not the total number of nephrons.

Neurogenic bladder is a functional *lower urinary tract* obstruction caused by an *interruption of the nerve supply* to the bladder. Upper motor neuron lesions result in *hyperreflexive bladder* and uncoordinated contractions. Lower motor neuron lesions result in underactive, hypotonic, or atonic bladder function. *Overactive bladder* (OAB) is an uncontrollable or premature contraction resulting in urgency with or without incontinence, frequency, and nocturia. *Underactive bladder* (UAB) occurs when the duration or strength of contraction is inadequate to empty the bladder and results in distention and incontinence. Detrusor sphincter *dyssynergia* is failure of the urethrovesical junction smooth muscle to release urine during micturition and causes a functional obstruction.

Because of disordered neural sensation, symptoms are difficult to assess. Management involves catheterization, drugs, or surgery to relieve obstruction. Any infection must be treated with appropriate antibiotics.

2. **Describe kidney stones.**
Study pages 742 and 743; refer to Figure 29-2.

Kidney stones are caused by supersaturation of stone-forming substances, change in urine pH, or urinary tract infections (UTIs). *Calcium* is a common constituent of renal stones; about 80% of stones, or ***renal calculi,*** are composed of *calcium* oxalate, calcium phosphate, or a combination of the two. Another stone, the struvite stone (which makes up 15% of stones), is composed of magnesium and ammonium phosphate. Uric acid stones (which accounts for about 7% of stones) may be seen with gout. Cystine stones are rare.

A *colicky pain* occurs as the rhythmic contractions of the ureter attempt to dislodge and advance the sharp-edged stone. The accumulation of urine behind the stone causes infection or damage to organs. This consequence of obstruction depends on the location of the obstruction. If the *obstruction is high* and complete, *glomerular filtration* may be affected. The pain may be in the *flank* or between the last rib and the lumbar vertebrae, or it may radiate into the groin, depending on the stone's location. The pain may be accompanied by nausea and vomiting.

Treatment involves dilution of stone-forming substances by a high fluid intake, extraction of larger stones by endoscopy, and fragmentation of stones by ultrasonic lithotripsy. Some smaller stones may pass spontaneously.

3. Describe renal and bladder tumors.
Study pages 746 and 747; refer to Figure 29-4 and Tables 29-3 and 29-4.

Renal adenomas are benign and uncommon, but they may become malignant and are, therefore, usually removed surgically. **Renal cell carcinoma,** the most common renal neoplasm, usually occurs in men between the ages of 50 and 60 years. The tumors usually occur unilaterally and spread through the lymph nodes and blood vessels to the lungs, liver, and bones.

The manifestations are hematuria, flank pain, palpable flank mass, and weight loss. These *signs and symptoms* are infrequent; when they occur, they *indicate* an *advanced stage of disease.* Treatment is usually surgical removal of the affected kidney, combined with use of chemotherapy. Radiation therapy and biologic response modifiers may be useful.

Bladder tumors represent about 1% of all malignant tumors and are the fifth most common malignancy. The development of bladder cancer is most common in men older than 60 years. Transitional cell carcinoma is the most common bladder malignancy.

The risk of primary bladder cancer is greater among individuals who smoke or work in the chemical, rubber, and textile industry and among women who take large amounts of phenacetin (an analgesic). *Bladder cancer results* from a *genetic alteration* in normal bladder epithelium. Metastasis is usually to lymph nodes, liver, bones, and lungs. Secondary bladder cancer develops by invasion of cancer from bordering organs, such as cervical carcinoma in women and prostatic carcinoma in men.

Bladder tumors may be asymptomatic or accompanied by hematuria. Advanced cancers are associated with pelvic pain and *frequent* day or night *urination.* Treatment depends on the type and size of the lesion and involves transurethral resection, chemotherapy, or immunotherapy; radical cystectomy may be required for invasive tumors.

4. Identify the predisposing risk factors and the most likely pathogens responsible for UTIs.
Study page 747.

The most common route in the development of acute UTI is by an *ascending infection* and are complicated by abnormalities in the urinary tract. Common pathogens in these infections are the gram-negative rods, namely *Escherichia coli, Klebsiella, Staphylococcus saprophyticus, Proteus*, and *Pseudomonas*. Other possible infectious agents are gram-positive cocci, tubercular bacilli, and fungi.

5. Compare and contrast the signs, symptoms, and etiology of cystitis and pyelonephritis.
Study pages 747-750; refer to Figure 29-5 and Table 29-5.

Cystitis and Pyelonephritis

	Cystitis (Bladder)	Pyelonephritis (Kidney Tubules, Pelvis, and Interstitium)*
Location	Lower urinary tract	Upper urinary tract
Signs and symptoms	Low back or suprapubic pain, painful burning on urination, frequent voiding/urgency, hematuria, cloudy urine	Fever, chills, backache, abdominal pain, nausea, vomiting, urinary urgency and frequency, costovertebral tenderness, possible hypertension (HTN)
Etiology	Urinary obstruction, prostatitis, ascending infection with gram-negative rods ("honeymoon cystitis"), irritable bladder from sphincter dysfunction; interstitial "nonbacterial" cystitis is caused by an inflammatory autoimmune response	Inflammation or scarring of the interstitial tissue and tubules; causative organism is usually an ascending gram-negative rod but can be a fungus or virus; a risk factor is any urinary obstruction or infection that causes urine reflux or residual urine

*Acute pyelonephritis involves an infection that exhibits inflammation of the pelvis, calyces, and medulla. Chronic pyelonephritis is persistent or recurrent autoimmune infection usually associated with an obstructive pathologic condition; it can lead to renal failure.

6. Describe the types of glomerulonephritis, their features, manifestations, and treatment.
Study pages 750-753; refer to Figures 29-6 and 29-7 and Tables 29-6 through 29-8.

Glomerulonephritis is a group of diseases of the glomerulus that are caused by immune responses, toxins or drugs, vascular disorders, hepatitis, immune deficiency viruses, and other systemic diseases, including diabetes mellitus and systemic lupus erythematosus. Glomerular damage generally occurs from the activation and products of the biochemical mediators of inflammation, namely complement, leukocytes, and fibrin. Damage begins after *antibodies against glomerular basement membrane or antigen-antibody complexes* have localized in the glomerular capillary wall. Complement is deposited with the antibodies. *Complement* activation attracts neutrophils and monocytes. The neutrophils and monocytes further the inflammatory reaction by releasing *lysosomal enzymes* that damage glomerular walls and increase glomerular capillary wall permeability. Membrane damage can lead to platelet aggregation and degranulation wherein platelets release *vasoactive amines*. Changes in membrane permeability permit the passage of protein molecules and red blood cells into the urine, thereby causing proteinuria and *hematuria*. The *coagulation system* may also be activated, leading to fibrin deposition in Bowman capsule; this substance reduces renal blood flow and depresses glomerular filtration.

Depending on the cause, extent, and degree of damage to the glomerulus, increased or decreased filtration results. Mild proteinuria and hematuria occur during the early years of the disease. Later, after 10 or 20 years, renal insufficiency develops and is followed by nephrotic syndrome and an accelerated progression to end-stage renal failure.

The diagnosis of glomerular disease is confirmed by a urinalysis that shows: (1) hematuria with red blood cell casts and (2) proteinuria that exceeds 3 g to 5 g per day. The basic principles for the treatment of glomerulonephritis are related to treating the primary disease, preventing or minimizing immune responses, and correcting accompanying problems such as edema, HTN, and hyperlipidemia.

Common Types of Glomerulonephritis

Type	Features
Poststreptococcal (group A beta-hemolytic streptococci)	Diffuse; subepithelial deposits of immune immunoglobulin G (IgG) and complement complexes; phagocytic infiltration; occlusion of glomerular capillary blood flow; decreased glomerular filtration
Rapidly progressive or crescentic* (nonspecific response to glomerular injury)	Diffuse; accumulation of fibrin or cells proliferate into Bowman capsule to form crescents and occlude glomerular filtration; antiglomerular basement membrane antibodies damage tissue and lead to renal failure
Minimal change disease or lipoid nephrosis (usually idiopathic)	Diffuse fusion of epithelial processes; loss of negative charge in basement membrane and increased permeability lead to proteinuria and nephrotic syndrome
Focal glomerulosclerosis (usually idiopathic)	Pathology similar to that of minimal change disease
Membranous nephropathy (usually can be associated with systemic disease)	Diffuse thickening of glomerular capillary wall from deposits of antibody and idiopathic complement; increased permeability with proteinuria and nephrotic syndrome
Membranoproliferative (usually idiopathic, associated with activation of complement pathways)	Diffuse; mesangial cell proliferation; thickened basement membrane; subendothelial deposits of immune complex occlude glomerular capillary blood flow and decrease glomerular filtration
IgA nephropathy (usually idiopathic)†	Focal; some diffuse lesions; mesangial cell proliferation with IgA deposits; release of inflammatory mediators with crescent formation; sclerosis; interstitial fibrosis; decreased GFR

*Goodpasture syndrome is a type of crescentic glomerular nephritis associated with antibody formation against both pulmonary capillary and glomerular basement membrane.
†IgA nephropathy is the most common type of glomerulonephritis in developed countries, especially in Asia.
Note: Membranous, focal, and minimal change diseases are associated with nephrotic syndrome.

7. Identify and explain key features of nephrotic syndrome.
Study pages 753 and 754; refer to Table 29-9.

In **nephrotic syndrome,** there is increased glomerular permeability and *protein leakage* of 3.5 g or more in the urine per day across an injured glomerular filtration membrane. Genetic defects that affect the function and structure of the glomerular capillary wall can cause nephrotic syndrome. Systemic diseases implicated in secondary nephrotic syndrome include diabetes mellitus, amyloidosis, systemic lupus erythematosus, and Henoch-Schönlein purpura.

The key features of **nephrotic syndrome** are *proteinuria, edema, hypoalbuminemia, hyperlipidemia, lipiduria,* and *vitamin D deficiency*. Proteinuria occurs with protein leakage from the serum into the urine and excretion. In **nephritic syndrome,** immune injury to the glomerulus, *hematuria* occurs because the glomerular pore size is large enough to allow RBCs and protein to pass into the filtrate.

This process *reduces blood oncotic pressure;* water leaves the capillaries more easily, and tissue edema follows. The *edema is soft, pitting, and generalized.* Hypoalbuminemia develops as albumin leaks through the capillaries and depletes its serum level. Hyperlipidemia occurs as the liver responds to the hypoalbuminemia by synthesizing replacement albumin. While synthesizing albumin, the liver also synthesizes lipoproteins in large amounts; therefore, hyperlipidemia develops. As tubular cells that contain fat are sloughed into the urine, lipiduria can be seen. Also, free fat from hyperlipidemia leaks across the glomerulus. Hypocalcemia develops in response to loss of vitamin bound to circulatory globulin. Loss of protein immunoglobulins increases susceptibility to *infection* in nephrotic syndrome. Treatment involves a normal-protein, low-fat diet; salt restriction; diuretics; and steroids.

8. Define and identify the common etiologies for prerenal, intrarenal, and postrenal injuries.
Study pages 754-756; refer to Figure 29-8 and Tables 29-10 through 29-12.

Acute renal injury is the rapid deterioration of renal function with accompanying elevation of BUN and plasma creatinine; oliguria also develops. The etiology may be either *prerenal* (before the kidney) because of renal hypoperfusion, *intrarenal* (within the kidney) from renal functional impairment, or *postrenal* (after the kidney) following obstruction of urinary flow.

The diagnosis and degree of renal injury can be described by the acronym RIFLE. R = risk (GFR decreases 25%), I = injury (GFR decreases 50%), F =failure (GFR decreases 75%), L = loss, and E = end-stage kidney disease. The progression of injury with recovery of renal function occurs in three phases: initiation, maintenance, and recovery. The *initiation phase* is reduced profusion or toxicity in which injury is evolving. The *maintenance phase* is the period of established injury and dysfunction after the initial event has been resolved. It can last from weeks to months. During the *recovery phase,* the injury is repaired and normal function is reestablished. *Diuresis* is common in this phase and is accompanied by a decline in serum creatinine and urea concentrations and an increase in creatinine clearance.

The primary goal is to maintain life until renal function returns. Management involves correcting fluid and electrolyte imbalances, acid-base imbalances, treating infections, and providing nutrients.

Causes of Acute Renal Injury

Prerenal	Intrarenal	Postrenal
Hypovolemia	Prolonged renal ischemia	Ureteral obstructions
Hemorrhage, plasma volume deficit, water and electrolyte loss	Nephrotoxins	Edema, tumors, stones, clots
Hypotension	Glomerulopathies	Bladder outlet obstruction
Cardiac failure or shock, massive pulmonary emboli, interruption of renal artery flow	Intratubular obstructions or necrosis, bilateral pyelonephritis	Prostatic hyperplasia, urethral strictures, neurogenic bladder

9. Describe chronic renal injury; identify the systemic manifestations of uremia.
Study pages 756-761; refer to Figure 29-8 and Tables 29-13 through 29-15.

Symptoms and signs of **chronic kidney injury** usually do not develop until GFR and renal function *decline to 25% of normal.* Normal GFR is greater than 90 mL/min; with mild kidney damage, GFR is 60 mL/min-89 mL/min; with moderate kidney damage, 30 mL/min-59 mL/min; and with severe kidney damage, 15 mL/min-29 mL/min. The chronic alteration is primarily caused by loss of *nephron mass.* The disease is associated with HTN, diabetes mellitus, or intrinsic kidney disease.

Two factors, proteinuria and angiotension II, advance kidney disease. *Proteinuria* contributes to tubulointerstitial injury by accumulating in the interstitial space and activating mediators that promote progressive fibrosis. *Angiotension II* promotes glomerular HTN and hyperfiltration caused by efferent arteriolar vasoconstriction, and thus *systemic HTN*.

The **uremic state** is characterized by a decline in renal function and the accumulation of *toxins in the blood* and associated systemic manifestations identified in the following table. If the *lesions are tubular*, electrolyte imbalances, volume depletions, and metabolic acidosis occur. In *glomerular lesions*, hematuria and nephrotic syndrome develop.

Manifestations of Uremia

Skeletal	Cardiopulmonary	Integumentary	Hematologic
Bone demineralization	HTN	Pruritus	Anemia
	Congestive heart failure (CHF)	Pigmentation	Bleeding
	Stroke	Pallor	Infection
	Pericarditis		Suppressed immunity
	Pulmonary edema		
Metabolic	**Gastrointestinal**	**Neurologic**	**Reproductive**
Acidosis	Diarrhea	Fatigue	Infertility
Hyperuricemia	Nausea	Attention deficit	Decreased libido
Hypocalcemia	Vomiting	Irritability	Impotence
Hyperkalemia	Anorexia	Peripheral neuropathy	Amenorrhea
Hyperlipidemia	Urinous breath	Seizure	
		Stupor	
		Coma	

Note: If chronic renal failure cannot be managed with diet, diuretics, and fluid restriction, then dialysis or transplantation becomes necessary.

PRACTICE EXAMINATION

Multiple Choice

Circle the correct answer for each question:

1. Renal function tests include:
   a. the urinalysis.
   b. BUN and serum creatinine.
   c. SGOT/SGPT.
   d. Both a and b are correct.
   e. a, b, and c are correct.

2. Which substance is an abnormal constituent of urine?
   a. urea
   b. glucose
   c. sodium chloride
   d. creatinine

3. The presence of albumin in the urine would indicate probable damage to:
   a. glomeruli.
   b. renal columns.
   c. collecting tubules.
   d. pyramids.
   e. None of the above is correct.

4. Upper urinary tract obstruction:
   a. can cause hydroureter.
   b. increases the force of detrusor contraction.
   c. predisposes an individual to hypotension.
   d. increases postvoid residual volume.

5. Renal calculi may be composed of:
   a. calcium oxalate.
   b. uric acid.
   c. cholesterol.
   d. All of the above are correct.
   e. Both a and b are correct.

6. Which can be characteristic of ureteral stones?
   a. severe pain in the back
   b. severe pain in the abdomen
   c. nausea and vomiting
   d. All of the above are correct.
   e. Both a and c are correct.

7. Which are predisposing factors for acute UTIs? (More than one answer may be correct.)
   a. congenital deformities of the urinary tract
   b. the sex of the patient
   c. decreased urine flow
   d. increased urine flow
   e. increased fluid intake

8. A common cause of both pyelonephritis and cystitis is:
   a. urinary calculi.
   b. invading, ascending microorganisms, such as *E. coli*.
   c. allergic reactions.
   d. heavy metals.

9. Uremia causes:
   a. polycythemia.
   b. retention of metabolic acids.
   c. low plasma calcium levels.
   d. increased erythropoiesis.
   e. Both a and d are correct.

10. Pyelonephritis is: (More than one answer may be correct.)
    a. an inflammation and infection of the urinary bladder.
    b. characterized by fever, chills, and flank pain.
    c. characterized by pyuria, bacteriuria, and hematuria.
    d. more common in young women than in young men.

11. Which renal condition usually has a history of recent infection with beta-hemolytic streptococci?
    a. pyelonephritis
    b. chronic renal failure
    c. nephrosis
    d. glomerulonephritis
    e. calculi

12. Which statement is *not* true concerning glomerulonephritis?
    a. Significant damage to the kidneys occurs during the body's response to an infection.
    b. Fever and flank pain occur.
    c. Complement activation attracts neutrophils.
    d. It is characterized by hematuria, proteinuria, and the presence of casts.
    e. Approximately 90% of individuals experience chronic disease.

13. Nephrotic syndrome is associated with _____ to plasma ______.
    a. increased glomerular permeability; urea
    b. decreased glomerular permeability; proteins
    c. decreased glomerular permeability; tubular filtrate
    d. increased glomerular permeability; proteins

14. Causes of acute renal injury include:
    a. cholecystitis.
    b. stones and strictures in kidneys or ureters.
    c. heart failure leading to poor renal perfusion.
    d. Both b and c are correct.
    e. a, b, and c are correct.

15. Which describe(s) a patient in acute renal injury? (More than one answer may be correct.)
    a. elevated serum creatinine
    b. leukocytosis
    c. low BUN
    d. fever
    e. oliguria

16. Which is *not* a characteristic of chronic renal injury?
    a. hyperkalemia
    b. anuria
    c. anemia
    d. pruritus
    e. acidosis

17. Chronic renal injury:
    a. may result from HTN.
    b. is usually the result of chronic inflammation of the kidney.
    c. may be treated with dialysis or transplants.
    d. All of the above are correct.
    e. Both a and c are correct.

18. An individual has elevated blood concentrations of urea and creatinine because of complete calculi blockage of one ureter. This condition is referred to as:
    a. prerenal disease.
    b. intrarenal disease.
    c. postrenal disease.
    d. preeclampsia.
    e. hypercalcemia.

19. Nephrotoxins, such as antibiotics, may be responsible for:
    a. acute tubular necrosis.
    b. acute glomerulonephritis.
    c. pyelonephritis.
    d. cystitis.

20. Uremia, as seen in chronic renal injury, would include:
    a. metabolic acidosis.
    b. elevated BUN and creatinine.
    c. cardiovascular disturbances.
    d. All of the above are correct.

21. The earliest symptom of chronic renal injury is:
    a. pruritus.
    b. oliguria.
    c. polyuria.
    d. decreased BUN.

22. In chronic renal failure, tubulointerstitial disease leads to:
    a. sodium retention.
    b. sodium wasting.
    c. no significant changes in sodium levels.
    d. increased phosphate excretion.

Matching

Match the condition with its characteristic:

_______ 23. Goodpasture syndrome

_______ 24. Hypovolemia

_______ 25. Uremia

a. prerenal failure
b. postrenal failure
c. chronic glomerulonephritis
d. pulmonary capillary and glomerular basement membrane antibodies
e. pruritus

Fill in the Blank

Complete the following table identifying the manifestations and contributing factors of nephrotic syndrome:

Characteristics of Nephrotic Syndrome

Manifestations	Contributing Factors
Proteinuria	
Hypoalbuminemia	
Edema	Hypoalbuminemia, decreased plasma oncotic pressure, sodium and water retention, increased aldosterone and ADH secretion, nonresponsiveness to atrial natriuretic peptides
Hyperlipidemia	
Lipiduria	

CASE STUDY 1

Ms. J. is a 26-year-old woman married for 3 years who has just returned from an outdoor camping trip with her husband. She presents with symptoms of dysuria with a burning sensation, urgency to urinate, and frequent urination. She said, "I have had similar symptoms three times over the last 2 years." Her reason for coming to the office today was being awakened by pubic and low back discomfort two nights ago. Her temperature was 98.6° F, BP was 114/64, P was 68, and RR was 12. Other than a tender abdominal pelvic area, the findings were unremarkable.

Notable laboratory results from a dipstick urinalysis, microscopic examination, and urine culture were as follows: color was dark yellow; trace blood; no casts; and bacteria and WBCs were too numerous to count, especially *E. coli*.

Given the laboratory results, what are the possible diagnoses and the likely final diagnosis and treatment?

CASE STUDY 2

Mr. and Mrs. C. returned from a weekend of downhill skiing to find that their 9-year-old son, Eddie, had bloody urine. About 2 weeks earlier, they had spent a week skiing, during which time Eddie had a severe sore throat that was not treated because his teenage sitter did not take him to a physician.

Eddie was taken to his pediatrician where his mother stated, "He has had no energy or appetite for the past 10 days and has complained of back pain." His physical examination demonstrated a temperature of 101° F and a blood pressure of 140/102. Eddie's urinalysis showed blood, protein, and RBC casts with an elevated specific gravity. BUN and serum creatinine also were elevated.

What do you think is the likely cause of Eddie's symptoms and signs? What do you think the pediatrician will do?

30 Alterations of Renal and Urinary Tract Function in Children

FOUNDATIONAL OBJECTIVE

a. Describe fluid balance in children; explain the implications of imbalances.
Review page 730.

MEMORY CHECK!

- Infants and young children have both a larger ratio of body water to body weight than adults and *decreased ability to remove excess water and solutes*. Risk for metabolic acidosis is increased during the first few months of life because *mechanisms for excreting acid and retaining bicarbonate are immature*. Children have *limited ability to concentrate urine* because of higher renal blood flow and shorter tubular length. Fluid and electrolyte balance is sensitive to the slightest changes in any of these factors.

LEARNING OBJECTIVES

After studying this chapter, the learner will be able to do the following:

1. Describe the common congenital/structural anomalies that occur within the renal and urologic system.
Study pages 764-766; refer to Figures 30-1 through 30-3.

Structural defects range from minor, easily correctable anomalies to those that are incompatible with life. **Horseshoe kidney** is a single U-shaped kidney that develops from *fusion of the kidneys* as they descend from the midline. The kidney may be asymptomatic or associated with hydronephrosis, stone formation, or infection. **Hypospadias,** with or without chordae and its band of fibrous tissue that *deviates* or bows the *penis ventrally,* and **epispadias** result in the placement of the urethral meatus on the *dorsal surface of the penis.* Hypospadias, with the urethral meatus opening ventrally on the penis, is the more common penile defect, and it is usually easily corrected with surgery. Epispadias is a more complex problem because it *can extend into the bladder.* It has a lower incidence in girls than in boys. The urethral meatus is located ventrally in females and often has an accompanying cleft. This can also be surgically corrected, but requires a more involved intervention.

Exstrophy of the bladder is a defect wherein the bladder and associated urinary tract structures are *exposed to the surface of the body.* This defect involves the abdominal wall and the pubic bone. Three fourths of the defects are in males. This defect allows urine to leak from the ureters onto the abdominal wall, leading to excoriation of the skin and the persistent odor of urine. The exposed bladder mucosa becomes edematous, bleeds easily, and is painful. Surgical repair of both the bladder and the pelvic bone requires several stages, the first during the first few days of life. Neoplastic changes have been associated with exstrophy of the bladder.

Congenital urethral valves consist of thin membranes of tissue that *occlude the urethral lumen* and obstruct urinary flow in males. Another bladder outlet obstruction can be a polyp arising from the prostatic urethra that causes obstruction and impairs renal embryogenesis. Both must be resected early.

Ureteropelvic junction (UPJ) obstruction is a *blockage* at the point where the *renal pelvis transitions into the ureter.* It is the most common cause of hydronephrosis in the neonate. Any infection must be treated, and recurrent infections may require surgical repair.

Renal aplasia is the absence of one or both kidneys. A **hypoplastic kidney** may be small and functionally normal or underdeveloped and functionally abnormal. The bilateral form is a common cause of chronic renal failure. **Renal dysplasia** is associated with abnormal differentiation of the renal collecting system. **Polycystic kidney disease** is an autosomal *dominant inherited disorder* occurring in about 1 in 1000 live births. The affected kidney has large fluid-filled cysts of the tubules and collecting ducts. **Unilateral renal agenesis** occurs in approximately 1 in 1000 births and has little or no effect on function if one of the kidneys is normal. **Bilateral agenesis**, or *Potter syndrome,* is usually associated with other anomalies, including facial defects; affected infants rarely live more than a few hours.

2. Indicate glomerular disorders in children.
Study pages 766 and 767.

Glomerulonephritis and **nephrotic syndrome** in children have pathophysiologic mechanisms similar to those observed in adults. **Glomerulonephritis** is an inflammation of the glomeruli characterized by hematuria, edema, and hypertension. It is often immune mediated and follows upper respiratory tract infections caused by group A beta-hemolytic streptococci. Immunoglobulin A (IgA) nephropathy is characterized by deposition mainly of IgA in glomerular capillaries and mesangium. *Deposits of IgA cause immune injury to the glomerulus that is usually reversible.*

Nephrotic syndrome is a symptom complex characterized by proteinuria, hypoproteinemia, hyperlipidemia, and edema. Metabolic, biochemical, or physiochemical disturbances in the glomerular basement membrane lead to markedly increased permeability to protein. Greater susceptibility to infection is common.

3. Describe hemolytic-uremic syndrome, its pathophysiology, and its treatment.
Study pages 767 and 768.

Hemolytic-uremic syndrome is associated with a viral or bacterial illness. The antecedent infection, upper respiratory or gastrointestinal, causes endothelial injury to the glomerular arterioles. This event triggers the inflammatory cascade, resulting in platelet aggregation and fibrin clot formation that *narrows the arterioles. Anemia* results when *erythrocytes* and platelets *are damaged* while passing through *narrowed and inflamed glomerular arterioles* and are later removed by the spleen. This same thrombocyte and fibrin clot mechanism activates the fibrinolytic cascade that prompts the release of damaged platelets from the arterioles. The spleen also removes, these damaged platelets. Thrombocytopenia eventually results.

Classic symptoms of hemolytic-uremic syndrome are pallor, bruising or purpura, and oliguria that may be accompanied by fever, vomiting, bloody diarrhea, abdominal pain, and jaundice. Central nervous system involvement, seizures, and lethargy may be features of severe disease.

Treatment is supportive and includes transfusions of red blood cells and platelets to treat the anemia and thrombocytopenia. Dialysis may be needed to regulate fluids and electrolytes until renal function returns to normal. Most children with this syndrome recover, but some experience renal failure.

4. Characterize childhood urinary tract infections (UTIs).
Study page 768.

UTIs are rare in newborns, and when they do occur, they are usually caused by bacteria from the *bloodstream* that settles in the *urinary tract.* UTIs in children are most common in 7- to 11-year girls as a result of perineal bacteria, especially *Escherichia coli*, ascending the urethra. Any abnormal urinary tract is particularly susceptible to infection. The bladder alone is infected in **cystitis.** The infection ascends to one or both kidneys in **pyelonephritis.** Urinary tract anomalies must be surgically corrected to prevent frequent recurrent infections.

5. Identify the structural cause of vesicoureteral reflux, and explain the potential effects on renal function.
Study pages 768 and 769; refer to Figures 30-4 and 30-5.

Primary vesicoureteral reflux is caused by the congenital malpositioning of a ureter or ureters into the bladder that allows *retrograde urine* flow up the ureters. If the urine contains microorganisms and can reach the renal parenchyma, chronic infection and scarring may result. The combination of *reflux and infection* can cause pyelonephritis. This condition is classified by a grading system, with grade I reflux the mildest and grade V the most severe. **Secondary vesicoureteral reflux** occurs because an infection causes mucosal edema and interferes with the *antireflux mechanisms of the urinary tract.* It is also associated with malformations of the ureterovesical (UV) junction, increased intravesical pressures, or surgery of the UV junction.

Symptoms associated with vesicoureteral reflux include fever, recurrent UTIs, and poor feeding. Diagnosis is confirmed by a radiologic procedure that allows visualization of reflux during voiding. Treatment goals are to prevent infection and to protect and preserve renal function. Recurrent infection and grade V status are indications for surgical repair.

6. Characterize nephroblastoma (Wilms tumor).
Study pages 769 and 770; refer to Table 30-1.

Nephroblastoma, or **Wilms tumor**, is a rare embryonic tumor arising from undifferentiated mesoderm. The peak age of diagnosis is 2 to 3 years, with an incidence of approximately 500 cases yearly in the United States. Nephroblastoma may occur as a sporadic phenomenon, or it may be inherited. The inherited form is an *autosomal dominant* disorder, but is rare. The inactivation of the tumor suppressor gene *WT1* is likely. Other congenital genitourinary anomalies have been associated with nephroblastoma in 18% of children.

Children with nephroblastoma may be asymptomatic or may present with vague abdominal pain, hematuria, fever, or hypertension. Diagnosis is made by locating the tumor and assessing its site with radiologic procedures. Depending on the stage of the tumor, resection, chemotherapy, radiation therapy, or a combination of these modalities may be required.

7. Define primary and secondary incontinence; discuss their likely causes and common approaches to management.
Study pages 770 and 771; refer to Table 30-2.

Incontinence, or involuntary urination after voluntary bladder control should exist, can be classified in two categories; **primary incontinence** occurs when a child has never obtained continence, and **secondary incontinence** occurs when a child has had and then loses bladder control. Secondary incontinence is also termed acquired enuresis. The origin may be neurologic, anatomic, or functional. Diabetes that increases the normal urinary output and renal failure that impairs the kidney's concentrating ability may cause this disorder. Incontinence shows a *familial tendency. Psychological problems* have been related to incontinence in some cases and must be considered a legitimate cause in the absence of organic findings. *Incontinence may be associated with sleep apnea.*

Management depends on cause and may involve a combination of interventions, such as medication, limited fluid intake, behavior modification, alarms, and periodic awakening during sleep. Psychological counseling also may benefit the child and family.

PRACTICE EXAMINATION

True/False

1. Exstrophy of the bladder occurs because of birth trauma.
2. Vesicoureteral reflux is caused by a congenitally malpositioned entry of the ureter or ureters into the bladder.
3. Children are at no greater risk for fluid and electrolyte imbalances than adults.
4. Grade V vesicoureteral reflux can be medically managed.
5. Polycystic kidney disease is an autosomal dominant disorder.
6. Secondary enuresis occurs when the child has never been continent.

Multiple Choice

Circle the correct answer for each question:

7. Nephrotic syndrome in children manifests as:
   a. proteinuria.
   b. hyperlipidemia.
   c. lipiduria.
   d. All of the above are correct.
   e. None of the above is correct.
8. Poststreptococcal glomerulonephritis in children:
   a. is a noninfectious renal disease.
   b. causes hypotension.
   c. causes dehydration.
   d. Both b and c are correct.
9. Infants *cannot* concentrate urine because of:
   a. shorter tubular length.
   b. increased tubular weight.
   c. increased blood flow to the kidneys.
   d. Both a and c are correct.
   e. a, b, and c are correct.
10. Vesicoureteral reflux causes urine to _____ up the ureters and places the young child at risk for _____.
   a. retrograde; glomerulonephritis
   b. retrograde; nephrotic syndrome
   c. retrograde; pyelonephritis
   d. retrograde; cystitis
11. Which manifestation may be associated with vesicoureteral reflux?
   a. recurrent UTIs
   b. poor growth
   c. irritability
   d. Both a and b are correct.
   e. a, b, and c are correct.
12. Children are at risk for hemolytic uremic syndrome after:
   a. upper respiratory tract infection.
   b. vomiting or diarrhea.
   c. viral infections.
   d. All of the above are correct.
13. Organic causes of incontinence may include:
   a. congenital abnormalities of the urinary tract.
   b. a neurologic origin.
   c. diabetes insipidus.
   d. All of the above are correct.
14. Children with incontinence may be managed by:
   a. sleep interruption.
   b. psychotherapy.
   c. diet.
   d. All of the above are correct.
15. Which characterizes IgA nephropathy?
   a. no systemic immunologic disease
   b. Injury to the glomerulus is usually reversible.
   c. gross hematuria
   d. All of the above are correct.
   e. Both a and b are correct.
16. Identify the sequence of events in hemolytic uremic syndrome that cause anemia.

a. 1, 3, 4	(1) The damaged cells are removed from the circulation by the spleen.
b. 2, 4, 1	(2) The endothelial lining of the glomerular arterioles becomes swollen.
c. 3, 1, 2	(3) Narrowed vessels damage erythrocytes.
d. 2, 3, 1	(4) Split products of fibrin appear in the urine and serum.

17. Which factor influences the prognosis of a child with nephroblastoma?
    a. the child's height
    b. genetics
    c. stage
    d. congenital anomalies
    e. b, c, and d are correct.

18. What causes neonate bladder outlet obstruction?
    a. polyps arising from the prostatic urethra
    b. congenital urethral valves
    c. impaired renal embryogenesis
    d. Both b and c are correct.
    e. a, b, and c are correct.

Matching

Match the description with the structural abnormality:

_______ 19. Small, normally developed kidney

_______ 20. Facial anomalies

_______ 21. Urethral opening on the dorsal surface of the penis; a cleft along the ventral urethra in girls

_______ 22. Results from abnormal differentiation of renal tissue

_______ 23. Bladder mucosa exposed through a fissure in the abdominal wall

_______ 24. Urethral meatus opening on the ventral side of the penis

_______ 25. Obstruction of the renal collection system

a. hypospadias
b. epispadias
c. bladder exstrophy
d. hypoplastic kidney
e. renal dysplasia
f. bilateral agenesis

Fill in the Blank

Complete the following table describing childhood urinary structural abnormalities:

Childhood Urinary Structural Abnormalities

Type	Characteristics
Hypospadias	
Epispadias and exstrophy of the bladder	
Bladder outlet obstruction	
Ureteropelvic junction disorder	
Hypoplastic/dysplastic kidney	
Renal agenesis	
Polycystic kidneys	

CASE STUDY

A 3-year-old girl is brought to the emergency department of a local hospital because she has bloody stools. Her mother says, "She had diarrhea and vomiting 2 weeks ago after a weekend of outdoor camping." The parents believe their daughter has been well since the gastrointestinal illness, until yesterday when bloody stools began. They indicated that she has not urinated at all today. Her physical assessment reveals pallor and bruising. A urine collection bag is placed on the child; however, she does not void while in the emergency department. A complete blood count reveals low Hgb, Hct, and platelet count.

From the laboratory values, what diagnosis is likely? What treatment will the girl require?

31 Structure and Function of the Reproductive Systems

FOUNDATIONAL OBJECTIVES

After reviewing this chapter, the learner will be able to do the following:

1. **Describe the hormonal stimulation of the reproductive systems; note the characteristics of puberty.**
   Review pages 774-777; refer to Figures 31-1 through 31-3 and Table 31-1.

2. **Describe female external and internal genitalia; identify the female sex hormones and their effects.**
   Review pages 777-780 and 782-784; refer to Figures 31-4 through 31-8 and Table 31-1.

3. **Describe the phases of the menstrual cycle, noting its differential hormonal effects.**
   Review pages 784-787; refer to Figure 31-9 and Tables 31-2 and 31-3.

4. **Characterize the structure of female breast tissue and its cyclical hormones; describe breast lymphatic drainage.**
   Review pages 787-789; refer to Figures 31-10 and 31-11.

5. **Identify male external and internal genitalia.**
   Review pages 789-792; refer to Figures 31-12 through 31-16.

6. **Describe spermatogenesis and the effects of male sex hormones.**
   Review pages 792 and 793; refer to Figures 31-17 and 31-18.

7. **Identify changes in the female and male reproductive systems that occur with advancing age.**
   Review pages 794 and 795; refer to Figure 31-19.

PRACTICE EXAMINATION

Multiple Choice

Circle the correct answer for each question:

1. Gonadotropin-releasing hormone (GnRH) reaches the anterior pituitary gland and causes the release of which of the following? (More than one answer may be correct.)
   a. growth hormone (GH)
   b. follicle-stimulating hormone (FSH)
   c. antidiuretic hormone (ADH)
   d. luteinizing hormone (LH)
   e. oxytocin

2. Which is *not* a structure of the female external genitalia?
   a. vagina
   b. clitoris
   c. vestibule
   d. labia minora
   e. labia majora

3. A new menstrual cycle involves a rise in the levels of:
   a. LH.
   b. GH.
   c. estrogen.
   d. progesterone.
   e. FSH.

4. Progesterone:
   a. stimulates lactation.
   b. increases uterine tube motility.
   c. thins the endometrium.
   d. maintains the thickened endometrium.
   e. causes ovulation.

5. The ovaries produce:
   a. ova, estrogen, and oxytocin.
   b. ova only.
   c. ova and estrogen.
   d. testosterone and semen.
   e. None of the above is correct.

6. During which days of the menstrual cycle does the endometrium achieve maximum development?
   a. 2 to 6
   b. 7 to 12
   c. 14
   d. 20 to 24
   e. 26 to 28

7. Hormones necessary for the growth and development of female breasts are:
   a. estrogens and progesterone.
   b. oxytocin and ADH.
   c. androgens and steroids.
   d. gonadocorticoids.
   e. relaxin.

8. The structure that releases a mature ovum is the:
   a. corpus albicans.
   b. graafian follicle.
   c. primary follicle.
   d. corpus luteum.
   e. infundibulum.

9. A major duct of the female reproductive system is the:
   a. suspensory tube.
   b. uterosacral duct.
   c. broad duct.
   d. mesovarian duct.
   e. uterine tube.

10. Prostate is to the accessory gland as gonad is to the:
    a. ejaculatory duct.
    b. ovary.
    c. bulbourethral gland.
    d. accessory gland.
    e. urethra.

11. Cells that produce testosterone are called:
    a. interstitial endocrinocytes.
    b. testicular endocrine cells.
    c. sustentacular cells.
    d. spermatogonia.
    e. None of the above is correct.

12. The function of testosterone consists of:
    a. development of male gonads.
    b. bone and muscle growth.
    c. influencing sexual behavior.
    d. growth of testes.
    e. All of the above are correct.

13. Immediately after the sperm cells leave the ductus epididymis, they enter the:
    a. ejaculatory duct.
    b. ductus deferens.
    c. urethra.
    d. seminiferous tubules.
    e. None of the above is correct.

14. A substance produced in the reproductive system mainly by the bulbourethral glands is:
    a. fructose.
    b. HCl.
    c. mucus.
    d. an alkaline, viscous fluid.

15. Which structure(s) produce(s) a secretion that helps maintain the motility of spermatozoa? (More than one answer may be correct.)
    a. prostate
    b. penis
    c. Cowper (bulbourethral) glands
    d. interstitial tissues
    e. All of the above are correct.

16. Semen is:
    a. vaginal secretions needed to activate sperm.
    b. the product of the testes.
    c. the sperm and secretions of the seminal vesicles, prostate, and bulbourethral gland.
    d. responsible for engorgement of the erectile tissue in the penis.
    e. the secretion that causes ovulation in the female.

17. The vulva consists of the:
    a. labia majora and labia minora.
    b. clitoris.
    c. vaginal orifice.
    d. Both a and b are correct.
    e. a, b, and c are correct.

18. The major difference between female and male hormone production is:
    a. LH is without effect in the male.
    b. GnRH does not cause the release of FSH in the male.
    c. hormonal production is relatively constant in the male.
    d. Both a and b are correct.
    e. None of the above is correct.

19. The primary spermatocyte has:
    a. 46 chromosomes.
    b. the same number of chromosomes as a sperm.
    c. 23 chromosomes.
    d. a diploid number of chromosomes.
    e. Both a and d are correct.

20. During the follicular/proliferative phase of the menstrual cycle:
    a. vascularity of breast tissue increases.
    b. vascularity of breast tissue decreases.
    c. progesterone constricts the ducts.
    d. Both b and c are correct.

21. Most of the lymphatic drainage of the female breast occurs through the:
    a. axillary nodes.
    b. internal mammary nodes.
    c. subclavian nodes.
    d. brachial nodes.
    e. anterior pectoral nodes.

Matching

Match the aging reproductive changes with the term or response:

_______ 22. Primary follicles resist gonadotropin stimulation

_______ 23. Corpus luteum fails to develop

_______ 24. Less effective erection

_______ 25. First menstruation

a. menarche
b. premenopause
c. menopause
d. vasomotor flush
e. vasocongestive response
f. luteal/secretory phase
g. follicular/proliferative phase

Fill in the Blank

Complete the following table comparing the effects of estrogen and progesterone on female structures:

Effects of Estrogen and Progesterone

Structure	Estrogen Effects	Progesterone Effects
Breasts	Growth of ducts; promotes prolactin effects	Growth of lobules and alveoli; inhibits prolactin effects
Vaginal mucosa		
Cervical mucosa		
Fallopian tube		
Uterine muscle		
Endometrium	Stimulates growth, increases number of progesterone receptors	Activates glands and blood vessels, decreases number of estrogen receptors

32 Alterations of the Reproductive Systems, Including Sexually Transmitted Infections

FOUNDATIONAL OBJECTIVES

a. Identify the female and male reproductive structures.
Review pages 777-780, 782, 783, and 789-792.

MEMORY CHECK!

- The female *external genitalia* collectively are called the *vulva* and comprise the structures externally visible: the mons pubis, the labia majora, the labia minora, the clitoris, and the vestibule. The urethral meatus, the vaginal opening, and two sets of glands—Skene glands and Bartholin glands—open onto the vestibule. The *internal organs* of the female reproductive system are two ovaries, two fallopian tubes or uterine tubes, the uterus, and the vagina. The ovaries are the primary female reproductive organs. They are located on both sides of the uterus and are suspended and supported by ligaments.
- The fallopian tubes extend from the ovaries to the uterus and open into the uterine cavity, thus providing a direct communication between the peritoneal cavity and the uterine cavity. The uterus lies centrally in the pelvis and is divided structurally into the body, or corpus, and the cervix. The inner layer, the endometrium, consists of surface epithelium, glands, and connective tissue. The *endometrium is shed during menstruation*. At the lowest portion of the corpus is the internal os of the cervix. The external os is at the lower end of the cervix. The canal of the cervix provides a direct communication from the cavity of the uterine body through the internal os and the external os to the vagina.
- The vagina extends from the cervix of the uterus to the vaginal opening. Thus, there is continuous *communication from outside the body to the peritoneal cavity* through the reproductive system structures.
- The male reproductive structures are the penis; the testes in the scrotal sac; the duct system, which includes the epididymis, the vas deferens, the ejaculatory ducts, and the urethra; and the accessory glands, which include the seminal vesicles, the prostate, and the bulbourethral glands.
- The testes are divided internally into lobules that contain the seminiferous tubules and Leydig cells. *Sperm production takes place in the seminiferous tubules; Leydig cells secrete testosterone*. On the posterior portion of each testis is a coiled duct, the epididymis. The head of the epididymis is connected with the seminiferous tubule of the testis, and its tail is continuous with the vas deferens. The vas deferens is the excretory duct of the testis. It extends to the duct of the seminal vesicle and joins with it to form the ejaculatory duct. The ejaculatory duct joins *the urethra*, which *is the common passageway to outside the body for both sperm and urine*. The accessory glands communicate with the duct system. The prostate surrounds the neck of the bladder and the upper urethra. Its glandular ducts open into the urethra. The bulbourethral glands, or Cowper's glands, are located near the urethral meatus. The penis is composed of three elongated cylindrical masses of erectile tissue, which comprise the shaft of the penis. The inner, ventral mass is the corpus spongiosum, which contains the urethra. The two outer, dorsal, parallel masses are the corpus cavernosa. The distal end of the penis or the glans is covered by the prepuce, or foreskin.

b. Describe the relationships of hormones to the normal menstrual cycle.
Review pages 783 and 784; refer to Figure 31-9 and Tables 31-2 and 31-3.

MEMORY CHECK!

- The three phases of the menstrual cycle are *the follicular/proliferative phase, the luteal/secretory phase, and menstruation*. During menstruation, the functional layer of the *endometrium disintegrates* and is discharged through the vagina. Menstruation is followed by *the follicular/proliferative phase*. During this phase, the anterior pituitary gland secretes follicle-stimulating hormone *(FSH)*, which causes cells of the *endometrium to proliferate*. By the time the ovarian follicle is mature, the endometrial lining is restored. At this point, ovulation occurs.
- Ovulation marks the beginning of *the luteal/secretory phase* of the menstrual cycle. The ovarian follicle begins its transformation into a corpus luteum. Luteinizing hormone (LH) from the anterior pituitary stimulates the corpus luteum to secrete *progesterone*, which initiates the secretory phase of endometrial development. If conception occurs, the nutrient-laden endometrium is ready for implantation. If *conception* and *implantation do not occur*, the corpus luteum degenerates and ceases its production of progesterone and estrogen. Without progesterone or estrogen to maintain it, the endometrium enters the ischemic phase and *disintegrates*. Then, menstruation occurs, *marking the beginning of another cycle*.

c. Characterize the structure and development of the female breast.
Review pages 787-789; refer to Figures 31-10 and 31-11.

MEMORY CHECK!

- The female breast is composed of 15 to 20 pyramid-shaped lobes, which are separated and supported by Cooper ligaments. Each lobe contains 20 to 40 lobules, which subdivide into many functional units called acini. Each *acinus* is lined with a layer of *epithelial cells* capable of *secreting milk* and a layer of *subepithelial cells* capable of *contracting* to squeeze *milk from the acinus*. The acini empty into a network of lobular collecting ducts that reach the skin through openings in the nipple. The lobes and lobules are surrounded and separated by muscle strands and fatty connective tissue. An extensive capillary network surrounds the acini. *Lymphatic draining* of the breast occurs largely through the *axillary nodes*.
- The nipple is a pigmented, cylindrical structure that has multiple openings. The *areola* is the pigmented, circular area around the nipple. A number of sebaceous glands are located within the areola and aid in lubrication of the nipple during lactation. The nipple's smooth muscle is innervated by the sympathetic nervous system.
- During childhood, breast growth is latent, and growth of the nipple and areola keeps pace with body surface. At the onset of puberty in the female, *estrogen secretion stimulates mammary growth*. Full differentiation and development of breast tissue are mediated by a variety of hormones, including estrogen, progesterone, prolactin, growth hormone, thyroid hormone, insulin, and cortisol.
- During the reproductive years, the breast undergoes cyclic changes in response to *changes in* the levels of *estrogen and progesterone* associated with the menstrual cycle. Because the length of the menstrual cycle does not allow for complete regression of new cell growth, breast growth continues at a slow rate until approximately age 35 years. The number of acini increases with each cycle, so epithelial tissue proliferation is under the influence of hormones as long as secretion occurs.

LEARNING OBJECTIVES

After studying this chapter, the learner will be able to do the following:

1. Distinguish between delayed or absent and precocious puberty.
Study pages 799 and 800.

In 95% of cases of **delayed puberty**, hormonal levels are normal and the hypothalamic-pituitary-gonadal axis is intact, but maturation occurs slowly. **Precocious puberty** can be defined as sexual maturation before age 6 years in black girls or age 7 years in white girls and before 9 years in boys. The first sign of puberty in girls is breast development, which begins by age 13. Normally, boys tend to mature later than girls, around 14 to 15 years of age.

2. Distinguish among various menstrual disorders and their hormonal alterations or causes; identify manifestations of premenstrual syndrome (PMS).
Study pages 801-805; refer to Figures 32-1 through 32-3 and Tables 32-1 and 32-2 (See next page).

PMS is the cyclic recurrence in *the luteal phase* of the menstrual cycle of physical, psychologic, or behavioral changes distressing enough to impair interpersonal relationships or usual activities. It has been estimated that 5% to 10% of menstruating women have severe to disabling premenstrual symptoms, and 3% to 8% of these women have exaggerated feelings of depression with psychosocial impairment known as **premenstrual dysphoric disorder (PMDD)**. PMS/PMDD is believed to be the end result of *abnormal tissue response to the normal hormone changes of the menstrual cycle*. Fluctuating estrogen and progesterone levels may trigger this biologic response.

A predisposition to PMS runs in families and likely results from genetics or environmental factors. Some evidence supports a relationship between the severity and frequency of premenstrual symptoms and the presence of perfectionism, increased stress, poor nutrition, lack of exercise, low self-esteem, and history of sexual abuse or family conflict. Depression, anger, irritability, and fatigue have been reported as the most prominent and the most distressing symptoms; physical symptoms seem less prevalent and problematic.

Treatment for PMS is symptomatic. After a trial of nonpharmacologic therapies that include dietary changes, various medications, such as selective serotonin reuptake inhibitors, may be added to the treatment plan, even if their efficacy in the treatment of PMS is questionable.

Menstrual Disorders

Disorder	Alteration
Primary dysmenorrhea	Excessive endometrial prostaglandin F (PGF) production causes painful menstruation, increases myometrial contractions, and constricts blood
Secondary dysmenorrheal	Results from endometriosis, pelvic adhesions, uterine fibroids, and adenomyosis
Amenorrhea*	
Primary	Menarche failure; no menstruation by 14 years of age with no secondary sex characteristics or the absence of menstruation by 16 years of age regardless of the presence of secondary sex characteristics
Secondary	Menstruation ceases following menarche; anovulation
Dysfunctional uterine bleeding (DUB)	Progesterone deficiency or estrogen excess; an imbalance between progesterone and estrogen
Heavy or irregular bleeding caused by disturbance of menstrual cycle	Estrogen proliferates endometrium, whereas progesterone limits it; large mass of tissue is available for heavy, irregular bleeding
Polycystic ovarian syndrome (PCOS) DUB and amenorrhea	Related to hypertension, hyperinsulinemia, and dyslipidemia; leads to infertility, hirsutism, acne, endometrial hyperplasia, cardiovascular disease, and diabetes mellitus

*Causes of amenorrhea include altered gonadotropin levels, altered ovarian hormone secretion, Turner syndrome, congenital and acquired central nervous system (CNS) defects, and anatomic malformations of the reproductive system.

3. Describe pelvic inflammatory disease (PID).
Study pages 805-807; refer to Figures 32-4 and 32-5.

PID is an acute inflammatory process caused by *infection*. PID involves organs of the upper genital tract, uterus, fallopian tubes or uterine tubes, or ovaries. In its most severe form, the entire peritoneal cavity may be involved. Infection of the fallopian tubes is **salpingitis;** infection of the ovaries is **oophoritis**. Most cases of PID are caused by sexually transmitted microorganisms that *ascend* from the vagina to the uterus, fallopian tubes, and ovaries.

PID is considered a *polymicrobial infection* with the majority of cases being caused by gonorrheal or chlamydial microbes, such as anaerobes and facultative organisms. These organisms may induce a response that causes necrosis with repeated infections and may predispose a woman to PID. After one episode of pelvic infection, 15% to 25% of women experience long-term *sequelae such as infertility, ectopic pregnancy, chronic pelvic pain, and pelvic adhesions*. The incidence of complications increases markedly with repeated infections.

The clinical manifestations of PID are variable. Subclinical infections occur in 67% to 75% of women with salpingitis. The first sign of the ascending infection may be the gradual onset of low bilateral abdominal pain often characterized as dull and steady. Symptoms are more likely to develop during or immediately after menstruation. The *pain of PID may worsen* with walking, jumping, or intercourse. Other manifestations of PID are difficult or painful urination and irregular bleeding. Treatment involves bed rest, avoidance of intercourse, and combined antibiotic therapy. Hospitalization is required in 25% to 40% of women with PID for intravenous administration of antibiotics and treatment of peritonitis or tubo-ovarian abscess.

4. Define and cite causes of vaginitis, cervicitis, vulvitis, and bartholinitis.
Study pages 807 and 808; refer to Figure 32-6.

Vaginitis is an infection of the vagina most often caused by sexually transmitted pathogens and *Candida albicans*. Because the acidic nature of vaginal secretions during the reproductive years provides protection against a variety of sexually transmitted pathogens, variables that alter the vaginal pH may predispose a woman to infection. The use of *antibiotics* may destroy *Lactobacillus acidophilus*, which helps maintain an acidic vaginal pH. Thus, there may be an *overgrowth* of *C. albicans*, which could cause a *yeast vaginitis*.

Cervicitis is an inflammation of the cervix usually caused by one or more sexually transmitted pathogens. If a mucopurulent exudate drains from the external os, the condition is *mucopurulent cervicitis*.

Vulvovestibulitis is an inflammation of the skin of the vulva and often of the perianal area. Vulvitis can be caused by contact with soaps, detergents, lotions, hygienic sprays, menstrual pads, perfumed toilet paper, nonabsorbent or tight-fitting clothes, or by candidal microbes.

Bartholinitis is an inflammation of one or both of the ducts that lead from the vaginal opening to the Bartholin glands. The causes of bartholinitis are microorganisms that infect the lower female reproductive tract; this disorder is usually preceded by cervicitis, vaginitis, or urethritis. Infection or trauma causes inflammatory changes that narrow the distal portion of the duct, leading to *obstruction and stasis of glandular secretions* and causing further inflammation.

5. Describe pelvic organ prolapse.
Study pages 808-810; refer to Figures 32-7 and 32-8 and Table 32-3.

The bladder, urethra, and rectum are supported by the endopelvic fascia and perineal muscles. This muscular and fascial tissue *loses tone and strength* with aging and may fail to maintain the pelvic organ in the proper position. Trauma, such as childbirth or pelvic surgery, damages or weakens the supporting structures.

Cystocele is descent of the bladder and the anterior vaginal wall *into the vaginal canal*. A cystocele may cause the woman to lose urine when she laughs, sneezes, coughs, or does anything that strains the abdominal muscles. Cystocele is usually accompanied by **urethrocele**, or *sagging of the urethra*. Urethrocele is usually caused by the shearing effect of the fetal head on the urethra during childbirth. A **rectocele** is the *bulging of the rectum and posterior vaginal wall into the vaginal canal*. Treatment includes isometric exercises to strengthen muscles; estrogens to improve tone and vascularity of fascial support; a pessary device to hold the uterus, bladder, and bowel in position; and possible surgery.

6. Characterize the benign growths and proliferative conditions of the female reproductive system; indicate treatments.
Study pages 810-813; refer to Figures 32-9 through 32-12.

Benign Lesions of the Female Reproductive System

Lesion	Cause	Manifestations	Treatment
Ovarian cysts			
Follicular cyst	Ovarian follicle fails to release ovum; fluid not reabsorbed from degenerating follicle	Pelvic and abdominal pain, bloatedness, menstrual irregularities	Usually regresses spontaneously
Corpus luteum cyst	A persistent corpus luteum secretes progesterone	Pelvic pain, amenorrhea with subsequent heavy bleeding	Usually regresses spontaneously
Endometrial polyps	Estrogen stimulation	Premenstrual or intermenstrual bleeding	Forceps removal
Leiomyomas (smooth tumors)	Unknown; hormonal fluctuations alter size	Abnormal or increased uterine bleeding, pain, pressure	Gonadotropin-releasing hormone (GnRH) agonist, oral contraceptives
Adenomyosis (endometrial tissue in the myometrium)	Repeated pregnancies	Dysmenorrhea, uterine enlargement and tenderness	Surgical resection

Benign Lesions of the Female Reproductive System—Cont'd

Lesion	Cause	Manifestations	Treatment
Endometriosis (endometrial tissue)	Depressed cytotoxic T cells tolerate ectopic tissues genetics	Ectopic tissue respond to hormonal stimulation bleeding causes pelvic adhesions and pain, infertility	Drug suppression of ovulation, laparoscopic removal of ectopic implants

Note: Dermoid cysts are ovarian teratomas having malignant potential and should be removed. Ovarian torsion may occur as a complication of ovarian cysts.

7. Characterize the malignant tumors of the female reproductive system; identify treatments.
Study pages 813 and 815-818; refer to Figures 32-13 through 32-16 and Tables 32-4 through 32-6.

Malignant Tumors of the Female Reproductive System

Tumor	Causes/Risk Factors	Manifestations	Treatment
Cervical cancer*	Sexually transmitted human papillomavirus (HPV), early sexual activity, multiple sex partners, smoking, poor nutrition	Asymptomatic; vaginal bleeding or discharge, grade of epithelial thickness enables precursor lesion diagnosis	Premalignant—cryosurgery, electrosurgery Invasive—hysterectomy, lymphadenectomy, chemotherapy, irradiation
Vaginal cancer	Previous cervical cancer, nonsteroidal estrogen exposure in utero	Asymptomatic; vaginal bleeding or discharge	Similar to that for cervical cancer
Vulvar cancer	HPV in younger women, vaginal or cervical dysplasia, smoking	Visible appearance	Surgery, irradiation, chemotherapy
Endometrial cancer	Obesity, high-fat diet, no pregnancies, late menopause, hypertension, diabetes	Vaginal bleeding	Curettage, hysterectomy, irradiation, chemotherapy, progestins
Ovarian cancer	Advancing age, family history, history of breast or colon cancer, frequency of ovulation	A silent—systemic manifestations, pain, and abdominal swelling; increased serum CA-125, postmenopausal bleeding	Surgery and staging, irradiation when small and confined lesion, chemotherapy when extensive

Note: Treatments for these malignancies depend on the clinical staging, the extent of metastasis, and the age of the individual. Each lesion can be managed by surgery, radiation, or chemotherapy; a combination of all these modalities may be necessary as well as lymphadenectomy.

8. Define terms used in female sexual dysfunction.
Study pages 818 and 819; refer to Table 32-7.

Inhibited sexual desire may be a biologic manifestation of depression, alcohol or other substance abuse, prolactin-secreting pituitary tumors, or testosterone deficiency. Beta-adrenergic blockers used for heart disease also may inhibit sexual desire.

Vaginismus is an involuntary muscle spasm in response to attempted penetration. Common causes include prior sexual trauma, fear of sex, and organic disorders.

Anorgasmia is the inability of the woman to reach or achieve orgasm. Drugs such as narcotics, tranquilizers, antidepressants, and antihypertensive medications can inhibit orgasm.

Dyspareunia, or painful intercourse, is common. Inadequate lubrication may make penetration or intercourse unpleasant. Drugs with a drying effect—such as antihistamines, certain tranquilizers, and marijuana—and disorders such as diabetes, vaginal infections, and estrogen deficiency can decrease lubrication. Other causes of dyspareunia include infections and anatomic constraints around the introitus or the vulva.

Infertility is the inability to conceive after 1 year of unprotected intercourse and affects approximately 15% of all couples. Important causes of infertility in the female are *malfunctions of the fallopian tubes,* the ovaries, and the *reproductive hormones,* and thyroid disease. *Endometriosis* also may contribute to infertility.

9. By site, describe common disorders of the male reproductive system.

Study pages 819-826; refer to Figures 32-17 through 32-32.

Urethritis is an inflammatory process usually caused by sexually transmitted microorganisms. Nonsexual origins of urethritis are inflammation or infection as a result of urologic procedures, insertion of foreign bodies into the urethra, anatomic abnormalities, and trauma.

Symptoms of urethritis include urethral tingling or itching or a burning sensation during urination. Frequency, urgency, and purulent or clear mucus-like discharge from the urethra may occur. Treatment is appropriate antibiotic therapy for infectious urethritis and avoidance of mechanical irritation.

Urethral stricture is a narrowing of the urethra because of *scarring*. The scars may be congenital, but are more likely to result from trauma or untreated or severe urethral infections.

Symptoms include urinary frequency and hesitancy, diminished force and size of the urinary stream, dribbling after voiding, and nocturia. Treatment is usually surgical and may involve urethral dilation, urethrotomy, or a variety of other surgical techniques.

Phimosis and **paraphimosis** are both disorders in which the penile foreskin, or prepuce, is "too tight" to be moved easily over the glans penis. In phimosis, the *foreskin cannot be retracted back over the glans;* in paraphimosis, the foreskin is retracted and *cannot be moved forward to cover the glans*. Phimosis can occur at any age and is most commonly caused by poor hygiene and chronic infection. Circumcision, if needed, is performed after infection has been eradicated. In paraphimosis, surgery must be performed to prevent necrosis of the glans due to constriction of blood vessels.

Peyronie disease is a *fibrotic condition that causes lateral curvature* of the penis during erection. The problem usually affects middle-aged men and is associated with painful erection, painful intercourse for both partners, and poor erection distal to the involved area. There is no definitive treatment for Peyronie disease. Spontaneous remissions occur about 50% of the time. Pharmacologic therapies that increase oxygenation may hasten resolution. Surgical resection of the fibrous plaque followed by grafting has been successful.

Balanitis is an inflammation of the glans penis and usually occurs in conjunction with an inflammation of the prepuce. *It is associated with poor hygiene* and phimosis. The accumulation under the foreskin of glandular secretions, sloughed epithelial cells, and *Mycobacterium smegmatis* can irritate the glans directly or lead to infection. Balanitis is most commonly seen in men with poorly controlled diabetes mellitus and candidiasis. Antimicrobials are used to treat infection, and circumcision can prevent recurrences.

Penile cancer is rare in the United States. Although the exact etiology is unknown, cancer of the penis is likely a result of chronic irritation caused by *smegma* beneath a phimotic foreskin.

Varicocele, hydrocele, and spermatocele are common intrascrotal disorders. **Varicocele** is an abnormal dilation of a vein within the spermatic cord, and most occur on the left side. They may be painful or tender. They occur in 10% to 15% of males, frequently after puberty. The cause of varicocele is incompetence or congenital *absence of valves in the spermatic veins* that normally prevent backflow of blood. Thus, blood pools in the veins rather than flowing into the venous system. Decreased blood flow through the testis interferes with spermatogenesis and can cause infertility.

A **hydrocele** is a collection of fluid *within the tunica vaginalis* and is the most common cause of scrotal swelling. Hydroceles in infants are congenital malformations that often resolve spontaneously by 1 year of age. Hydroceles in adults may be caused by an imbalance between the secreting and absorptive capacities of scrotal tissues.

The **spermatocele** is a cyst located between the head of the epididymis and the testis that usually is asymptomatic or produces mild discomfort that is relieved by scrotal support. Neither hydroceles nor spermatoceles are associated with infertility.

Cryptorchidism is a condition in which one or both *testes fail to descend into the scrotum.* It is the most common congenital condition involving the testes. In approximately 75% to 90% of infants with cryptorchidism, the testes descend into the scrotum by 1 year of age. The cause of cryptorchidism is not clear, but it may result from a developmental delay, a defect of the testis, deficient maternal gonadotropin stimulation, or some mechanical factor that prevents descent of the testis through the inguinal canal.

Untreated cryptorchidism is associated with lowered sperm count and impaired fertility. Undescended testes are susceptible to neoplastic processes. Treatment often begins with administration of human chorionic gonadotropin. If hormonal therapy is not successful, the testis is located and moved into the scrotum surgically.

Torsion of the testis is a condition wherein the testis rotates on its vascular pedicle; this position interrupts its blood supply. Onset may be spontaneous, or torsion may follow physical exertion or trauma. If the torsion cannot be reduced manually, surgery must be performed within 6 hours after the onset of symptoms to preserve normal testicular function.

Orchitis is an acute inflammation of the testes and is uncommon except as a complication of systemic infection or as an extension of an associated epididymitis. *Mumps* is the most common infectious cause of orchitis and usually affects postpubertal males. The onset is sudden and occurs 3 to 4 days after the onset of parotitis. Irreversible damage to spermatogenesis occurs in about 30% of affected testes.

Treatment is supportive and includes bed rest, scrotal support, elevation of the scrotum, hot or cold compresses, and analgesic agents for relief of pain. Appropriate antimicrobial drugs should be used for bacterial orchitis. Corticosteroids are indicated in proven cases of nonspecific granulomatous orchitis.

Testicular cancers are rare, accounting for approximately 1% of all male cancers; yet they are the most common solid tumor of young adult men. The cure rate is greater than 95% if any relapse is diagnosed and treated.

The etiology of testicular neoplasms is unknown. Because young men are affected most often, it is believed that high levels of androgens may contribute to carcinogenesis. A genetic predisposition exists. Cryptorchidism also is statistically associated with the development of testicular cancer. Apparently, the *undescended testis* has a developmental defect or *undergoes gradual involution and degeneration over time,* which may contribute to neoplastic changes.

Painless testicular enlargement is usually the first sign of testicular cancer. Enlargement is gradual and may be accompanied by a sensation of testicular heaviness or a dull ache in the lower abdomen. Occasionally, acute pain occurs because of rapid growth; then, there may be hemorrhage and necrosis. Besides surgery, treatment involves irradiation and chemotherapy, singly or in combination. Orchiectomy does not affect sexual function.

Epididymitis, or inflammation of the epididymis, generally occurs in sexually active young males. In young men, the usual cause is a sexually transmitted microorganism. In men older than 35 years, intestinal bacteria and *Pseudomonas aeruginosa, which is* found in UTIs and prostatitis, may also cause epididymitis. The pathogenic microorganism reaches the epididymis by ascending the vas deferens from an infected urethra or bladder. *Chemical epididymitis* may result from inflammation caused by urine reflux into ejaculatory ducts; it is usually self-limiting.

Acute and severe scrotal or inguinal pain is caused by inflammation of the epididymis and surrounding tissues. The individual may have pyuria and bacteriuria and a history of urinary symptoms, including urethral discharge. Complications of epididymitis include abscess formation, infarction of the testis, recurrent infection, scarring of epididymal endothelium, and infertility. Treatment includes antibiotic therapy for the infection and various measures to provide symptomatic relief. The individual's sexual partner should be treated with antibiotics if the causative microorganism is a sexually transmitted pathogen.

10. Distinguish among benign prostatic hyperplasia (BPH), prostatitis, and prostatic cancer.

Study pages 826-831, 833, and 835-837; refer to Figures 32-28 through 32-36.

BPH, formerly called *benign prostatic hypertrophy,* causes problems as enlarged prostatic tissue compresses the prostatic urethra. More than half of all men between 60 and 69 years of age have prostatic enlargement. During the third decade of life, the prostate reaches adult size. Between 40 and 45 years of age, benign hyperplasia begins and continues slowly until death. Theories of BPH focus on aging and androgen/estrogen ratios, the role of *chronic inflammation,* and autocrine/paracrine *growth-stimulating and growth-inhibiting factors*. These factors create an increase in prostate volume and tissue remodeling. The remodeled stroma promotes inflammation.

BPH begins in the *periurethral glands*, which are the inner glands or layers of the prostate. As nodular hyperplasia and cellular hypertrophy progress, the compressed prostatic urethra usually, but not always, causes bladder outflow obstruction.

Symptoms include the *urge* to urinate frequently, some *delay* in starting urination, *incomplete emptying, nocturia, and decreased force* of the urinary stream. Over a period of several years, the bladder is unable to empty all of the urine, and urine retention becomes chronic. Progressive bladder distention causes sacculations or diverticular outpouchings of the bladder wall. The ureters may be obstructed as they pass through the hypertrophied detrusor muscle. Bladder or kidney infection can develop.

Digital rectal examination (DRE) and measurement of serum prostate-specific antigen (PSA) are conducted to determine hyperplasia. PSA levels, alone, cannot determine whether symptoms are because of BPH or prostate cancer. It is possible that changes in PSA levels over time, also called PSA velocity, are poor indicators of prostate cancer, leading to unnecessary biopsies. Cancer diagnosis is confirmed by biopsy. Lymphography, bone scans, magnetic resonance imaging (MRI), or computed tomography (CT) may be performed to determine the presence or absence of metastasis.

Prostatitis is an inflammation of the prostate usually limited to a few of the gland's excretory ducts. Prostatitis is categorized as acute bacterial prostatitis, chronic bacterial prostatitis, or nonbacterial prostatitis.

Acute bacterial prostatitis is an *ascending infection* of the urinary tract that tends to occur in men between the ages of 30 and 50 years, but also is associated with BPH in older men. Urinary tract bacteria are common causes of acute bacterial prostatitis.

Symptoms include dysuria and urinary frequency and lower abdominal and suprapubic discomfort. The individual also may have a slow, small urinary stream, an inability to empty the bladder, and the need to urinate frequently during the night. Systemic signs of infection include sudden onset of a high fever, fatigue, joint pain, and muscle pain. Long-term, broad-spectrum antibiotics may be required to resolve the infection and control its spread. Pain relievers, antipyretics, bed rest, and adequate hydration also are used therapeutically.

Chronic bacterial prostatitis is characterized by *recurrent urinary tract infections (UTIs)* and the persistence of gram-negative pathogenic bacteria. This prostatitis is the most common recurrent UTI in men.

Symptoms are variable and may be similar to those of acute bacterial prostatitis. The prostate may be only slightly enlarged, but fibrosis causes it to be firm and irregular in shape. Treatment of chronic bacterial prostatitis is difficult mainly because calculi and fibrosis block passage of antibiotics into prostatic tissues. If chronic bacterial prostatitis is not cured medically, a radical transurethral prostatectomy may be required.

Chronic nonbacterial prostatitis consists of prostatic inflammation without evidence of bacterial infection. Its etiology is unclear.

Men with nonbacterial prostatitis may complain of dull continuous or spasmodic pain in the suprapubic, rapubic, scrotal, penile, or inguinal area. The prostate gland generally feels normal upon palpation. There is no generally accepted treatment for nonbacterial prostatitis. Symptomatic relief is possible.

The incidence of **prostatic cancer** increases with advancing age. By age 85 years, the incidence is 1 in 6 for all American men. Prostatic cancer rarely occurs in men who are younger than 40 years. It is believed that both genetic/epigenetic and dietary influences play a role in the etiology of prostate cancer. *Androgens act as tumor promoters* through receptor mechanisms to enhance endogenous DNA carcinogens, including reactive oxygen species (ROS), *reactive estrogen metabolites and estrogen,* and environmental carcinogens. Also, there are changes in the balance between autocrine/paracrine growth-promoting and growth-inhibiting factors such as *insulin growth factors (IGFs).* Vasectomy has been identified as a possible risk factor for prostate cancer, because *free testosterone levels* rise after vasectomy. There is no clear evidence of a causal link between BPH and prostate cancer, even though they frequently occur together.

More than 95% of prostatic neoplasms are *adenocarcinomas,* and most occur in the periphery of the prostate. The aggressiveness of the neoplasm appears to be related to the degree of *differentiation,* rather than the size of the tumor. Local extension is usually *posterior,* although late in the disease the tumor may invade the rectum or encroach on the prostatic urethra and cause bladder outlet obstruction. Sites of distant metastasis occur via lymph and blood vessels and include the lymph nodes, bones, lungs, liver, and adrenals. The pelvis, lumbar spine, femur, thoracic spine, and ribs are the most common sites of bone metastasis.

Prostatic cancer often causes no symptoms until it is far advanced. The first manifestations of disease are slow urinary stream, hesitancy, incomplete emptying, frequency, nocturia, and dysuria. Unlike the symptoms of obstruction caused by BPH, the *symptoms* of obstruction caused by prostatic cancer *are progressive* and do not temporarily remit. Symptoms of late disease include bone pain at sites of bone metastasis, edema of the lower extremities, enlarged lymph nodes, liver enlargement, pathologic bone fractures, and mental confusion associated with brain metastases.

Transrectal ultrasound (TRUS), measurement of prostatic-specific antigen (PSA) in the blood (note PSA issues stated for BPH), and digital examination can validate the symptoms of prostatic cancer. Treatment options include hormonal therapy, immunotherapy, chemotherapy, radiation therapy, surgery, and any combination thereof. Symptomatic relief of urinary obstruction, bladder outlet obstruction, colon obstruction, and spinal cord compression may be required.

11. Describe sexual dysfunction in the male.
Study pages 837 and 838.

Male sexual dysfunction is the impairment of erection, emission, and ejaculation. Vascular disorders cause erectile dysfunction. Neurologic disorders can interfere with the important sympathetic, parasympathetic, and CNS mechanisms of erection, emission, and ejaculation. Men who are taking antihypertensives, antidepressants, antihistamines, antispasmodics, sedatives or tranquilizers, barbiturates, diuretics, sex hormone preparations, narcotics, or psychoactive drugs, or who consume ethyl alcohol experience sexual dysfunction. Treatments for organic sexual dysfunction include both medical and surgical approaches. For example, the drug Viagra (sildenafil) has the ability to counteract erectile dysfunction.

12. Differentiate between benign and malignant female breast disease; characterize galactorrhea.
Review pages 838-852 refer to Figures 32-37 through 32-45 and Tables 32-8 through 32-13.

Galactorrhea, or inappropriate lactation, is the persistent and sometimes excessive secretion of a milky fluid from the breast of a woman who is not pregnant or nursing an infant. Galactorrhea is not a breast disorder but, rather, a manifestation of pathophysiologic processes elsewhere in the body.

The most common cause is *nonpuerperal hyperprolactinemia,* or excessive prolactin in the blood unrelated to pregnancy or childbirth. This excess prolactin can be caused by any factor that stimulates prolactin secretion from the pituitary gland, that interferes with prolactin-inhibiting factor (PIF), which inhibits prolactin secretion (probable dopamine), or that interferes with pituitary receptors for PIF.

Benign breast entities are numerous and involve both ducts and lobules. They can be classified according to their future risk of causing breast cancer as: (1) nonproliferative breast lesions, (2) proliferative breast disease, or (3) atypical hyperplasia (atypia).

Breast cancer is the most common form of cancer in women and second to lung cancer as the most common cause of cancer death. It is a heterogenous disease with diverse molecular phenotypic and pathologic changes. Clinical breast examinations, mammography, thermography, MRI, percutaneous needle aspiration, biopsy or minimally invasive biopsy, hormone receptor assays, and gene expression profiling are used in evaluating breast alterations and cancer.

Benign/Malignant Female Breast Disorders

Disorder	Risks	Pathophysiology	Manifestations	Treatment
Proliferative lesions: Without atypia: • Epithelial hyperplasia • Sclerosing adenosis • Complex sclerosing lesions (radial scar)* • Papilloma* Fibroadenoma With atypia: • Atypical ductal and lobular hyperplasia	Puberty to lifetime; proliferative lesions without atypia generally demonstrate no added risk for cancer; proliferative lesions with atypia hyperplasia have increased risk for cancer development	Increased estrogen levels, alterations in estrogen-to-progesterone ratio; genetic alterations	Fluctuating lesion size; mobile multiple lesions; cysts are evident radiographically; possible nipple discharge; breast tenderness with menstrual cycle	Cyst drainage; surgical excision of mass or duct or breast segment, possible mastectomy (extend of surgery depends on atypia); pain relief with synthetic androgens
Breast cancer	Increase with age: Lifetime risk is 1 in 8 for non-Hispanic white women and less for others No term pregnancies, long reproductive life; ionizing radiation; high-fat diet; physical inactivity; alcohol ingestion; first-degree relatives with breast cancer	Estrogens (endogenous and exogenous) and their receptors have a proliferative effect on mammary gland epithelium—estrogens may increase susceptibility to environmental carcinogens, oxidative catabolism of estrogens generate ROS that cause genetic damage, transforming growth factor (TGF), IGF, epidermal growth factor (EGF), platelet-derived growth factor (PDGF); mutations of *BRCA1, BRCA2*, and other related genes (p53, Bcl-2, Her2, c-myc)	Painless or painful mass, skin retraction over lesion; nipple puckering and discharge; hemorrhage After metastasis: palpable axillary lymph nodes, bone pain, site-specific signs and symptoms; approximately 50% of breast cancers occur in the upper quadrant because of predominantly glandular tissue there	Surgery to remove lesion; irradiation to prevent metastasis; chemotherapy; hormones for hormone-dependent tumors; trastuzumab (antibody; Herceptin), antiestrogens (tamoxifen) antiestrogens, bone marrow transplantation; treatment depends on stage or extent

Note: Breast carcinogenesis involves uncontrolled cellular proliferation, alterations in cell signaling pathways, and aberrant apoptosis or loss of apoptosis as a consequence of accumulated genetic damage. Germline mutation or acquired somatic mutations due to environment carcinogens transform the phenotype. Changes in malignant cells are accompanied or preceded by alterations in the supporting myoepithelial and stromal cells because of genetic and epigenetic events. The final alteration, invasion of the stroma, likely is the result of loss of myoepithelial and stromal cells that maintain the basement membrane.

Ductal carcinoma in situ (DCIS) refers to a heterogenous group of lesions. These lesions are presumed to be malignant epithelial cells of the ductal system. The increase in the incidence of DCIS may reflect an increase in cancer or increased detection by mammography.

13. Describe male gynecomastia and breast cancer.
Study pages 856 and 857.

Gynecomastia is the overdevelopment of breast tissue in a male. Gynecomastia accounts for approximately 85% of all masses that develop in the male breast and affects approximately 35% of the male population. Incidence is greatest among adolescents and men older than 50 years.

Gynecomastia usually involves *an imbalance of the estrogen-testosterone ratio*. The ratio can be altered by tumor- and drug-induced *hyperestrogenism,* which raises the estrogen levels while testosterone levels remain normal. Gynecomastia also can be caused by increased breast tissue responsiveness to estrogen or decreased responsiveness to androgen. Estrogen-testosterone imbalances are associated with hypogonadism, Klinefelter syndrome, testicular neoplasms, cirrhosis of the liver, infectious hepatitis, chronic renal failure, chronic obstructive lung disease, hyperthyroidism, tuberculosis, and chronic malnutrition.

Hyperplasia results in a firm, palpable mass at least 2 cm in diameter and located beneath the areola. Identification and treatment of the cause likely will resolve the gynecomastia.

Breast cancer in males is uncommon. Risk factors include gynecomastia, chest irradiation, and family history. Incidence is greatest in men in their 60s.

Treatment protocols are similar to those for female breast cancer. Tamoxifen is used more often for males because a higher percentage of male tumors are hormone dependent. Breast cancer in males has a poor prognosis because men tend to delay seeking treatment.

14. Describe sexually transmitted infections (STIs) and their infectious agents and manifestations.
Study page 859; refer to Tables 32-14 through 32-16. (See color plates on pp. 860 and 861)

The etiology of an STI may be bacterial, viral, or parasitic. Although the majority of STIs can be treated, viral STIs are considered incurable. The increased incidence of STIs can be attributed to earlier onset of sexual activity, a greater number of lifetime sexual partners and high-risk sexual behaviors, such as lack of condom use, new sexual partners, illicit drug use, prostitution, and selection of high-risk sexual partners.

Complications of STIs include PID, infertility, ectopic pregnancy, chronic pelvic pain, neonatal morbidity and mortality, genital cancer, and transmission of human immunodeficiency virus (HIV).

Bacterial and Sexually Transmitted Infections

Disease and Infectious Agent	Manifestations
Gonorrhea *Neisseria gonorrhoeae*	Possibly asymptomatic; urethritis, cervicitis, mucopurulent discharge, anorectal infection, pharyngitis, conjunctivitis, ophthalmia
Syphilis *Treponema pallidum*	Primary: nonpainful chancre at site of invasion Secondary: systemic involvement with skin rash and lymphadenopathy Tertiary: gummas (granuloma)
Chancroid *Haemophilus ducreyi*	Papule erodes into painful ulcer, superficial exudate, painful lymphadenopathy
Urogenital infections Lymphogranuloma venereum *Chlamydia trachomatis*	Commonly associated with other STIs; purulent discharge, cervicitis, urethritis, proctitis, newborn conjunctivitis and pneumonia, tender lymph nodes, and inguinal buboes

Note: Treatment of bacterial and bacterial-like STIs is with appropriate antibiotics

Viral Sexually Transmitted Infections

Disease and Infectious Agent	Manifestations
Genital herpes Herpes simplex virus (HSV-1 or HSV-2) (latent virus)	Painful blister-like lesions on external genitalia and genital tract
Condylomata acuminata (warts) HPV	Soft, skin-colored single or clustered growths; asymptomatic

Note: Treatment for HSV is not curative, but oral and topical antiviral agents (acyclovir) are used to lower recurrence; HPV lesions are treated with topical agents and cosmetic surgery. A vaccine is now available to prevent HPV infection and cervical cancer.

Parasitic Sexually Transmitted Infections

Disease and Infectious Agent	Manifestations
Trichomoniasis *Trichomonas vaginalis*	Pain during intercourse, dysuria, spotting
Scabies *Sarcoptes scabiei*	Intense pruritus
Pediculosis pubic (crabs) *Phthirus pubis*	Pruritus

Note: Treatment is with antitrichomonal agents, scabicides, and prescription creams.

PRACTICE EXAMINATION

Multiple Choice

Circle the correct answer for each question:

1. Secondary amenorrhea is:
   a. failure to begin menstruation by age 20 years.
   b. menarche failure.
   c. increased myometrial vasculature constriction.
   d. the absence of menstruation following menarche.

2. What is the likely pathophysiology of PMS?
   a. Elevated prolactin values cause salt and water retention.
   b. Elevated aldosterone values cause salt and water retention.
   c. An abnormal nervous, immunologic, vascular, and gastrointestinal response to hormone fluctuations of the menstrual cycle likely occurs.
   d. Both a and b are correct.

3. Acute PID:
   a. primarily affects males.
   b. is usually caused by viruses.
   c. never causes peritonitis.
   d. involves the epididymis.
   e. may cause infertility or tubular pregnancy.

4. Anovulatory cycles having prolonged estrogen levels and absence of progesterone production are found in:
   a. cervical cancer.
   b. corpus luteum cysts.
   c. adenomyosis.
   d. endometrial hyperplasia.
   e. Both b and c are correct.

5. Depressed T cell function is associated with:
   a. follicular cysts.
   b. endometrial polyps.
   c. leiomyomas.
   d. adenomyosis.
   e. endometriosis.

6. A 42-year-old retired prostitute who became sexually active at age 14 is at risk for development of:
   a. endometriosis.
   b. cervical carcinoma.
   c. breast cancer.
   d. uterine carcinoma.

7. Polycystic ovary syndrome is:
   a. the most common cause of infertility in the United States.
   b. associated with hyperinsulinemia.
   c. sometimes a precursor of endometrial carcinoma.
   d. a, b, and c are correct.

8. Endometriosis:
   a. involves the ectopic endometrium responding to hormonal fluctuations of the menstrual cycle.
   b. occurs primarily in the pleural cavity.
   c. causes infertility in most women having the disorder.
   d. does not reoccur after treatment.

9. Phimosis is:
   a. thickening of the fascia in the erectile tissue of the corpora cavernosa.
   b. the condition in which a retracted foreskin cannot be moved forward.
   c. a condition in which the foreskin cannot be retracted.
   d. caused by poor hygiene and chronic infection.
   e. Both c and d are correct.

10. A varicocele is an intrascrotal disorder:
    a. that results in a collection of fluid within the tunica vaginalis.
    b. that occurs because of independent or congenitally absent valves in the spermatic veins.
    c. located between the head of the epididymis and the testis.
    d. that does not interfere with spermatogenesis.

11. Cryptorchidism is:
    a. underdevelopment of the testes.
    b. the absence of scrotal tissue.
    c. relieved by scrotal support.
    d. failure of testes to descend into the scrotum.
    e. an imbalance between secreting and absorptive capacities of scrotal tissues.

12. The infectious cause of orchitis is:
    a. streptococci.
    b. gonococci.
    c. chlamydial organisms.
    d. mumps virus.

13. Which organisms can cause epididymitis?
    a. *Enterobacteriaceae*.
    b. *Neisseria gonorrhoeae*.
    c. *Chlamydia trachomatis*.
    d. All of the above are correct.
    e. None of the above is correct.

14. In BPH, enlargement of periurethral tissue of the prostate causes:
    a. obstruction of the urethra.
    b. inflammation of the testis.
    c. decreased urinary outflow from the bladder.
    d. abnormal dilation of a vein within the spermatic cord.
    e. tension of the spermatic cord and testis.

15. Recurrent UTIs in the male cause:
    a. orchitis.
    b. balanitis.
    c. epididymitis.
    d. chronic bacterial prostatitis.
    e. nonbacterial prostatitis.

16. A symptom or sign of late-stage, metastatic prostatic cancer is:
    a. a slow urinary stream.
    b. frequency of urination.
    c. incomplete emptying.
    d. mental confusion associated with brain metastases.
    e. a, b, and c are correct.

17. Male sexual dysfunction may be caused by:
    a. infection around the introitus.
    b. diabetes mellitus.
    c. infected hymenal remnants.
    d. None of the above is correct.

Matching

Match the characteristic with the benign or malignant female breast disorder:

_______ 18. Fluctuating lesion size

_______ 19. Palpable axillary lymph node

_______ 20. Mutated gene on chromosome 13 or 17

a. fibrocystic disease
b. breast cancer

Match the Sexually Transmitted Infection with its causative agent:

_______ 21. Gonorrhea

_______ 22. Syphilis

_______ 23. Condylomata acuminata

_______ 24. Pediculosis pubis

_______ 25. Lymphogranuloma

a. *Haemophilus ducreyi*
b. *Mycoplasma hominis*
c. *Neisseria gonorrhoeae*
d. *Gardnerella vaginalis*
e. *Treponema pallidum*
f. HPV
g. *Sarcoptes scabiei*
h. *Phthirus pubis*
i. *Chlamydia trachomatis*
j. *Trichomonas vaginalis*

Fill in the Blank

Complete the following table comparing benign prostatic hyperplasia with prostatic cancer:

Characteristics	Benign Prostatic Hyperplasia	Prostatic Cancer
Involved site	Periurethral gland	Posterior periphery of gland
Causes		
Symptoms	Remitting: slow urinary stream, hesitancy, incomplete emptying, frequency, nocturia	
Subsequent course		Metastasis to bones (lumbar spine, pelvis, ribs) with pain, lower extremity edema, lymphadenopathy

CASE STUDY 1

B.J. is a 63-year-old retired white woman who is physically fit and socially active. She is the mother of two children and has high blood pressure and high cholesterol; both are controlled with medications. On her annual visit to her gynecologist, Dr. F., she reported that she recently had noted a serous, lightly blood-tinged vaginal discharge. Having been postmenopausal since age 52, she expressed concern about this discharge. She also reported that she had been trying to decrease the amount of the hormone replacement therapy (HRT) she had been using since her perimenopausal phase, which began at age 49. B.J. asked Dr. F., "What is going on here? I am too old to be having periods again." After the typical gynecologic exam including a Pap smear, Dr. F. suggested that B.J.'s recent self-regulating of her hormone therapy and a possible irritated vaginal wall could account for the discharge. Dr. F. prescribed a vaginal hormone cream to be used for 2 weeks and suggested that B.J. continue low-dose HRT. This approach did not stop the discharge, and so a few weeks later, an endometrial biopsy and culture of the discharge were done. Both had negative results, as did the Pap smear, so Dr. F. prescribed additional progesterone for 2 months. After 4 months of continual serous discharge that was becoming more blood tinged, B.J. again contacted Dr. F. and said, "This discharge is continual, getting bloodier, and cannot be normal. What do we need to do right now?"

What further diagnostic tests are indicated? After results of the further tests are available, what needs to be done?

CASE STUDY 2

Mrs. B., a 46-year-old woman, consulted her physician about the nature of a lump in one breast. About 3 months earlier, her spouse noticed a small lump in her left breast. This lump seemed to be growing and did not seem to fluctuate in size as other lumps had during her menses. Mrs. B. also noticed three small lumps in her right breast that did fluctuate in size. She stated, "I am in excellent health, I exercise daily, and I do not smoke nor drink alcohol."

Mrs. B. is the mother of two preteen children. After the birth of her last child, she took birth control pills for 8 years and then selected an alternative method of birth control. Onset of her menses occurred at age 10 years. Her family history reveals that her mother and one of three aunts died of breast cancer.

On examination, a 2-cm to 3-cm mass was palpated in the upper quadrant of her left breast. This mass was firm, fixed to the chest wall, and slightly tender to touch. The skin and nipple appeared normal. Under the left axilla, a node about the size of a pea was palpable. Three 1-cm to 2-cm soft, movable masses were palpated in Mrs. B.'s right breast.

Mammography confirmed the presence of a 3-cm mass in the left breast and four 1.5-cm masses in the right breast. Results of all other diagnostic procedures were negative.

What thoughts do you have concerning Mrs. B.'s examination and her risk factors?

33 Structure and Function of the Digestive System

FOUNDATIONAL OBJECTIVES

After reviewing this chapter, the learner will be able to do the following:

1. **List the parts of the alimentary canal sequentially from mouth to anus.**
   Refer to Figure 33-1.

2. **Describe the histology of the structural layers of the gastrointestinal tract.**
   Review page 871; refer to Figure 33-2.

3. **Describe the mouth and esophagus, noting specific structure, function, and secretions.**
   Review pages 873 and 874; refer to Figures 33-3 and 33-4.

4. **Describe the stomach, noting specific structure, function, and secretions.**
   Review pages 874-877; refer to Figures 33-5 through 33-9 and Table 33-1.

5. **Describe the small intestine, noting specific structure, function, and secretions.**
   Review pages 877-881; refer to Figures 33-10 through 33-12 and Table 33-1.

6. **Describe the structure and function of the large intestine, and identify normal intestinal flora and their activities.**
   Review pages 881-883; refer to Figure 33-13.

7. **Note the significance of splanchnic blood flow.**
   Review page 883; refer to Figures 33-6 and 33-13.

8. **Describe the structure, function, and secretions of the liver; identify the gallbladder-liver relationship.**
   Review pages 883-888; refer to Figures 33-14 through 33-19 and Table 33-3.

9. **Explain the relationship between cell types and function of the exocrine pancreas.**
   Review pages 888 and 890; refer to Figure 33-20 and Table 33-4.

10. **Identify age-related changes in gastrointestinal function.**
    Review page 890.

PRACTICE EXAMINATION

Multiple Choice

Circle the correct answer for each question:

1. The muscularis of the gastrointestinal tract is:
   a. skeletal muscle throughout the tract, particularly in the esophagus and large intestine.
   b. the layer that contains the blood capillaries for the entire wall of the tract.
   c. composed principally of keratinized epithelium.
   d. composed of circular fibers and longitudinal fibers.

2. The digestive functions performed by the saliva and salivary amylase, respectively, are:
   a. moistening and protein digestion.
   b. deglutition and fat digestion.
   c. peristalsis and polysaccharide digestion.
   d. lubrication and carbohydrate digestion.

3. The nervous pathway involved in salivary secretion requires stimulation of:
   a. receptors in the taste buds and somatic motor impulses to the salivary glands.
   b. receptors in the mouth, sensory impulses, and parasympathetic impulses to the salivary glands.
   c. taste receptors, sensory impulses, and somatic motor impulses to the salivary glands.
   d. pressoreceptors in blood vessels and autonomic impulses to the salivary glands.

4. Food would pass rapidly from the stomach into the duodenum if it were *not* for the:
   a. fundus.
   b. epiglottis.
   c. rugae.
   d. cardiac sphincter.
   e. pyloric sphincter.

5. The secretion of gastric juice:
   a. occurs only when swallowed food comes in contact with the stomach.
   b. is entirely under the control of the hormone gastrin.
   c. is entirely under the control of the hormone enterogastrone.
   d. is stimulated by the presence of saliva in the stomach.
   e. occurs in three phases: cephalic, gastric, and intestinal.

6. During nervous control of gastric secretion, the gastric glands secrete before food enters the stomach. This stimulus to the glands comes from:
   a. gastrin.
   b. impulses over somatic nerves from the hypothalamus.
   c. motor impulses from the cerebral cortex and cerebellum.
   d. parasympathetic impulses over the vagus nerve.

7. Pepsinogen:
   a. must be activated by HCl.
   b. is secreted by the chief cells.
   c. is a precursor to pepsin.
   d. All of the above are correct.

8. Beginning at the lumen of the tube, the sequence of layers of the gastrointestinal tract is:
   a. mucosa, submucosa, muscularis, serosa.
   b. submucosa, mucosa, serosa, muscularis.
   c. submucosa, mucosa, muscularis, skeletal muscle.
   d. serosa, muscularis, mucosa, submucosa.

9. Normally, when chyme leaves the stomach:
   a. the nutrients are ready for absorption into the blood.
   b. the amount of inorganic salts has been increased by the action of hydrochloric acid.
   c. its pH is neutral.
   d. the proteins have been partly digested into polypeptides.
   e. All of the above are correct.

10. Which layer of the small intestine includes microvilli?
    a. submucosa
    b. mucosa
    c. muscularis
    d. serosa

11. Which is *not* an example of mechanical digestion?
    a. chewing
    b. churning and mixing of food in the stomach
    c. peristalsis and mastication
    d. conversion of protein molecules into amino acids

12. Pancreatic juice is to trypsin as gastric juice is to:
    a. salivary amylase.
    b. pepsin.
    c. mucin.
    d. intrinsic factor.

13. Which part of the small intestine is most distal from the pylorus?
    a. jejunum
    b. pyloric sphincter
    c. duodenum
    d. cardiac sphincter
    e. common bile duct

14. The pancreas:
    a. lies mostly on the left side of the abdominal cavity, anterior to the stomach and the spleen.
    b. secretes all of its products directly into the bloodstream.
    c. is a gland with its duct ultimately opening into the duodenum.
    d. contains cells with endocrine function for the determination of secondary sex characteristics.
    e. is classified as a digestive exocrine gland and does not have endocrine functions.

15. The chief role played by the pancreas in digestion is to:
    a. secrete insulin and glucagon.
    b. churn the food and bring it into contact with digestive enzymes.
    c. secrete enzymes, which digest food in the small intestine.
    d. assist in absorbing the digested foods.

16. Among the structural features of the small intestine are villi, microvilli, and circular folds. Their function is to:
    a. liberate hormones.
    b. promote peristalsis.
    c. liberate digestive enzymes.
    d. increase the surface area for absorption.

17. The fate of carbohydrates in the small intestine is:
    a. digestion to monosaccharides.
    b. conversion to simple sugars by the activity of trypsin.
    c. hydrolysis to amino acids.
    d. conversion to glycerol and fatty acids.

18. The absorptive fate of the end products of digestion may be summarized by which of the following?
    a. Most fatty acids are absorbed into the blood; glucose and amino acids are absorbed into the lymphatic system.
    b. Amino acids and monosaccharides are absorbed into blood capillaries; most fatty acids are absorbed into lymph.
    c. Amino acids and fatty acids are absorbed into lymph capillaries; glycerol and glucose are absorbed into blood capillaries.
    d. Fatty acids are absorbed into blood capillaries; glycerol, glucose, and amino acids are absorbed into lymph.

19. A lobule of the liver contains a centrally located:
    a. vein with radiating hepatocytes and sinusoids.
    b. arteriole with radiating capillaries and Kupffer cells.
    c. hepatic sinus with radiating sinusoids.
    d. hepatic duct with radiating Kupffer cells and cords of hepatic cells.

20. An obstruction of the common bile duct would cause blockage of bile coming from:
    a. the gallbladder.
    b. the liver but not from the gallbladder.
    c. both the liver and the gallbladder.
    d. the pancreatic duct but not from the gallbladder.

21. The human adult liver does *not:*
    a. store glycogen.
    b. produce erythrocytes.
    c. convert ammonia to urea.
    d. produce blood coagulation proteins.

22. The chyme that enters the large intestine is converted to feces by activity of:
    a. specific mucosal enzymes.
    b. gastric and duodenal hormones.
    c. bacteria and water reabsorption.
    d. the microvilli, villi, and circular muscles.

Matching

Match the substance/structures with its/their function:

_______ 23. Splanchnic organs

_______ 24. Kupffer cells

_______ 25. Cholecystokinin

a. stimulate(s) gallbladder to eject bile
b. activate(s) pepsinogen
c. trap(s) bacteria
d. increase(s) gastrointestinal mobility
e. act(s) as blood reservoir for heart and lungs
f. stimulate(s) liver to secrete bile

Fill in the Blank

Complete the following table describing the digestive enzymes and their substrates, products, and absorption routes:

Digestive Enzyme Actions and Food Absorption Routes

Food Type	Enzymes	Products	Absorption Routes
Starch	Salivary amylase	Polysaccharides	
Polysaccharides	Pancreatic amylase	Lactose, maltose, sucrose	
Lactose, maltose, sucrose			
Proteins			
Peptones, proteoses			
Small polypeptides, dipeptides			
Unemulsified fats			

34 Alterations of Digestive Function

FOUNDATIONAL OBJECTIVE

a. Describe the structure and function of the gastrointestinal tract and accessory organs of digestion.
Review pages 871 and 873-890; refer to Figure 33-1.

MEMORY CHECK!

- The gastrointestinal system includes the: (1) oral structures (mouth, salivary glands, pharynx), (2) alimentary tract (esophagus, stomach, small intestine, large intestine, appendix, anus), and (3) accessory organs of digestion (liver, gallbladder, bile ducts, pancreas). The function of the alimentary tract is to *digest* masticated food, to *absorb* digestive products, and to *excrete* the digestive residue and certain waste products excreted by the liver through the bile duct.
- The alimentary tract has four layers: mucosa, submucosa, muscularis, and serosa. The mucosal layer consists of epithelial cells lining the lumen's surface, supporting connective tissue called the *lamina propria*, and a unique thin, muscular layer called the *muscularis mucosae*. The structure of the inner mucosal layer varies to provide specialized function at each part of the tract. The esophagus is lined by stratified squamous epithelium, which enables masticated food to glide rapidly from the mouth to the stomach. The stomach has a thick glandular mucosa, which provides mucus, acid, and proteolytic enzymes to help digest food. The small intestinal mucosa has a villous structure to provide a large surface of cells for active absorption. The large intestinal mucosa is lined by abundant mucus secreting cells that facilitate storage and evacuation of the residue. Beneath the mucosa is the submucosa, which gives structural support to the tract because of its abundant collagenous tissue. The muscle layer contracts rhythmically to move materials through the alimentary tract. The serosal layer is a thin, smooth membrane present on the outer surface of the alimentary tract. It keeps the tortuous loops of bowel from becoming tangled and is continuous with the mesentery. The mesentery is a connective tissue attachment of the bowel to the abdominal wall; it contains blood vessels, lymphatics, and nerves.
- A wave of muscle contraction carries a bolus of swallowed food down the esophagus, where a sphincter at the lower end of the esophagus prevents regurgitation. Contractions in the stomach mix the food and push the partially digested contents into the duodenum. The muscle of the pylorus only partially closes the outlet to the stomach, so intestinal contents can regurgitate into the stomach if the small intestine is not emptying properly. Normally, movement of luminal contents in the small intestine is more rapid in the upper small intestine and slows as chyme moves distally. Contents pass from the ileum into the colon, where reverse proximal movement is partially prevented by the ileocecal valve. Water is absorbed in the colon, and the contents become solid; the solid residue is moved to the left side of the colon and rectum. When the rectum becomes distended, an urge for defecation develops.
- The liver and the pancreas are glandular organs with excretory ducts emptying into the duodenum at a site called the *ampulla of Vater*. The excretory ducts of the liver are called *bile ducts*. The gallbladder is a storage reservoir connected to the bile ducts by the cystic duct.
- Most of the blood from the abdominal organs is carried to the liver via the *portal vein*. Therefore, the glandular cells of the liver *filter* blood before it returns to the heart via the *hepatic vein* and *vena cava*. Because portal blood has little oxygen left after passing through the abdominal organs, oxygenated blood is supplied to the liver by the hepatic artery. The bulk of the liver is composed of *hepatocytes,* which are aligned in cords with sinusoids between the cords to diffuse the blood from the portal areas to the central vein. Between adjacent hepatocytes are tiny canaliculi that carry bile produced by the hepatocytes to the portal area, where they empty into epithelium-lined bile ducts. In the sinusoids, waste products and nutrients are removed and metabolized by the hepatocytes. The metabolites may be returned to the blood, stored in the hepatocytes, or excreted into bile canaliculi. The liver also contains many mononuclear cells, or *Kupffer cells,* that line the sinusoids. They *phagocytize* particulate material from the blood. Metabolically, the liver: (1) produces bile salts, (2) excretes bilirubin, (3) metabolizes nitrogenous substances, (4) produces serum proteins, and (5) detoxifies drugs and poisons.

Continued

MEMORY CHECK!—Cont'd

- The gallbladder is a distention of the common bile duct that becomes a *bile storage reservoir*. The gallbladder empties its contents into the duodenum after meals, when *bile* salts are needed for *fat absorption*. This reservoir function is not essential, because the gallbladder can be removed without loss of digestive function.
- The pancreas is a long, narrow glandular organ lying horizontally and retroperitoneally in the midabdomen region. The pancreatic duct runs the length of the pancreas and empties into the duodenum after joining the bile duct. The bulk of the pancreas is made up of *glands that secrete digestive enzymes* into the pancreatic duct. When activated by intestinal juices, these enzymes digest carbohydrate, fat, and protein. Pancreatic enzymes are essential for life. Scattered among the pancreatic glands are clusters of endocrine cells known as the *islets of Langerhans,* which *produce insulin* and other hormones.
- The digestive process begins in the mouth, where a carbohydrate-splitting enzyme or *amylase* from the salivary glands mixes with food during mastication. In the stomach, proteolytic *pepsin and hydrochloric acid* are added to speed the digestive process. The greatest volume of *digestive enzymes originates from the pancreas* and is added to the digesting mixture of food in the duodenum. In addition, bile salts secreted by the liver and stored in the gallbladder are added to emulsify lipids into small water-soluble micelles. The *final phase* of the digestive process occurs at the *surfaces of small intestinal epithelial cells*. Complex endocrine and nervous mechanisms coordinate the timing of the secretion of digestive enzymes, hydrochloric acid, and bile salts. The sight of food may cause salivation and gastric secretions because of nervous stimulation. Distention of the stomach releases gastrin, which stimulates acid production and gastric emptying. Movement of food into the duodenum causes the pancreas to secrete more fluid and enzymes and the gallbladder to release bile. The products of both enter the duodenum.

LEARNING OBJECTIVES

After reviewing this chapter, the learner will be able to do the following:

1. Describe the common terms used in identifying the manifestations of gastrointestinal dysfunction.
Study pages 894-898; refer to Figure 34-1 and Table 34-1.

Anorexia is no desire to eat despite physiologic stimuli that would normally produce hunger. Anorexia is a nonspecific symptom often associated with nausea, abdominal pain, and psychological stress. Disorders of other systems besides the digestive system are accompanied by anorexia. These include cancer, heart disease, and renal disease.

Vomiting (emesis) is the forceful emptying of stomach and intestinal contents, referred to as chyme, through the mouth. The vomiting reflex is stimulated by the presence of ipecac or copper salts in the duodenum, severe pain, or distention of the stomach or duodenum. Torsion or trauma affecting the ovaries, testes, uterus, bladder, or kidney also elicits vomiting.

Vomiting occurs when the stomach is full of gastric contents and the diaphragm is forced high into the thoracic cavity by strong abdominal muscle contractions. The higher intrathoracic pressure forces the upper esophageal sphincter to open, and chyme is discharged from the mouth. Spontaneous vomiting not preceded by nausea or retching is called **projectile vomiting**. This vomiting is caused by direct stimulation of the vomiting center because of neurologic lesions involving the brain stem. The metabolic consequences of vomiting are fluid, electrolyte, and acid-base disturbances.

Nausea and retching usually precede vomiting. **Nausea** is a subjective experience associated with many different conditions. **Retching** is a strong involuntary effort to vomit. In retching, the lower esophageal sphincter and body of the stomach relax, but the duodenum and antrum of the stomach go into spasm. The reverse peristalsis forces chyme from the stomach and duodenum up into the esophagus. Because the upper esophageal sphincter is closed, chyme does not enter the mouth. As the abdominal muscles relax, the contents of the esophagus drop back into the stomach. This process may be repeated several times before vomiting occurs.

Constipation is difficult or infrequent defecation involving decreased numbers of bowel movements per week, hard stools, and difficult evacuation. Constipation is often caused by unhealthy dietary and bowel habits combined with inadequate exercise and low fluid intake. It also can occur as a result of intestinal immobility or obstruction disorders.

Conditions associated with constipation include congenital megacolon, hyperthyroidism, pelvic hiatal hernia, multiple sclerosis, spinal cord trauma, cancer, cerebrovascular disease, and irritable bowel syndrome.

Diarrhea is increased frequency of defecation accompanied by changes in *fecal fluidity and volume*. In **osmotic diarrhea,** the presence of nonabsorbable substances in the intestine causes water to be drawn into the lumen by osmosis. The excess water and the nonabsorbable substances increase stool weight and volume. This causes *large-volume diarrhea.* **Secretory diarrhea** is a form of large-volume diarrhea caused by excessive mucosal secretion of fluid and electrolytes. Excessive intestinal secretion is caused mostly by bacterial enterotoxins released by strains of *Escherichia coli* or exotoxins from *Clostridium difficile*. A lesion that impairs autonomic control of motility, such as diabetic neuropathy, can cause large-volume diarrhea. **Motility diarrhea** can be caused by resection of the small intestine, surgical bypass of an area of the intestine, or fistula formation between loops of the intestine. Absorption is impaired.

Small-volume diarrhea is usually caused by inflammatory disorders of the intestine or by fecal impaction from severe constipation. In the latter case, the diarrhea consists of mucus and fluid produced by the colon to lubricate the impacted feces and move it toward the anal canal. Systemic effects of prolonged diarrhea are dehydration, electrolyte imbalance, and weight loss.

Abdominal pain is observed in a number of gastrointestinal diseases. The causal mechanisms of abdominal pain are *mechanical, inflammatory, or ischemic*. Abdominal organs are sensitive to *stretching and distention, which can activate nerve endings* in both hollow and solid structures. Histamine, bradykinin, and serotonin, when released during inflammation, stimulate organic nerve endings and produce abdominal pain. The edema and vascular congestion that accompany inflammation also cause painful stretching. Any obstruction of blood flow because of distention of bowel obstruction or mesenteric vessel thrombosis produces ischemic pain.

Parietal pain arises from the parietal peritoneum and is more localized and intense than **visceral pain,** which arises from the organs themselves. **Referred pain** is *visceral pain* felt at some distance from a diseased or affected organ. Referred pain is usually well localized and occurs in the skin or deeper tissues, which share a central, common afferent pathway with the affected organ.

Numerous disorders cause **gastrointestinal tract bleeding**. Acute gastrointestinal bleeding is usually characterized by *hematemesis*, or the presence of blood in the vomitus; *hematochezia,* or frank bleeding from the rectum; or *melena,* which is dark, tarry stools. *Occult bleeding* is slow, chronic blood loss that results in iron deficiency anemia as iron stores in the bone marrow are slowly depleted. Occult bleeding can be detected only by testing for blood in the stool or vomitus.

2. Compare and contrast the various disorders of digestive motility.

Study pages 898-903; refer to Figures 34-2 through 34-5 and Tables 34-2 through 34-4.

Motility Disorders

Tissue	Causes	Manifestations	Treatment
Dysphagia (swallowing difficulty)	Esophageal obstruction, tumors, strictures or diverticula, impaired esophageal motility, neural dysfunction, muscular disease, achalasia (decreased ganglion cells in myenteric plexus, causing relaxation of cardiac sphincter)	Distention and spasm of esophagus after swallowing, regurgitation of undigested food	Anticholinergic drugs, dilation of esophageal sphincter, surgical separation of lower esophageal muscles
Gastroesophageal reflux disease (GERD)*	Increased abdominal pressure, duodenal ulcers, pyloric edema and strictures, hiatal hernia	Regurgitation of chyme within 1 hour of eating	Antacids, head elevation during sleep, proton pump inhibitors, laparoscopic fundoplication
Hiatal hernia (protrusion of upper stomach through diaphragm into thorax)	Congenitally short esophagus, trauma, weak diaphragmatic muscles at gastroesophageal junction, increased abdominal pressure	Gastroesophageal reflux, dysphagia, epigastric pain	Similar to that for GERD
Pyloric obstruction (narrow pylorus)	Peptic ulcer or carcinoma near pylorus	Epigastric fullness, nausea and pain, vomitus without bile	Manage symptoms, surgery for gastric carcinoma or fibrosis and scarring
Intestinal obstruction (impaired chyme flow through intestinal lumen)	Hernia (protuberance), telescoping of one part of intestine into another (intussusception), twisting (volvulus), inflamed colonic diverticula (herniation), tumor growth, loss of peristaltic activity (paralytic ileus), fibrous adhesions	Colicky pain to severe and constant pain; vomiting, diarrhea, constipation, dehydration, and hypovolemia; acidosis with their complications	Fluid and electrolyte replacement, suction to decompress and lumen, surgery for complete obstruction or strangulation

*Nonerosive reflux disease (NERD) exhibits heartburn symptoms without mucosal injury and symptoms.

3. **Describe the pathogenesis of acute and chronic gastritis.**
   Study page 903.

Gastritis is a common inflammatory disorder of the gastric mucosa that may be acute or chronic and affects the fundus or antrum or both. *Anti-inflammatory drugs* are known to cause **acute gastritis,** which erodes the epithelium, probably because they inhibit prostaglandins that normally stimulate the secretion of protective mucus. Alcohol, histamine, digitalis, and metabolic disorders, such as uremia, are contributing factors for gastritis.

The clinical manifestations of acute gastritis can include vague abdominal discomfort, epigastric tenderness, and bleeding. Healing usually occurs spontaneously within a few days. Discontinuing injurious drugs, using antacids, or decreasing acid secretion with drugs facilitates healing.

Chronic gastritis is a progressive disease that tends to occur in elderly individuals. This gastritis causes thinning and degeneration of the stomach wall.

Chronic *fundal* gastritis is the most severe type, because the gastric mucosa degenerates extensively. The loss of chief cells and parietal cells diminishes secretion of pepsinogen, hydrochloric acid, and intrinsic factor. *Pernicious anemia* develops because intrinsic factor is unavailable to facilitate vitamin B12 absorption. Chronic fundal gastritis becomes a risk factor for *gastric carcinoma*, particularly in individuals in whom pernicious anemia develops. A significant number of individuals with chronic fundal gastritis have antibodies to parietal cells, intrinsic factor, and gastric cells in their sera, suggesting an autoimmune mechanism in the pathogenesis of the disease.

Chronic *antral* gastritis is more common than fundal gastritis. It is not associated with decreased hydrochloric acid secretion, pernicious anemia, or the presence of parietal cell antibodies. *Helicobacter pylori* is a major etiologic factor associated with the inflammation seen in chronic gastritis. The long-standing inflammatory process and gastric atrophy may develop without a history of abdominal distress. Individuals may report vague symptoms, including anorexia, fullness, nausea, vomiting, and epigastric pain. Gastric bleeding may be the only clinical manifestation of gastritis.

4. **Compare duodenal, gastric, and stress ulcers; identify the complications of surgical management of ulcers.**
   Study pages 903, 904, and 907; refer to Figures 34-6 through 34-8 and Table 34-5.

A **peptic ulcer** is a break or ulceration in the protective mucosal lining of the lower esophagus, stomach, or duodenum. Such breaks expose submucosal areas to gastric secretions and autodigestion.

Risk factors for peptic ulcer disease are smoking and habitual use of nonsteroidal anti-inflammatory drugs *(NSAIDs) or alcohol, rapid emptying that depletes bicarbonate levels, and high serum gastrin levels.* Some chronic diseases, such as emphysema, rheumatoid arthritis, and cirrhosis, are associated with the development of peptic ulcers. Infection of the gastric and duodenal mucosa with *H. pylori* causes peptic ulcers. Studies of life stress and ulcer disease are inconclusive regarding causation of peptic ulcers.

Postgastrectomy syndromes are a group of signs and symptoms that occur after gastric resection/surgery. They are caused by alterations in motor and control functions of the stomach and upper small intestine. The manifestations include dumping syndrome, alkaline reflux gastritis, afferent loop obstruction, diarrhea, weight loss, anemia, and bone disorders.

Dumping syndrome is the rapid emptying of *hypertonic chyme* from the surgically reduced and smaller stomach into the small intestine 10 to 20 minutes after eating. **Alkaline reflux gastritis** is stomach inflammation caused by reflux of bile and alkaline pancreas secretions that contain proteolytic enzymes that disrupt the mucosal barrier. Clinical manifestations include nausea, vomiting in which the vomitus contains bile, and sustained epigastric pain that worsens after eating and is not relieved by antacids.

Features of Ulcers

Feature	Duodenal	Gastric	Stress
Age incidence	25–50 years	50–70 years	Related to severe illness, trauma, sepsis, neural injury
Sex prevalence	Men	No sex difference	
Stress factors	Average	Increased	Increased
Acid production	Increased	Normal to low	Increased
Ulcerogenic drugs	Heavy use of alcohol and tobacco, NSAIDs	Moderate use of alcohol and tobacco	
Associated gastritis	Seldom	Common	
*Helicobacter pylori**	Usually present	May be present	
Pain	Pain-food-relief, common nocturnal pain, remission exacerbations	Pain-food-relief, uncommon nocturnal chronic, uncommon remission and exacerbations	Asymptomatic until hemorrhage or perforation

Features of Ulcers—Cont'd

Feature	Duodenal	Gastric	Stress
Hemorrhage	Common	Less common	Very common (most frequent complication)
Malignancy	Almost never	Possible	

*H. pylori's urease leads to formation of ammonia, which is toxic to mucosal cells, and the phospholipases of these organisms damage mucosa. Also, *H. pylori* infection stimulates gastrin production, which increases acid secretion.
Note: Medical treatment is directed at inhibiting or buffering acid secretions to relieve symptoms and promote healing. Antacids, dietary management, anticholinergic histamine blockers, and physical and emotional rest are used to accomplish relief and promote healing. *H. pylori* infection is treated with a combination of antibiotics and bismuth.

Afferent loop obstruction is a problem caused by volvulus, hernia, adhesion, or stenosis in the duodenal stump on the proximal side of the surgical procedure. The symptoms of afferent loop obstruction include intermittent severe pain and epigastric fullness after eating. Postgastrectomy **diarrhea** appears to be related to rapid gastric emptying of large amounts of high-carbohydrate liquids. **Weight loss** often follows gastric resection because the stomach is less able to mix, churn, and break down food. **Anemia** after gastrectomy results from iron, vitamin B12, or folate deficiency. **Bone disorders** are related to altered calcium levels, which increase the risk of fractures and bone deformity.

5. Define malabsorption syndrome and maldigestion; characterize pancreatic insufficiency and lactase and bile salt deficiency.
Study pages 907 and 908.

Malabsorption syndromes interfere with nutrient absorption in the small intestine; the intestinal mucosa fails to absorb or transport the digested nutrients into the blood. *Malabsorption* is the result of mucosal disruption caused by gastric or intestinal resection, vascular disorders, or intestinal disease. *Maldigestion* is failed or faulty digestion because of deficiencies of chemical enzymes in the intestinal lumen or mucosa.

Pancreatic insufficiency occurs because of deficient production of lipase, amylase, trypsin, or chymotrypsin by the pancreas. Causes of pancreatic insufficiency include chronic pancreatitis, pancreatic carcinoma, pancreatic resection, and cystic fibrosis. *Fat maldigestion* is the chief problem. A large amount of fat in the stool is the most common sign of pancreatic insufficiency.

Lactase deficiency inhibits the breakdown of lactose or milk sugar into monosaccharides and therefore prevents lactose digestion and absorption across the intestinal wall. Lactase deficiency is most common in African Americans, Hispanics, and Native Americans. The *undigested lactose* remains in the intestine, where bacterial fermentation *causes gases to form.* The osmotic gradient in the intestine also increases, causing irritation and *osmotic diarrhea.*

Conjugated bile acids or bile salts are necessary for the digestion and absorption of fats. When bile from the liver enters the duodenum, the bile salts aggregate with fatty acids and monoglycerides to form micelles. Micelle formation solubilizes fat molecules and allows them to pass through the unstirred layer at the brush-border. Advanced liver disease that causes **bile salt deficiency,** obstruction of the common bile duct, intestinal immotility, and diseases of the ileum all lead to *poor intestinal absorption of fat and of the fat-soluble vitamins,* A, D, E, and K. Increased fat in the stool leads to diarrhea and decreased plasma proteins. The loss of fat-soluble vitamins causes night blindness, bone demineralization, and bleeding abnormalities.

6. Compare ulcerative colitis to Crohn disease.
Study pages 908-910; refer to Table 34-6.

Ulcerative Colitis and Crohn Disease

Feature	Ulcerative Colitis	Crohn Disease
Family history	Less common	More common
Location of lesions	Large intestine; no "skip" lesions, mucosal layer involved	Large or small intestine, "skip" lesions common, entire intestinal wall involved
Granulomas	Rare	Common
Anal and perianal fistulas and abscesses	Rare	Common
Narrowed lumen and possible obstruction	Rare	Common

Continued

Ulcerative Colitis and Crohn Disease—Cont'd

Feature	Ulcerative Colitis	Crohn Disease
Abdominal pain	Common, mild to severe	Common, moderate to severe
Diarrhea	Common	Common
Bloody stools	Common	Less common
Abdominal mass	Rare	Common
Small intestinal malabsorption	Rare	Common
Cancer risk	Increased	Increased

7. Distinguish between diverticular disease and appendicitis.
Study page 910; refer to Figure 34-9.

Diverticula are herniations or saclike outpouchings of mucosa through the muscle layers of the colon wall. **Diverticulosis** is *asymptomatic* diverticular disease. **Diverticulitis** represents *symptomatic* inflammation. The most common site of diverticula is the sigmoid colon at weak points in the colon wall where arteries penetrate the muscularis. Habitual consumption of a low-residue diet reduces both fecal bulk and the diameter of the colon. According to the law of Laplace, wall pressure increases as the diameter of the lumen decreases. Pressure within the narrow lumen can increase enough to *rupture the diverticula* and cause *abscess formation* or peritonitis. An increase of dietary fiber intake often relieves symptoms. Surgical resection may be required if there are severe complications.

Appendicitis is an inflammation of the vermiform appendix. *Obstruction of the lumen* with feces, tumors, or foreign bodies followed by bacterial infection is the most likely cause of appendicitis. The obstructed lumen does not allow drainage of the appendix, and as mucosal secretion continues, intraluminal pressure rises. The increased pressure decreases mucosal blood flow, and the *appendix becomes hypoxic.* The mucosa ulcerates, promoting bacterial inflammation and edema. Gangrene develops from thrombosis of the luminal blood vessels, followed by perforation.

Epigastric or periumbilical pain is the typical symptom of an inflamed appendix. Right lower quadrant pain and *rebound tenderness* are associated with extension of the inflammation to the surrounding tissues. Nausea, vomiting, and anorexia follow the onset of pain. Leukocytosis and a low-grade fever are common. Perforation, peritonitis, and abscess formation are the most serious complications of appendicitis.

Appendectomy is the treatment for simple or perforated appendicitis.

8. Characterize irritable bowel syndrome (IBS)
Study page 911.

IBS is a functional disorder without specific structural or biochemical alterations. It manifests as *diarrhea or constipation* or both. Diarrhea is present in individuals having rapid colonic transit whereas those having bloating and constipation have delayed transit times. It is estimated that 7% to 20% of the world's population is afflicted with IBS. Other symptoms are anxiety, depression, and chronic fatigue syndrome.

The causal mechanisms are multiple and related to dysregulation of the *"brain-gut axis,"* the role of serotonin, activation of the immune system, or alterations in autonomic or central nervous system information processing. Intestinal infections and low-grade inflammation have been associated with symptoms of IBS. Food antigens or food borne pathogens may activate the mucosal immune system or mediate hypersensitivity. Psychosocial factors and stress influence brain-gut interreactions. There is no cure for IBS. Treatment of symptoms may include laxatives and fiber, antidiarrheals, low-dose antidepressants, visceral analgesics, and serotonin agonists or antagonists.

9. Distinguish between acute and chronic arterial insufficiencies.
Study pages 911 and 912.

Acute occlusion of mesenteric artery blood flow results from dissecting aortic *aneurysms or emboli arising from cardiac alterations.* The ischemic and damaged intestinal mucosa cannot produce enough *mucus to protect itself from digestive enzymes.* Mucosal alteration causes fluid to move from the blood vessels into the bowel wall and peritoneum. Fluid loss causes hypovolemia and further decreases the intestinal blood flow. As intestinal infarction progresses, shock, fever, bloody diarrhea, and leukocytosis develop. Abdominal pain may be severe. Bacteria invade the necrotic intestinal wall, causing gangrene and peritonitis.

Chronic mesenteric insufficiency can develop from any condition that decreases arterial blood flow. Elderly individuals with arteriosclerosis are particularly susceptible. Colicky abdominal pain after eating is the cardinal symptom of chronic mesenteric insufficiency. Progressive vascular obstruction eventually causes continuous abdominal pain and necrosis of the intestinal tissue. Chronic segmental ischemia may lead to strictures and destruction.

Diagnosis of mesenteric artery occlusion is based on clinical manifestations and laboratory findings. After angiography, a vasodilating agent may be injected to improve circulation. Surgery is required to remove necrotic tissue or repair sclerosed vessels.

10. Characterize the disorders of overnutrition and undernutrition.
Study pages 912-915; refer to Figure 34-10.

Overnutrition, or excessive caloric intake, leads to **obesity**, or excessive body fat, which is associated with three leading causes of death: *cardiovascular disease, cancer,* and *diabetes mellitus*. Obesity also is a risk factor for breast, cervical, endometrial, and liver cancers in women. Obese men are at greater risk for prostatic, colon, and rectal cancers than nonobese men.

Obesity, defined as a body mass index (BMI = kg/m^2) greater than 30, is evidenced by an increased fat cell mass. Neuroendocrine regulation of appetite, eating behavior, energy metabolism, and body fat mass is controlled by a dynamic circuit of signaling molecules from the periphery acting on the hypothalamus. An imbalance in this system is usually associated with excessive caloric intake in relation to exercise and caloric expenditure; the consequence is weight gain and obesity. Obesity is associated with increased circulating plasma levels of leptin, insulin, ghrelin, and peptide YY and decreased levels of adiponectin.

Leptin, a product of the obesity gene (Ob gene), is a hormone. Leptin acts on the hypothalamus to suppress appetite and regulates body weight in a fairly narrow range. There are two forms of adipose distribution. **Central obesity** occurs when body fat is localized around the abdomen and upper body resulting in an *apple shape*; it is the form found in men. **Peripheral obesity** occurs when body fat is around the thighs and buttocks, resulting in *pear shape*; it is found in women.

Obesity is a chronic disease treated by correction of metabolic abnormalities, individual weight-reduction diets, and exercise. Additional treatments include psychotherapy, behavioral modification, medications, and gastric bypass or gastric banding.

Undernutrition affects many young adults and adolescents in the United States and is manifested by two complex and related eating disorders: anorexia nervosa and bulimia nervosa. **Anorexia nervosa** is characterized by a refusal to eat because of distorted body image perceptions that one is too fat even if actually underweight. As the disease progresses, fat and muscle depletion give the individual a skeletal appearance. The *loss of 25% to 30%* of ideal body weight can eventually lead to death caused by starvation-induced cardiac failure. Treatment objectives for anorexia nervosa include reversing the compromised physical and psychologic states, promoting insights and knowledge about the disorder, and modifying food habits to restore weight.

Bulimia nervosa is characterized by *binging* or the consumption of normal to large amounts of food followed by *self-induced vomiting* or purging of the intestines with laxatives. Although individuals with bulimia are afraid of gaining weight, their weight usually remains within normal range. Because of the negative connotations of vomiting and purging, individuals who have bulimia often binge and purge secretly. Bulimics may binge and purge as often as 20 times a day. Continual vomiting of acidic chyme can cause pitted teeth, pharyngeal and esophageal inflammation, and tracheoesophageal fistulas. Overuse of laxatives can cause rectal bleeding.

Starvation (extreme malnutrition) can be either short term or long term. Therapeutic *short-term starvation* is part of many weight-reduction programs, whereas therapeutic *long-term starvation* is used in medically controlled environments to facilitate rapid weight loss in morbidly obese individuals. Short-term starvation consists of several days of total dietary abstinence or deprivation. Glucose is the preferred energy source for cells. Once all available energy has been absorbed from the intestine, glycogen in the liver is converted to glucose through glycogenolysis, or the splitting of glycogen into glucose. This process peaks within 4 to 8 hours after glycogenolysis, and gluconeogenesis in the liver begins by the formation of glucose from noncarbohydrate molecules. Both of these processes deplete stored nutrients, which thus cannot meet the body's energy needs indefinitely. Proteins continue to be catabolized in gluconeogenesis to a minimal degree to provide carbon for the synthesis of glucose.

Poverty or chronic disease—such as cardiovascular, pulmonary, hepatic, and digestive disorders, malabsorption syndromes, and cancer—can cause pathologic long-term starvation. The main characteristics of long-term starvation are *decreased dependence on gluconeogenesis and increased use of products of lipid and pyruvate metabolism for cellular energy sources.* Once the supply of adipose tissue is depleted, proteolysis begins. The breakdown of muscle protein is the last process to supply energy for life. Death results from severe alteration in electrolyte balance and loss of renal, pulmonary, and cardiac function

Cachexia is physical *wasting* with loss of weight and muscle atrophy, fatigue, and weakness. Inflammatory mediators associated with advanced cancer, AIDS, tuberculosis, and other chronic progressive diseases contribute to cachexia. Cachexia is not the same as starvation. A healthy individual's body can adjust to starvation by slowing metabolism; in cachexia, the body does not make this adjustment.

Adequate ingestion of appropriate nutrients is the obvious treatment for starvation. Starvation caused by chronic disease, long-term illness, or malabsorption is treated with enteral or parenteral nutrition.

11. Describe the complications of liver dysfunction.
Study pages 915-919; refer to Figures 34-11 through 34-14 and Table 34-7.

The complications of liver disease include portal hypertension, ascites, hepatic encephalopathy, jaundice, and hepatorenal syndrome. (See the following table.)

Liver Disease Complications

Complication	Cause(s)	Manifestations
Portal hypertension	Obstruction or impeded blood flow in portal venous system or vena cava cirrhosis, viral hepatitis, parasitic infection hepatic vein thrombosis, right heart failure	Esophageal and stomach varices, with vomiting of blood, splenomegaly, ascites
Ascites	Portal hypertension and reduced serum albumin levels increase capillary hydrostatic pressure, which pushes water into the peritoneal cavity; cirrhosis, heart failure, constrictive pericarditis, abdominal malignancies, nephritic syndrome, malnutrition	Abdominal distention, displaced diaphragm, dyspnea, peritonitis
Hepatic encephalopathy	Blood that contains toxins, such as ammonia, is shunted from gastrointestinal tract to systemic circulation, toxins reach brain	Subtle changes in cerebral function, confusion, tremor of hands, stupor, convulsions, coma
Jaundice	Hyperbilirubinemia	Dark urine, light-colored stools, yellow discolorization of sclera and skin, anorexia, malaise, fatigue, pruritus
Hemolytic (unconjugated bilirubin)	Excessive hemolysis of red blood cells because of immune reactions, infections, toxic substances, or transfusions of incompatible blood	
Obstructive (conjugated bilirubin)	Obstruction of bile flow by gallstones or tumor prevents flow into duodenum, drugs	
Hepatocellular (conjugated and unconjugated bilirubin)	Intrahepatic disease, obstruction by bile calculi, genetic enzyme defects, infections	
Hepatorenal syndrome	Decreased blood volume; intrarenal vasoconstriction due to failure of the liver to remove excessive vasoactive substances from the blood	Oliguria, sodium and water retention, hypotension, blood urea nitrogen (BUN) and creatinine increases

12. Compare the types of viral hepatitis.
Study pages 919-921; refer to Table 34-8.

The clinical manifestations of the different types of hepatitis are similar and usually consist of three phases: prodromal, icteric, and recovery. The **prodromal phase** of hepatitis begins about 2 weeks after exposure and ends with the appearance of jaundice. Fatigue, anorexia, malaise, nausea, vomiting, headache, hyperalgia, cough, and low-grade fever precede the onset of jaundice. The infection is highly transmissible during this phase.

The **icteric phase** begins about 1 to 2 weeks after the prodromal phase and lasts 2 to 6 weeks. The icteric phase is the actual phase of illness. The liver is enlarged, smooth, and tender, and percussion over the liver causes pain.

The posticteric or **recovery phase** begins with resolution of jaundice at about 6 to 8 weeks after exposure. In most cases, liver function returns to normal within 2 to 12 weeks after the onset of jaundice.

Characteristics of Viral Hepatitis

	Hepatitis A (HAV)	Hepatitis B (HBV)	Hepatitis D (HDV)	Hepatitis C (HCV)	Hepatitis E (HEV)
Transmission route	Fecal-oral, parenteral, sexual	Parenteral, sexual	Parenteral, fecal-oral, sexual	Parenteral	Fecal-oral
Incubation period (days)	30	60–180	30–180	35–60	15–60
Carrier state?	No	Yes	Yes	Yes	No

Characteristics of Viral Hepatitis—Cont'd

	Hepatitis A (HAV)	Hepatitis B (HBV)	Hepatitis D (HDV)	Hepatitis C (HCV)	Hepatitis E (HEV)
Severity	Mild	Severe, may be prolonged	Severe	Unknown	Severe in pregnant women
Chronic hepatitis?	No	Yes	Yes	Yes	No
Prophylaxis	Hygiene, immune serum globulin	Hygiene, HBV vaccine	Hygiene, HBV vaccine	Hygiene, screening blood	Hygiene, safe water

Note: Treatment is supportive; physical activity is restricted; low-fat and high-carbohydrate diet is recommended; and interferon is useful in B, C, and D types.

Fulminant hepatitis is a clinical syndrome resulting in severe impairment or necrosis of liver cells and potential liver failure. It may occur as a complication of hepatitis C or hepatitis B and is compounded by infection with the delta virus. The hepatic necrosis is irreversible. Treatment of fulminant hepatitis is supportive, and many affected individuals die. Liver transplantation may be lifesaving. Survivors usually do not experience cirrhosis or chronic liver disease.

13. Describe cirrhosis and contrast the various types.
Study pages 921-923; refer to Figure 34-15.

Cirrhosis is an irreversible inflammatory disease that disrupts liver structure and function. Structural changes result from fibrosis, which is a consequence of inflammation to liver failure.

Cirrhosis of the Liver

Type	Cause	Manifestations
Alcoholic cirrhosis	Toxic effects of chronic and excessive alcohol intake; alcohol is oxidized by the liver to acetaldehyde, which damages hepatocytes	Typical*; decreased sexual function
Primary biliary cirrhosis	Unknown, possibly an autoimmune mechanism that scars ducts	Typical*; circulating IgG
Secondary biliary cirrhosis	Obstruction by neoplasms, strictures, or gallstones scar the ducts proximally	Typical*
Nonalcoholic fatty liver disease	Associated with obesity, high levels of cholesterol and triglycerides, metabolic syndrome, type 2 diabetes mellitus	Typical*

*Typical manifestations include hepatomegaly, splenomegaly, ascites, and jaundice. Serologic studies reveal elevations of enzymes and bilirubin, decreased albumin, and prolonged prothrombin time.

14. Compare cholelithiasis with cholecystitis.
Study pages 923 and 924; refer to Figure 34-16.

Gallstone formation is termed **cholelithiasis,** whereas inflammation of the gallbladder or cystic duct is known as **cholecystitis.** Gallstones are of two types: cholesterol and pigmented. Cholesterol stones are more common. Cholesterol gallstones form in bile that is supersaturated with cholesterol produced by the liver. Usually within the gallbladder, supersaturation sets the stage for cholesterol crystal formation and aggregation into "macrostones." If the stones become lodged in the cystic or common duct, they cause pain and cholecystitis. Pigmented stones are created by the binding of unconjugated bilirubin with calcium. Risk factors for cholelithiasis include obesity, middle age, female gender, American Indian ancestry, and gallbladder, pancreatic, or ileal disease.

Cholecystitis can be acute or chronic and is almost always caused by the lodging of a gallstone in the *cystic duct*. Obstruction causes distention and inflammation of the gallbladder, followed by decreased blood flow, ischemia, necrosis, and possible perforation.

Abdominal pain and *jaundice* are the cardinal manifestations of *cholelithiasis*. Vague symptoms include heartburn, flatulence, epigastric discomfort, and fatty food intolerances. *Biliary colic pain* can be intermittent or steady and is located in the *right upper quadrant* with radiation to the mid-upper back. Jaundice indicates that the stone is located in the *common bile duct*. Fever, leukocytosis, rebound tenderness, and abdominal muscle guarding are common findings. Serum bilirubin and alkaline phosphatase values may be elevated.

Laparoscopic cholecystectomy is the preferred treatment for gallstones that cause obstruction or inflammation.

Alternative treatments are the administration of drugs that dissolve the stones and ultrasonic lithotripsy.

15. Describe the pathogenesis of pancreatitis.
Study pages 924 and 925.

Pancreatitis, or inflammation of the pancreas, is a relatively rare but potentially serious disorder. It is believed that **acute pancreatitis** develops because of an injury or disruption of the pancreatic ducts or acini that permits leakage of pancreatic enzymes into pancreatic tissue. The *leaked enzymes initiate autodigestion* and acute pancreatitis. Bile reflux into the pancreas occurs if gallstones obstruct the *common bile duct*; the refluxed bile also injures pancreatic tissue. The acinar cell metabolizes ethanol, which generate toxic metabolites that injure pancreatic acinar cells, causing inflammation. Toxic enzymes also are released into the bloodstream and cause injury to vessels and other organs, such as the lungs and kidneys.

Chronic pancreatitis is caused mostly by alcohol abuse. The abuse results in structural fibrosis that impairs pancreatic function.

Mild to severe epigastric or midabdominal pain is the cardinal symptom of acute pancreatitis. The pain is caused by distention of pancreatic ducts and capsule, chemical irritation and inflammation of the peritoneum, and irritation or obstruction of the biliary tract. Fever and leukocytosis accompany the inflammatory response. Hypermotility or paralytic ileus secondary to the pancreatitis or peritonitis causes nausea and vomiting. Elevated *serum amylase and lipase* are diagnostic features, along with elevated urine amylase. Hypotension and shock often occur because plasma volume is lost as enzymes and kinins released into the circulation increase vascular permeability and dilate vessels. The results are hypovolemia, hypotension, and myocardial insufficiency.

The goal of treatment for acute pancreatitis is to stop the process of autodigestion and prevent systemic complications. Parenteral fluids are given to restore blood volume and prevent hypotension and shock. Severe, unremitting pancreatitis may require peritoneal lavage or surgical drainage of the pancreas to remove toxic exudates.

16. Characterize the various cancers of the digestive system.
Study pages 925-931; refer to Figures 34-17 through 34-20 and Tables 34-9.

Cancers of the Digestive System

Type	Risk Factors	Manifestations
Esophagus: Squamous cell carcinoma Adenocarcinom	Malnutrition, alcohol, tobacco, chronic reflux	Chest pain, dysphagia
Stomach: Adenocarcinoma Squamous cell carcinoma	Dietary salty foods, nitrates, nitrosamines, gastric atrophy, *H. pylori*–associated gastritis	Anorexia, malaise, weight loss, upper abdominal pain, vomiting, occult fecal blood, symptoms of organ involved in metastasis from stomach
Colorectal: Adenocarcinoma (left colon grows in ring; right colon grows in mass)	Chromosomal deletions, polyps, diverticulitis, ulcerative colitis, diet high in refined carbohydrate (CHO), low-fiber/high-fat diet	Pain, anemia, bloody stool, mass—right colon; obstruction—left colon; distention, elevated carcinoembryonic antigen (CEA)
Liver: Hepatocarcinoma Cholangiocarcinoma	HBV, HCV, HDV, cirrhosis, intestinal parasites, aflatoxin	Pain, anorexia, bloating, weight loss, portal hypertension, ascites, ±jaundice, elevated serum proteins and enzymes
Gallbladder: Secondary metastases Adenocarcinoma Squamous cell carcinoma	Cholelithiasis	Steady pain, diarrhea, anorexia, vomiting, weight loss
Pancreas: Adenocarcinoma	Chronic pancreatitis, cigarette smoking, alcohol, diabetic women	Weight loss, weakness, nausea, vomiting, abdominal pain, depression, ± jaundice, possible hypoglycemia if an insulin-secreting tumor

Note: The usual treatment for gastric, gallbladder, and pancreatic cancer is essentially surgical. Esophageal cancer is treated with a combination of irradiation and chemotherapy. Liver neoplasms are treated by surgery and chemotherapy. Colorectal cancer treatment consists of surgery, irradiation, and chemotherapy.

PRACTICE EXAMINATION

Multiple Choice

Circle the correct answer for each question:

1. During vomiting, there is:
   a. forceful diaphragm and abdominal muscle contractions, airway closure, esophageal sphincter relaxation, and deep inspiration.
   b. deep inspiration, airway closure, forceful diaphragm and abdominal muscle contractions, and esophageal sphincter relaxation.
   c. airway closure, forceful diaphragm and abdominal muscle contractions, deep inspiration, and esophageal sphincter relaxation.
   d. esophageal sphincter relaxation, forceful diaphragm and abdominal muscle contractions, deep inspiration, and airway closure.

2. IBS:
   a. is a structural disorder.
   b. manifests diarrhea when colonic transit is delayed.
   c. can be cured by using laxatives.
   d. is related to dysregulation of the "brain-gut axis."

3. Osmotic diarrhea is caused by:
   a. lactase deficiency.
   b. bacterial enterotoxins.
   c. ulcerative colitis.
   d. Crohn disease.
   e. Both c and d are correct.

4. Melena is:
   a. bloody vomitus.
   b. gaseous bowel distention.
   c. blood in the stool.
   d. loss of appetite.
   e. black, tarry stools.

5. A common manifestation of hiatal hernia is:
   a. gastroesophageal reflux.
   b. diarrhea.
   c. belching.
   d. postprandial substernal pain.
   e. Both a and d are correct.

6. Gastroesophageal reflux is:
   a. caused by rapid gastric emptying.
   b. excessive lower esophageal sphincter functioning.
   c. associated with abdominal surgery.
   d. caused by spontaneously relaxing lower esophageal sphincter.

7. Intestinal obstruction causes:
   a. decreased intraluminal tension.
   b. hyperkalemia.
   c. decreased nutrient absorption.
   d. Both a and b are correct.
   e. a, b, and c are correct.

8. Peptic ulcers may be located in the:
   a. stomach.
   b. esophagus.
   c. duodenum.
   d. colon.
   e. a, b, and c are correct.

9. Gastric ulcers:
   a. may lead to malignancy.
   b. occur at a younger age than duodenal ulcers.
   c. always have increased acid production.
   d. exhibit nocturnal pain.
   e. Both a and c are correct.

10. Duodenal ulcers:
    a. occur four times more often in females than in males.
    b. may be complicated by hemorrhage.
    c. are associated with sepsis.
    d. may cause inflammation and scar tissue formation around the sphincter of Oddi.

11. In malabsorption syndrome, flatulence and abdominal distention are likely caused by:
    a. protein deficiency and electrolyte imbalance.
    b. undigested lactose fermentation by bacteria.
    c. fat irritating the bowel.
    d. impaired absorption of amino acids and accompanying edema.

12. The characteristic lesion of Crohn disease is:
    a. found in the ileum.
    b. precancerous.
    c. granulomatous.
    d. malignant.
    e. Both a and c are correct.

13. Low-residue diets and chronic constipation play a role in the pathogenesis of:
    a. appendicitis.
    b. diverticulitis.
    c. ulcerative colitis.
    d. Crohn disease.
    e. cholecystitis.

14. A 14-year-old boy has been admitted to the emergency room with acute-onset abdominal pain in the lower right quadrant. Abdominal rebound tenderness is intense, and he has a fever and leukocytosis. This individual most likely is suffering from:
    a. acute appendicitis.
    b. diverticulitis.
    c. ulcerative colitis.
    d. cholelithiasis.
    e. cholecystitis.

15. Leptin:
    a. promotes insulin resistance.
    b. binds to insulin receptors.
    c. suppresses hunger/appetite at the hypothalamus.
    d. a, b, and c are correct.
    e. None of the above is correct.

16. Short-term starvation involves:
    a. glycogenolysis.
    b. gluconeogenesis.
    c. proteolysis.
    d. Both a and b are correct.
    e. a, b, and c are correct.

17. The most common manifestation of portal hypertension is:
    a. rectal bleeding.
    b. cirrhosis.
    c. intestinal bleeding.
    d. duodenal bleeding.
    e. vomiting of blood from esophageal bleeding.

18. Hepatic encephalopathy is manifested by:
    a. ascites.
    b. splenomegaly.
    c. dark urine.
    d. oliguria.
    e. cerebral dysfunction.

19. Which would be consistent with a diagnosis of viral hepatitis? (More than one answer may be correct.)
    a. elevated aspartate transaminase (AST) serum enzymes
    b. decreased serum albumin levels
    c. prolonged coagulation times
    d. increased serum bilirubin levels
    e. decreased alanine transaminase (ALT) serum enzymes

20. Which viral hepatitis is *not* associated with a chronic state or a carrier state?
    a. hepatitis A
    b. hepatitis B
    c. hepatitis C
    d. serum hepatitis
    e. hepatitis D

21. Which type of jaundice is caused by the increased destruction of erythrocytes?
    a. obstructive
    b. hemolytic
    c. hepatocellular
    d. Both b and c are correct.

22. Which most often causes biliary cirrhosis?
    a. malnutrition
    b. alcoholism
    c. hepatitis A or C
    d. autoimmunity
    e. biliary obstruction

23. Symptoms of cholelithiasis include all of the following *except*:
    a. nausea and vomiting.
    b. right upper quadrant tenderness.
    c. jaundice.
    d. decreased serum bilirubin levels.
    e. abdominal distress.

24. In pancreatitis:
    a. the tissue damage likely results from release of pancreatic enzymes.
    b. high cholesterol intake is causative.
    c. that is chronic, diabetes is uncommon.
    d. bacterial infection is the etiologic cause.

25. Predisposing factors in the development of colon cancer include all of the following *except*:
    a. familial polyposis.
    b. ulcerative colitis.
    c. low-fiber/high-fat diet.
    d. high-fiber diet.
    e. diet high in refined CHO.

Fill in the Blank

Complete the following table describing the manifestations of gastrointestinal bleeding:

Manifestations of Gastrointestinal Bleeding

Manifestations	Characteristics
Acute bleeding	
Occult bleeding	

CASE STUDY 1

Dr. R. is a 55-year-old male professor whose department chair is an unrelenting "harasser." Dr. R.'s family investments have failed, and his early planned retirement is no longer possible. Persistent upper abdominal pain for the last 2 months has persuaded him that he needs a diagnostic workup.

At the physician's office, Dr. R. reveals a history of smoking one pack of cigarettes a day for 25 years. His eating habits are irregular. However, he states, "My pain is more intense right after eating and if I use an antacid, the pain lessens." He often takes aspirin for headaches and to relieve rheumatoid stiffness while golfing. His family history and remaining personal history are unremarkable except that he has lost 10 pounds during the previous 6 weeks.

Which type of peptic ulcer do you, suspect? How could your suspicion be confirmed?

CASE STUDY 2

At a physician's office, D.K., a 33-year-old man states, "I have had several days of increasing fatigue and loss of appetite, and now I have a fever and abdominal and muscle discomfort." He admits to intravenous drug use.

Physical examination reveals right upper quadrant tenderness with hepatomegaly; a nonpalpable spleen; fever; no jaundice, rashes, nor ecchymoses; no ascites; no blood on rectal exam; no joint involvement; and no confusion or neurologic symptoms.

What laboratory tests would you choose and why? What information obtained from the history, physical examination, and laboratory results differentiates one possible diagnosis from another?

35 Alterations of Digestive Function in Children

FOUNDATIONAL OBJECTIVE

a. Describe the structure and function of the gastrointestinal tract and accessory organs of digestion.

MEMORY CHECK!
• See Foundational Objective "a" in Chapter 34.

LEARNING OBJECTIVES

After studying this chapter, the learner will be able to do the following:

1. Describe the pathophysiology and treatment associated with cleft lip and palate.
Study pages 938 and 939; refer to Figure 35-1.

Cleft lip is caused by *incomplete fusion* of the *nasomedial or intermaxillary process* during the fourth month of fetal development and occurs in approximately 1 in 1000 births. The defect in cleft lip is usually beneath one or both nostrils and may involve the external nose, nasal cartilages, nasal septum, and alveolar processes. It also may be associated with a flattening and broadening of the facial features, probably because of the absence of constraining structures that are omitted by the cleft.

Cleft palate occurs in approximately 1 in 2500 births and is often associated with cleft lip but can occur alone. The defect may affect only the *uvula* and *soft palate,* but may extend forward toward the nostrils through the hard palate. If it extends through the *hard palate,* open communication between the structures of the nasopharynx and the oral cavity leads to sinusitis and otitis media.

Cleft lip and cleft palate are caused by gene-environmental interactions. A major difficulty seen with these defects is *poor feeding.* The infant with isolated cleft lip, but an intact palate may feed without great difficulty. On the other hand, cleft palate may significantly interfere with feeding. Bottle-feeding may require a large, soft nipple with an oversized opening. Breastfeeding may be impossible for some infants with cleft palate without a prosthesis for the roof of the mouth.

Treatment is surgical correction that is usually accomplished in stages. Supportive therapy may include prosthodontics, orthodontics, and speech therapy.

2. Describe the structural defects of esophageal atresia and tracheoesophageal fistula (TEF).
Study pages 939 and 940; refer to Figure 35-2.

Congenital malformations of the esophagus occur in approximately 1 in 3000 to 4500 births. **Esophageal atresia** is a condition wherein the esophagus ends in a blind pouch and may be accompanied by a connection between the esophagus and the trachea called a TEF. These conditions develop from aberrant differentiation of the trachea at 4 to 6 weeks of embryonic development. The blind esophageal pouch in atresia fills rapidly with secretions or food and overflows; regurgitated food and fluid may be aspirated into the lungs. Thirty percent of children with this anomaly have other associated congenital defects, particularly cardiovascular defects.

Diagnosis is confirmed by the inability to pass a catheter through the esophagus. Treatment is surgical correction.

3. Describe the structural defect and pathophysiology associated with pyloric stenosis.
Study page 940.

Pyloric stenosis is an obstruction of the pylorus caused by hypertrophy of the pyloric sphincter. The cause is unknown. Obstruction becomes evident between 1 to 2 weeks and 3 to 4 months of age. Males are affected more often than females, and whites are more often affected than Asians or blacks. Pyloric stenosis is seen more often in full-term than in premature infants.

Generally, stenosis is manifested in a previously healthy infant who begins to have *marked forceful vomiting* at 2 to 3 weeks of age that does not resolve. Weight loss and fluid and electrolyte imbalances follow and may end in death if there is no intervention. A small, movable mass at the site of the hypertrophic pylorus may be palpable in the right upper quadrant of the abdomen.

Sonography shows hypertrophied pyloric muscles and a narrowed pyloric channel. Treatment usually involves surgical release of the hypertrophic fibers or pyloromyotomy after stabilization of the infant's fluid and electrolyte balance.

4. Describe intestinal malrotation.
Study page 941.

In **intestinal malrotation of the colon,** there is incomplete rotation around the superior mesenteric artery during fetal development. Additionally, an abnormal membrane or periduodenal band (Ladd band) may press on the duodenum and obstruct it. Intestinal twisting, or *volvulus,* around the rudimentary mesentery angulates and obstructs the intestinal lumen and can occlude the superior mesenteric artery, causing *infarction of the entire midgut.*

Fever, pain, scanty or bloody stools, and diarrhea are seen in infants with intestinal malrotation of the colon. In older children, the condition may be asymptomatic, being discovered during unrelated abdominal surgery, or may cause nausea after meals, vomiting, or abdominal pain. Treatment involves laparoscopic or open surgery to reduce the volvulus.

5. Describe meconium ileus; note other intestinal obstructions or malformations.
Study pages 941 and 942.

Meconium is a substance of intestinal secretions and amniotic fluid that fills the entire intestine before birth, forms the first stools of the newborn, and is usually passed during the first 12 to 72 hours after birth. **Meconium ileus** is an intestinal obstruction caused by the meconium in the newborn. Peristalsis fails to propel meconium through the ileum, and impaction occurs. The cause is usually *a lack of digestive enzymes during fetal life,* which is associated with cystic fibrosis. Abdominal distention usually develops during the first days of life, and the infant, unable to pass meconium, begins to vomit. Infants with cystic fibrosis (CF) may have signs of pulmonary involvement.

The treatment in cases without volvulus or perforation is a hyperosmolar enema performed using fluoroscopy to evacuate the meconium. If evacuation is not possible, the meconium is removed surgically.

Other obstructions involve the duodenum, jejunum, and ileum, which are caused by atresia, congenital aganglionic megacolon, and acquired obstructive disorders. *Meckel diverticulum* is a congenital malformation of the gastrointestinal tract involving all layers of the small intestinal wall, usually in the ileum. *Malformations* of the anus and rectum range from mild congenital stenosis to complex deformities and are classified as imperforate anus.

6. Describe congenital aganglionic megacolon, or Hirschsprung disease.
Study page 942; refer to Figures 35-3 and 35-4.

Congenital aganglionic megacolon, or **Hirschsprung disease**, is a condition associated with failure of the *parasympathetic nervous system* to produce intramural ganglion cells in the enteric nerve plexuses. This failure of innervation causes a section of the colon to be *immotile* and creates a functional intestinal obstruction in the affected area. This section becomes distended with feces, thus the name "megacolon." Eighty percent of these disorders are limited to the rectal end of the sigmoid colon. Hirschsprung disease accounts for one third of all intestinal obstructions in infants and occurs in 1 in 5000 births, with a greater incidence in males.

Clinical manifestations are mild to severe chronic constipation, although diarrhea may be the first sign because only liquid may pass the aganglionic section. Severe edema of the colon begins to obstruct blood and lymphatic flow, causing *enterocolitis* and tissue destruction. Bacteria can infiltrate the bowel wall from the lumen and may cause gram-negative sepsis. Severe fluid and electrolyte imbalance caused by diarrhea may become life threatening.

Diagnosis is confirmed by rectal biopsy that demonstrates the aganglionic bowel. Definitive treatment consists of resection of the aganglionic segment and constant attention to bowel hygiene thereafter.

7. Describe intussusception.
Study pages 943 and 944; refer to Figure 35-5.

Intussusception is the *telescoping or invagination* of one portion of the intestine into another, which causes an intestinal obstruction. The most commonly affected area is the ileum, which invaginates into the cecum through the ileocecal valve. Intussusception generally occurs between 5 and 7 months of age and is the most common obstruction in infants.

The telescoping bowel *obstructs blood and lymphatic flow,* leading rapidly to edema and compression and obstructing chyme flow. Abdominal tenderness and distention develop as the obstruction becomes more acute. Classic symptoms include colicky abdominal pain, vomiting, and bloody stools. Diagnosis is made from clinical manifestations and is confirmed by ultrasonography. Reduction of the intussusception must be done immediately and is often performed using an air enema to push the invaginated bowel segment from its intussusception. Some children require surgery to correct the intussusception or related complications. This condition is fatal if untreated.

8. Describe the pathophysiology and potential complications related to gastroesophageal reflux (GER).
Study page 944.

GER is the return of gastric contents into the esophagus because of poor function of the *lower esophageal sphincter*. GER is more common in premature than in term newborn infants and usually decreases by 6 to 12 months of age. Delayed maturation of the sphincter and impaired hormonal response mechanisms are likely causes. Other factors include the location of the gastroesophageal junction and the angle of the junction between the esophagus and the stomach.

Clinical manifestations include forceful vomiting within the first week of life (85%), *aspiration pneumonia* in one third of those affected, and poor weight gain. **Esophagitis** may result from exposure of the esophagus to acidic gastric contents, which may cause either strictures or anemia from prolonged occult blood loss.

Diagnosis may be confirmed by endoscopy or esophageal pH probe studies that demonstrate an abrupt drop in esophageal pH during the reflux episodes. Mild GER resolves without treatment, although some children require small and frequent feedings to help reduce reflux. Pharmacologic therapies include medication to increase lower gastrointestinal motility, gastric emptying time, and decrease gastric acidity. Surgical correction or fundoplication is rarely required but may be performed if medical management is ineffective.

9. Describe the gastrointestinal and digestive abnormalities associated with CF.
Study page 944; refer to Table 35-1.

CF is an autosomal recessive disease. The classic triad of the pathophysiology of CF is: (1) *pancreatic enzyme deficiency* leading to maldigestion, (2) *overproduction of mucus in the respiratory tract* leading to chronic obstructive pulmonary disease, and (3) *elevations of sodium and chloride in sweat*. Viscous exocrine secretions tend to obstruct glandular ducts.

Approximately 85% of children with CF have pancreatic insufficiency. The lack of pancreatic enzymes results in maldigestion of proteins, carbohydrates, and fats, leading to chronic malnutrition. Pancreatic ducts also may be blocked with viscous secretions that eventually may damage pancreatic cells and lead to diabetes mellitus.

Pancreatic enzyme function may be estimated by 72-hour fecal fat measurement; fecal content of trypsin and chymotrypsin also may be measured. Pancreatic enzyme replacement may be administered with meals, and a high-calorie, high-protein diet is required.

10. Describe gluten-sensitive enteropathy.
Study pages 944-946; refer to Figure 35-6.

Gluten-sensitive enteropathy, formerly called *celiac sprue* or *celiac disease*, is an autoimmune disease that damages small intestinal villous epithelium upon ingestion of *gluten,* the protein components of *cereal grains.* It has been associated with other immune disorders, including diabetes and thyroid disease. The disease occurs mostly in whites.

Diarrhea and failure to thrive are early signs in most infants with the disorder. The stools are pale, bulky, greasy, and foul smelling; they may contain oil droplets. Vomiting and abdominal pain are prominent in infants, but unusual in older children. Anorexia is prevalent, and growth is usually diminished. Consequences of malabsorption, such as rickets, tetany, frank bleeding, or anemia, may be obvious.

An intestinal biopsy is required to detect the classic mucosal changes caused by gluten-sensitive enteropathy. Serum gluten immunoglobulin A (IgA) antibodies also may be measured.

Treatment requires immediate and permanent institution of a diet free of wheat, rye, barley, oats, and malt. *Lactose* (milk sugar) is also excluded because lactose intolerance is presumed. Infants are given vitamin D, iron, and folic acid supplements to treat deficiencies.

11. Compare kwashiorkor with marasmus; describe failure to thrive (FTT) in infants or children.
Review page 995.

Kwashiorkor and **marasmus** are types of malnutrition in children. They are collectively known as **protein energy malnutrition (PEM)**. Both are states of long-term starvation. Kwashiorkor is a severe *protein deficiency*, and marasmus is a severe *deficiency of all nutrients*. Both are problems in impoverished populations.

In kwashiorkor, protein synthesis is reduced in all tissues. Physical and mental growth is stunted. The lack of sufficient plasma proteins results in generalized edema. The liver swells with stored fat because no hepatic proteins are synthesized to form and release lipoproteins. Kwashiorkor also causes malabsorption, reduces bone density, and impairs renal function.

In marasmus, metabolic processes including liver function are preserved, but growth is severely retarded. Caloric intake is too low to support protein synthesis for growth or the storage of fat. Muscle and fat wasting occur. Anemia is common and may be severe.

FTT is the inadequate physical growth of an infant or child and has either an *organic or nonorganic cause*. Organic FTT is caused by genetic, anatomic, or pathophysiologic factors. Nonorganic FTT is caused by nutritional deficits associated with inadequate nurturing.

Management of organic FTT from consists of treating the cause. Management of nonorganic FTT involves the immediate total care of the infant or child.

12. Describe necrotizing enterocolitis (NEC).
Study text pages 947-949.

NEC is a disorder of neonates, particularly premature infants. Reduced mucosal blood flow leading to *hypoxic injury to intestinal mucosa* is thought to be the cause. This injury allows bacteria to invade the mucosa and submucosa, and release of inflammatory mediators causes necrosis and even perforation of the intestinal wall.

Treatments include cessation of feeding, gastric section to decompress the intestines, fluid and electrolyte maintenance, and antibiotic administration to control sepsis. Surgical resection is the treatment of choice for intestinal perforation.

13. Describe childhood diarrhea.
Study text page 948.

Diarrhea in children is similar to that in adults. *Prolonged diarrhea* is more dangerous in children because they have much smaller fluid reserves than adults. Therefore, *dehydration* can develop rapidly. *Infectious diarrhea* in newborns is usually associated with nursery epidemics involving gram-negative pathogens and staphylococci. *Acute diarrhea* in children is most synonymous with acute viral or bacterial gastroenteritis and tends to be self limiting. *Chronic diarrhea*—diarrhea persisting more than 4 weeks—is caused by abnormal colonic motility, *lactose intolerance,* parasitic infestation, impaired absorption, and antibiotic use.

14. Describe physiologic jaundice of the newborn.
Study pages 948 and 949.

Physiologic jaundice of the newborn is usually a transient, benign icterus that occurs during the first week of life in otherwise healthy, full-term infants. It is caused by mild unconjugated (indirect reacting) *hyperbilirubinemia.* A high level of indirect hyperbilirubinemia (15 mg/dL) is considered pathologic. There is a risk of brain damage, **kernicterus,** because the bilirubin passes into brain cells and is toxic with persistent high indirect hyperbilirubinemia.

Physiologic jaundice is usually treated with ultraviolet light. *Pathologic jaundice* requires an exchange transfusion.

15. Identify other childhood liver disorders.
Study text pages 949-951.

Biliary atresia is a congenital malformation of the bile ducts that obstructs bile flow causing jaundice, cirrhosis, and liver failure. Acute **hepatitis** is usually caused by a virus, and hepatitis A (caused by hepatitis A virus [HAV]) is the most common form of childhood hepatitis. Chronic hepatitis B (HBV) or C (HCB) usually is caused by perinatal transmission. **Cirrhosis** results from fibrotic scarring of the liver and is rare in children, but it can develop in most forms of chronic liver disease. **Portal hypertension** in children is usually caused by extrahepatic obstruction; thrombosis of the portal vein is the most common cause and leads to in splenomegaly.

16. Identify common metabolic disorders injurious to the liver.
Refer to Table 35-2.

The three most common metabolic disorders that cause liver damage in children are *galactosemia* (galactose cannot be converted to glucose), *fructosemia* (fructose, sucrose, or honey cannot be metabolized), and *Wilson disease* (impaired copper transport in blood). All three are inherited as genetic traits and permit the accumulation of toxins in the liver.

PRACTICE EXAMINATION

True/False

1. Pyloric stenosis is caused by the prolapse of gastric tissue into the pylorus and results in edema and obstruction.
2. TEF is often associated with esophageal atresia.
3. Poor weight gain associated with GER may be ignored because it is a self-limiting disorder.
4. Intussusception involves a blind pouch in the esophagus.
5. Kernicterus is present in physiologic jaundice of the newborn.
6. A small, movable mass may be palpable in the right upper quadrate of the abdomen.
7. Diabetes mellitus may be a complication of CF.
8. The pharmacologic approach to GER includes pancreatic enzyme replacement.
9. Congenital aganglionic megacolon is the result of faulty innervation of the colon.
10. The pharmacologic approach to CF includes the administration of medications that increase lower gastrointestinal motility in an effort to aid the passage of large, bulky stools.
11. Rectal biopsy is useful in the diagnosis of aganglionic megacolon.

Fill in the Blank

12. ________________ has been attributed to impaired hormonal response.
13. In congenital aganglionic megacolon, the first sign may be ________________.
14. A pH probe will demonstrate a(n) ________________ in esophageal pH during a period of reflux.
15. Cleft palate is often complicated by communication between the ________________ and ________________ cavities.
16. ________________ may be a complication of CF.

Matching

Match the description with the alteration:

17. Involves the parasympathetic nervous system
18. Acute onset of abdominal pain and distention
19. Accompanying cardiovascular defects
20. May cause development of enterocolitis
21. Food regurgitation
22. May contribute to aspiration pneumonia
23. Incompetent lower esophageal sphincter
24. Bloody stools
25. Enema may be treatment

a. congenital aganglionic megacolon
b. TEF
c. intussusception
d. GER
e. esophageal atresia

Fill in the Blank

Complete the following table identifying the secretory dysfunction, manifestations, and complications of the pathophysiologic triad of CF:

Cystic Fibrosis Characteristics

Involved Organ	Secretory Dysfunction	Manifestations	Complications
Sweat glands			
Pancreas			
Lungs	Overproduction of viscid mucus in bronchi and bronchioles	Obstruction of bronchioles causing bronchiolectasis, bronchiectasis, and lung infection	Hemoptysis, pneumothorax, cor pulmonale, respiratory failure

CASE STUDY

Baby B is a male term infant born vaginally to a 21-year-old white woman; he is her first child. Three weeks after birth, he began to vomit without apparent reason. At the pediatrician's office, his mother states, "He eats well and has gained weight until now. But now he vomits right after eating."

What is Baby B's likely problem, and what can be done?

36 Structure and Function of the Musculoskeletal System

FOUNDATIONAL OBJECTIVES

After reviewing this chapter, the learner will be able to do the following:

1. **Identify the structural elements and function of bone.**
   Review pages 954, 955, 957 and 958; refer to Figure 36-1 and Tables 36-1 through 36-3.

2. **Describe the features of compact and spongy bone; classify bones.**
   Review pages 959 and 960; refer to Figures 36-2 through 36-4.

3. **Describe the process of bone remodeling and healing.**
   Review page 962; refer to Figure 36-5.

4. **Classify joints structurally and functionally; characterize articular cartilage.**
   Review pages 962-965; refer to Figures 36-6 through 36-11.

5. **Describe the arrangements of muscle fiber in a skeletal muscle; explain the structure and function of a motor unit.**
   Review pages 965 and 967-970; refer to Figures 36-12 through 36-15 and Tables 36-4 and 36-5.

6. **Describe skeletal muscle contraction at the molecular level.**
   Review pages 970-972; refer to Figure 36-16 and Table 36-5.

7. **Identify the energy sources for muscular contraction.**
   Review pages 972 and 973; refer to Table 36-6.

8. **Indicate the types of skeletal muscle contractions and the interaction among groups of muscles.**
   Review pages 973 and 974; refer to Figure 36-17.

9. **Describe the relationship between tendons and ligament.**
   Review page 974; refer to Figure 36-18.

10. **Describe the changes in the musculoskeletal system that accompany normal aging.**
    Review pages 974 and 975.

PRACTICE EXAMINATION

Multiple Choice

Circle the correct answer for each question:

1 Tendons: (More than one answer may be correct.)
   a. are composed of collagen.
   b. restrict movement.
   c. have parallel rows of fibroblasts.
   d. provide stability during movement.
   e. line body cavities.

2. Sialoprotein:
   a. promotes resorption.
   b. binds calcium.
   c. stabilizes the basement membrane of bones.
   d. promotes calcification.

3. The diaphysis is the:
   a. rounded end of a long bone.
   b. shaft of a long bone.
   c. lattice framework of a spongy bone.
   d. surface of a synovial cavity.

4. A function of the epiphyseal plate that is *not* a function of the articular cartilage is to:
   a. enable articulation of bones.
   b. enable bone to increase in length.
   c. repair damaged bone tissue.
   d. provide sensory nerves to bone.

5. The remodeling of bone is done by basic multicellular units that consist of bone precursor cells. Precursor cells:
   a. differentiate into osteoclasts and osteoblasts.
   b. are located on free surfaces of bone and along vascular channels.
   c. Neither a nor b is correct.
   d. Both a and b are correct.

6. Identify the sequence of bone healing in fractures and surgical injuries.
   a. 2, 1, 3, 4, 5
   b. 3, 1, 2, 4, 5
   c. 3, 2, 1, 4, 5
   d. 1, 2, 3, 4, 5
   e. 1, 2, 3, 5, 4

   (1) procallus formation
   (2) callus formation
   (3) hematoma formation
   (4) callus replacement with lamellar or trabecular bone
   (5) periosteum and endosteum remodeling

7. Joints are classified functionally and structurally. Which is a proper functional and structural relationship?
   a. amphiarthrosis/fibrous
   b. diarthrosis/synovial
   c. synarthrosis/synchondrosis
   d. diarthrosis/fibrous
   e. synarthrosis/cartilaginous

8. In older individuals, the bone remodeling cycle:
   a. is faster because osteoclastic activity is enhanced.
   b. is enhanced because mineralization increases.
   c. has more precursor cells.
   d. has fewer bone cells because the bone marrow becomes infiltrated with fat.
   e. Both a and b are correct.

9. Which is *not* included in a motor unit?
   a. muscle fibers
   b. motor nerve axons
   c. anterior horn cell
   d. upper motor neuron

10. The perimysium is to a fasciculus as:
    a. periosteum is to a bone.
    b. a muscle is to the epimysium.
    c. a myofibril is to a muscle fiber.
    d. the epimysium is to the endomysium.
    e. a muscle cell is to the endomysium.

11. Which is *not* a characteristic of type I muscle fibers?
    a. sparse capillary supply
    b. slow contraction speed
    c. high resistance to fatigue
    d. profuse capillary supply
    e. oxidative metabolism

12. Which protein is found in the thick myofilaments?
    a. actin
    b. myosin
    c. troponin
    d. tropomyosin
    e. a, c, and d are correct.

13. An important function of the transverse tubules is to:
    a. provide organic nutrients to muscle fibers.
    b. initiate fiber contraction.
    c. enable regeneration of muscle fibers.
    d. allow for intracellular calcium uptake.

14. The ion necessary for coupling is:
    a. sodium.
    b. calcium.
    c. potassium.
    d. magnesium.
    e. phosphate.

15. Aerobic respiration:
    a. permits the body brief periods during which it does not require oxygen.
    b. causes an increase in the amount of lactic acid.
    c. yields more molecules of ATP than anaerobic respiration.
    d. uses more glycogen to produce ATP than anaerobic respiration.
    e. leads to oxygen debt.

16. Repayment of oxygen debt:
    a. converts lactic acid to glycogen.
    b. replenishes ATP stores.
    c. replenishes phosphocreatine stores.
    d. Both b and c are correct.
    e. a, b, and c are correct.

17. The strength of muscle contraction depends on the:
    a. extent of the load.
    b. initial length of muscle fibers.
    c. recruitment of additional motor units.
    d. nerve innervation ratios.
    e. All of the above are correct.

18. Attempting to push an object that is too heavy to move is an example of a(n) _____ contraction.
    a. isotonic
    b. concentric
    c. flaccid
    d. tetanic
    e. isometric

19. Which does *not* happen with muscle as individuals grow older?
    a. Type II fibers may decrease.
    b. Mitochondrial volume decreases.
    c. The amount of RNA increases to compensate for decreased size of motor units.
    d. All of the above occur with advancing age.

Matching

Match the microscopic feature of bone with its description:

_______ 20. Volkmann canals

_______ 21. Trabeculae

_______ 22. Lamellae

a. small canals that connect bone cells
b. concentric rings
c. cavities where bone cells are housed
d. contains blood vessels
e. irregular meshwork

Match the microscopic feature of muscle fibers with its description:

_______ 23. Sarcomere

_______ 24. Sarcolemma

_______ 25. Sarcoplasmic reticulum

a. membrane covering the muscle cell
b. flattened, tubelike network
c. unit of contraction
d. calcium transport
e. tubules that run perpendicular to muscle myofibrils

Fill in the Blank

Complete the following table comparing bone remodeling with bone repair:

Bone Remodeling and Repair

Stage	Process
Remodeling (Minor Injuries)	
Phase 1	
Phase 2	
Phase 3	Osteoblasts lining the resorption cavity lay down new or secondary bone by forming a new haversian cavity in compact bone or new trabeculae in spongy bone
Repair (Fracture and Surgery)	
Hematoma formation	Blood leaks from torn blood vessel across the fracture line, causing a hematoma
Procallus formation	
Callus formation	
Callus replacement	
Remodeling	

37 Alterations of Musculoskeletal Function

FOUNDATIONAL OBJECTIVES

a. Describe the processes that maintain bone integrity.
Review text page 962; refer to Figure 36-5.

MEMORY CHECK!

- The internal structure of bone is maintained by a *remodeling process* in which existing bone is resorbed and new bone is laid down to replace it. Remodeling is accomplished by clusters of bone cells made up of bone precursor cells located on the free surfaces of bones and along the vascular channels and marrow cavities. The precursor cells differentiate into osteoclasts and osteoblasts.
- In *phase one* of the remodeling cycle, a stimulus such as a hormone, drug, vitamin, or physical stressor activates the osteoclasts. In *phase two*, the osteoclasts resorb bone and leave in its place an elongated cavity termed a resorption cavity. The resorption cavity in compact bone follows the longitudinal axis of the haversian system; whereas in spongy bone the resorption cavity parallels the surface of the trabeculae. In *phase three*, new bone or secondary bone is laid down by osteoblasts lining the walls of the resorption cavity. In compact bone, successive layers are laid down until the resorption cavity is reduced to a narrow haversian canal around a blood vessel. This process destroys old haversian systems and forms new haversian systems. New trabeculae are formed in spongy bone.
- The remodeling process just described is capable of repairing microscopic bone injuries, but gross injuries, such as fractures and surgical wounds, heal via a different process. In bone wound healing, the stages are as follows:
  1. *Hematoma formation* occurs when damaged vessels hemorrhage. Fibrin and platelets within the hematoma form a meshwork. Hematopoietic growth factors, such as platelet-derived growth factor and transforming growth factor, are involved in this stage.
  2. *Procallus formation* occurs as fibroblasts, capillary buds, and osteoblasts move into the wound and produce granulation tissue; this is the procallus. Enzymes and growth factors aid in this stage of healing.
  3. *Callus formation* occurs as osteoblasts in the procallus form membranous or woven bone. Enzymes increase the phosphate content, and the phosphate joins with calcium as a deposit of mineral that hardens the callus.
  4. *Osteoblasts continue to replace the callus* with either lamellar bone or trabecular bone.
  5. Synthesis of type I bone collagen predominates at this stage. This final remodeling stage is vital to ensure good mechanical properties for weight bearing and mobility.

b. Describe the types of joints.
Review pages 962-965; refer to Figures 36-6 through 36-11.

MEMORY CHECK!

- Joints are classified according to either the *degree of movement* they permit or the *connecting tissues* that hold them together. A joint is classified on the basis of movement, as: (1) a synarthrosis or an immovable joint, (2) an amphiarthrosis or a slightly movable joint, or (3) a diarthrosis or a freely movable joint. On the basis of connective structures, joints are classified as fibrous, cartilaginous, or synovial.
- A joint united directly to bone by fibrous connective tissues is called a *fibrous joint*. Generally, fibrous joints are *synarthrotic*, or immovable, but many fibrous joints allow some movement. The degree of movement depends on the distance between the bone and the flexibility of the fibrous connective tissue.
- There are two types of *cartilaginous joints*, or *amphiarthroses*. A *symphysis* is a cartilaginous joint in which bones are united by a pad or disk of fibrocartilage. The articulating surfaces are usually covered by a thin layer of hyaline cartilage and a thick pad of fibrocartilage, which acts as a shock absorber and stabilizer. Examples of symphyses are the symphysis pubis and the intervertebral disks. A *synchondrosis* is a joint in which hyaline cartilage connects

MEMORY CHECK!—Cont'd

the two bones. The joints between the ribs and the sternum are synchondroses. Slight movement at the synchondroses between the ribs and the sternum allows the chest to move outward and upward during breathing.

- *Synovial joints* or *diarthroses* are the most movable and complex joints in the body. A synovial joint consists of a fibrous joint capsule or articular capsule, a synovial membrane, a joint cavity or synovial cavity, synovial fluid, and an articular cartilage. The joint capsule consists of parallel, interlacing bundles of dense, white fibrous tissue. It has a rich supply of nerves, blood vessels, and lymphatic vessels. The nerves are sensitive to the rate and direction of motion, compression, tension, vibration, and pain.
- The *synovial membrane* is the smooth, delicate inner lining of the joint capsule. It lines the nonarticular portion of the synovial joint and any ligaments or tendons that traverse the joint cavity. The synovial membrane is capable of rapid repair and regeneration.
- The joint cavity or *synovial cavity* is an enclosed, fluid-filled space between the articulating surfaces of the two bones that enables the two bones to move against each other. Synovial fluid within the cavity lubricates the joint surfaces, nourishes the pad of the articular cartilage, and contains free-floating synovial cells and various leukocytes that phagocytose joint debris and microorganisms.
- *Articular cartilage* is a layer of hyaline cartilage that covers the end of each bone. The function of articular cartilage is to reduce friction and to distribute the weight-bearing forces.

c. Define terms associated with muscle fibers.
Review pages 965 and 967-970; refer to Figures 36-12 through 36-15 and Tables 36-4 and 36-5.

MEMORY CHECK!

- Each anterior horn cell, its axon, and the innervated muscle fibers are referred to as a *motor unit.* The motor unit behaves as a single entity and contracts as a whole when it receives an adequate electrical impulse. A *muscle fiber* is a single *muscle cell.* This long cell is cylindrical in structure and surrounded by a membrane capable of excitation and impulse propagation. The muscle fiber contains bundles of *myofibrils* in a parallel arrangement along the longitudinal axis of the muscle. The myofibrils contain *sarcomeres* that are the actual contracting units. The sarcomeres consist of *actin and myosin*, which are the contractile proteins.
- Besides the myofibrils, the major components of the muscle fiber are the *muscle membrane, sarcotubular system, sarcoplasm, and mitochondria.* The muscle membrane is a two-part membrane. It includes the sarcolemma, which contains the plasma membrane of the muscle cell, and the cell's basement membrane. At the motor nerve end plate, where the nerve impulse is transmitted, the sarcolemma forms the highly convoluted synaptic cleft. The protein systems of the sarcolemma transport nutrients and synthesize proteins. They also provide the sodium-potassium pumps and include the cell's cholinergic receptors. The basement membrane serves as the cell's microskeleton and maintains the shape of the muscle cell.
- The *sarcoplasm,* the cytoplasm of the muscle cell, contains numerous enzymes and proteins that are responsible for the cell's energy production, protein synthesis, and oxygen storage. Unique to the muscle is the *sarcotubular system*, which includes *the transverse tubules and the sarcoplasmic reticulum.* The sarcoplasmic reticulum is involved in calcium transport, which initiates muscle contraction at the sarcomere. The sarcoplasmic reticulum is composed of tubules that run parallel to the myofibrils and are termed sarcotubules. The transverse tubules are closely associated with the sarcotubules, run across the sarcoplasm, and communicate with the extracellular space. Both types of tubules allow for intracellular calcium uptake, regulation, and release during muscle contraction, as well as storage of calcium during muscle relaxation.

d. Identify the major events of muscle contraction and relaxation.
Review pages 970 and 972; refer to Figure 36-16.

MEMORY CHECK!

MAJOR EVENTS OF MUSCLE CONTRACTION AND RELAXATION

Excitation and Contraction

A nerve impulse reaches the end of a motor neuron and releases acetylcholine

↓

Acetylcholine diffuses across the neuromuscular junction and binds to acetylcholine receptors on the muscle fiber

↓

Stimulation of acetylcholine receptors initiates an impulse that travels along the sarcolemma, through the transverse tubules, and to the sarcoplasmic reticulum

↓

Calcium is released from the sarcoplasmic reticulum into the sarcoplasm; calcium binds to troponin molecules on the thin myofilaments

↓

Tropomyosin molecules shift to expose actin's active engagement sites

↓

Energized myosin cross-bridges of the thick myofilaments bind to actin and use their ATP energy to pull the thin myofilaments toward the center of each sarcomere

↓

As the thin myofilaments slide past the thick myofilaments, the entire muscle fiber shortens

Relaxation

↓

After the impulse passes, the sarcoplasmic reticulum begins actively pumping calcium back into the sarcoplasm

↓

As calcium leaves the troponin molecules of the thin myofilaments, tropomyosin returns to its position and blocks actin's active engagement sites

↓

Myosin cross-bridges cannot bind to actin and can no longer sustain the contraction

↓

The thick and thin myofilaments are no longer connected, so the muscle fiber returns to its longer, resting length

LEARNING OBJECTIVES

After studying this chapter, the learner will be able to do the following:

1. Compare the types of fractures; describe the causes, manifestations, and treatment of fractures.
Study pages 978-981; refer to Figure 37-1 and Table 37-1.

Fractures are classified as complete or incomplete and open or closed. In a **complete** fracture, the bone is broken all the way through; in an **incomplete** fracture, the bone is damaged, but remains in one piece. Complete or incomplete fractures also are considered open if the skin is broken or **closed** if it is not. A fracture wherein the bone breaks into two or more fragments is termed a **comminuted** fracture. Fractures also are classified according to the direction of the fracture line.

The signs and symptoms of a fracture include *unnatural alignment (deformity), swelling, muscle spasm, tenderness, pain, and impaired sensation.* The immediate pain of a fracture is severe and usually caused by the traumatic injury. Subsequent pain is often produced by muscle spasm. Numbness is caused by the pinching of a nerve by the trauma or by bone fragments. Range of motion in the joint is limited, and movement may evoke audible clicking sounds or crepitus.

Fracture treatment involves realigning the bone fragments to their normal or anatomic positions and then holding them in place so that bone union can occur. Several methods are available to reduce or align a fracture, including closed manipulation, traction, and open surgical reduction. Splints and plaster casts are used to immobilize and hold a reduction in place. Improper reduction or immobilization of a fractured bone may result in nonunion, delayed union, or malunion. (See the following table.)

Types of Fractures

Type of Fracture	Characteristic	Cause
Common Complete Fractures		
Open	Communicating wound between bone and skin	Moderate to severe energy that exceeds tissue tolerance
Oblique	Fracture line at 45-degree angle to long axis of bone	Angulation and compressive energy
Spiral	Fracture line encircling bone	Twisting energy with distal part of bone unable to move
Transverse	Fracture line perpendicular to long axis of bone	Energy directly toward bone
Impacted	Fracture fragments pushed into one another	Comprehensive energy directly to distal fragment
Pathologic	Fracture occurs at any point in the bone	Minor energy to already weakened bone
Common Incomplete Fractures		
Greenstick	Break of cortical bone on convex side of a bent bone only with spongy bone splintering	Minor direct or indirect energy in children or elderly
Stress	Microfracture	Bone is subjected to repeated stress beyond its strength; muscles are stronger than bone

2. **Define terms associated with skeletal system stress.** Study pages 981-986; refer to Figures 37-4 through 37-7 and Table 37-2.

Dislocation is the temporary displacement of two bones in which the two bone surfaces lose contact entirely. If the contact between the surfaces is only partially lost, the injury is called **subluxation**. Dislocations and subluxations are often accompanied by fracture. As the bone separates from the joint, it may bruise or tear adjacent nerves, blood vessels, ligaments, supporting structures, and soft tissue.

A *tear in a tendon* is a **strain**. Major trauma or excessive stress can tear a tendon at any site in the body. The tendons of the hands, feet, knee, upper arm, thigh, ankle, and heel are often injured sites. *Ligament tears* are known as **sprains**. Ligament tears and ruptures can occur at any joint but are most common in the wrist, ankle, elbow, and knees. A complete separation of a tendon or ligament from its attachment is an **avulsion**. An avulsion is the result of abnormal stress on the ligament or tendon and is commonly seen in young athletes, especially sprinters, hurdlers, and runners. Trauma can also cause painful inflammation of tendons, or **tendinopathy** (tendinitis), and of bursae, or **bursitis**. Besides trauma, causes of tendinopathy include crystal deposits, postural misalignment, and hypermobility in a joint. **Epicondylopathy** (epicondylitis) is inflammation of a tendon where it attaches to a bone. Examples of epicondylopathy are *tennis elbow*, which is an inflammation of the lateral epicondyle of the humerus, and medial epicondylopathy, also called *golfer's elbow*. Acute **bursitis** occurs primarily in the middle years and is caused by repeated trauma. Septic bursitis is caused by wound infection or bacterial infection of the skin overlying the bursae. The shoulder is the most common site of bursitis.

Muscle strain damages local muscle and is often the result of sudden, forced motion causing the muscle to become *stretched beyond its normal capacity.* Muscles are injured more often than tendons in young people; the opposite is true in older populations. Regardless of the cause of trauma, muscle cells are usually able to regenerate, although regeneration may take up to 6 weeks.

Myositis ossificans is a late complication of some muscle injuries. The basic problem seems to be the *inability of mesenchymal cells to differentiate* into osteoblastic stem cells and fibroblasts into bone-forming cells. Myositis ossificans is involved with muscles or tendons, ligaments, or bones near the injured muscle.

Rhabdomyolysis or *myoglobinuria* is manifested by excess myoglobin, an intracellular muscle protein, which passes into the urine. Muscle damage releases the myoglobin into the extracellular space and the bloodstream. Along with the release of myoglobin, creatine kinase and other enzymes are released in massive quantities. *Myoglobin precipitates in the kidney tubules* and obstructs flow through the nephron, producing injury. The risk of renal failure increases directly with elevated creatine kinase, potassium, and phosphorus values.

The most severe form of myoglobin release is often called *crush syndrome*. Less severe and more localized forms are known as *compartment syndromes,* which can lead to *Volkmann ischemic contracture* in the forearm or leg.

Malignant hyperthermia is an inherited muscle disorder characterized ay a hypermetabolic reaction to certain volatile anesthetics or succinylcholine that activates a prolonged release of intracellular calcium from the sarcoplasmic reticulum. This process causes hypermetabolism with extremely high body temperature, muscle rigidity, rhabdomyolysis, and death if not treated with dantrolene infusion.

3. Differentiate among osteoporosis, osteomalacia, Paget disease, and osteomyelitis.

Study pages 987-996; refer to Figures 37-8 through 37-16 and Tables 37-3 and 37-4.

Common Disorders of Bone

Disorder	Cause	Pathophysiology	Manifestations	Treatment
Osteoporosis	Decreased levels of estrogen and testosterone, reduced physical activity lessens muscle stress on bone, inadequate vitamins C and D, insufficient dietary magnesium and calcium, corticosteroid use	Reduced bone mass or density, imbalance in bone resorption and formation, alteration in the OPG/RANKL/ RANK system*	Pain and bone deformity, fracture, increased radiolucency	Weight-bearing exercise, dietary supplements, selective estrogen receptor modulators, intranasal parathyroid hormone, calcitonin, possible PTH and testosterone
Osteomalacia (adult) Rickets (children)	Deficiency of vitamin D lowers absorption of calcium from intestines	Inadequate and delayed mineralization; osteoid tissue is not mineralized	Pain, bone fractures, vertebral collapse, radiolucent bands perpendicular to bone surface pseudofracture	Serum calcium and phosphorus adjustments, vitamin D supplements, renal dialysis
Paget disease	Unknown, possible genetic and environmental	Excessive resorption of spongy bone followed by accelerated formation of softened bone	Thickening of bones, radiographic findings of irregular bone trabeculae with thickened and disorganized patterns	Infrequently required—bisphosphonates and calcitonin to slow resorption
Osteomyelitis	Most often a staphylococcal infection, contaminated open wound, or hematogenous bone infection	Acute inflammation of marrow and cortex; impaired blood supply leads to necrosis that forms a sequestrum and an involucrum that surrounds the infected bone	Acute and chronic inflammation, fever, pain, lymphadenopathy, necrotic bone on radiographic imaging	Antibiotics and débridement, surgical removal of exudates, hyperbaric oxygen therapy

*Osteoblasts and osteoclasts cooperate to maintain normal bone homeostasis. RANKL is a cytokine needed for the formation and activation of osteoclasts and increases bone loss. OPG decreases bone loss because when activated, it promotes bone formation. When RANKL binds to its receptor RANK on osteoclast precursor cells, it triggers their proliferation and increases bone resorption. *OPG acts as a decoy by binding to RANK,* preventing the binding of RANKL to RANK and thus preventing bone resorption.

4. Compare noninflammatory osteoarthritis (OA) to inflammatory rheumatoid arthritis (RA); characterize ankylosing spondylitis and gout.
Study pages 1045-1056; refer to Figures 37-16 through 37-23 and Tables 37-4 and 37-6.

Noninflammatory Osteoarthritis and Inflammatory Rheumatoid Arthritis

	Osteoarthritis (OA)	Rheumatoid arthritis (RA)
Pathologic feature	Noninflammatory (enzymatic lysis); loss of proteoglycans and collagen fibers from articular cartilage in synovial joints, bone sclerosis, bone spurs	Inflammatory; damage or destruction of synovial membrane, extends to articular cartilage joint capsule and surrounding ligaments and tendons, pannus
Onset age and sex distribution	>40 years, increases with age, equal sex distribution	Middle age, prevalence in females
Cause	Joint stress, congenital abnormalities, joint instability	Genetics, environmental microbes, autoimmunity, estrogen, released tumor necrosis factor-α and interleukin-1
Joints affected	Peripheral and central, weight-bearing	Phalangeal, wrists, knee
Joint fluid	Proteoglycans/fragments, normal mucin, few cells	Inflammatory exudates, poor mucin
Manifestations	Pain, stiffness, enlargement, tenderness, limited motion, muscle wasting, dislocation, deformity	Same as in OA with systemic involvement, subcutaneous nodules, deviation of joints, rheumatoid factor (RF), and circulating immune complexes

Ankylosing spondylitis is a chronic, inflammatory joint disease characterized by stiffening and fusion or ankylosis of the *spine and sacroiliac joints.* Like RA, ankylosing spondylitis is a *systemic, immune inflammatory disease*. The disease is strongly associated with the presence of histocompatibility antigen HLA-B27 on the chromosomes of affected individuals, suggesting a genetic predisposition to the disease. In ankylosing spondylitis, the *primary pathologic site is at the point where ligaments, tendons, and the joint capsule are inserted into bone* rather than in the synovial membrane as in RA. The end result of ankylosing spondylitis is fibrosis, ossification, and fusion of the joint.

The most common symptoms of early ankylosing spondylitis are low back pain and stiffness. The pain initially is insidious, but progressively becomes persistent. Forward flexion, rotation, and lateral flexion of the spine are restricted and painful. As the disease progresses, the individual becomes *increasingly stooped. The thoracic spine becomes rounded; the head and neck are flexed.* Many individuals may have peripheral joint involvement, uveitis or inflammation of eye structures, fibrotic changes in the lungs, cardiomegaly, aortic incompetence, amyloidosis, and Achilles tendinitis.

Treatment of individuals with ankylosing spondylitis consists of physical therapy to maintain skeletal mobility and prevent the natural progression of contractures. Anti-inflammatory and analgesic medications are prescribed to suppress some of the pain and stiffness and to facilitate exercise. Surgical procedures and radiotherapy are sometimes used to provide relief for individuals with end-stage disease or intolerable deformity.

Gout is a *metabolic disorder* that disrupts the body's control of uric acid production or excretion. High levels of *uric acid accumulate* in the blood and in other body fluids, including synovial fluid. When the uric acid, a breakdown product of purine nucleotides, reaches a certain concentration in fluids, it crystallizes.

When crystallization occurs in synovial fluid, painful inflammation of the joint develops. This condition is known as **gouty arthritis.** With time, crystal deposition in subcutaneous tissues causes the formation of small, white nodules, or **tophi,** and their inflammatory sequelae. **Tophaceous gout,** the chronic stage of disease, can begin as early as 3 years or as late as 40 years after the initial attack of gouty arthritis. Though the *tophi* themselves are painless, they often cause progressive stiffness and persistent aching of the affected joint. The helix of the ear is the most common site of tophi, which are the diagnostic lesions of chronic gout. Tophaceous deposits appear in other areas and produce irregular swellings of the fingers, hands, knees, and feet. Although the tophi themselves are painless, they often cause progressive stiffness and persistent aching of the affected joint.

The pathophysiology of gout is closely linked to *purine metabolism,* cellular metabolism of purines, and kidney function. *Uric acid is a breakdown product of purine nucleotides.* Some individuals with gout have an accelerated rate of purine synthesis, and others break down purine nucleotides at an accelerated rate. Both conditions result in an overproduction of uric acid.

Kidney function is involved in the pathophysiology of gout because most uric acid is eliminated from the body through the kidneys. Urate undergoes both reabsorption and excretion within the renal tubules. Sluggish urate excretion by the kidney may be caused by decreased glomerular filtration of urate or acceleration in urate reabsorption.

Acute gouty arthritis is treated with anti-inflammatory drugs. The individual should have a low-purine diet and high fluid intake to increase urinary output. Anti-hyperuricemic drugs can be given to reduce serum urate concentrations.

5. Describe secondary muscular dysfunction.
Study pages 1007 and 1008.

Muscular symptoms arise from causes unrelated to the muscle itself. These secondary muscular phenomena include contracture, stress-related muscle tension, and immobility.

Several conditions cause the muscle *fibers to shorten without contracting*; this condition is called a **contracture.** A physiologic muscle contracture occurs without muscle action potential in the sarcolemma and is explained as *failure of the calcium pump* even in the presence of plentiful ATP. A physiologic contracture occurs in McArdle disease, which is an enzyme deficiency, and malignant hyperthermia. The contracture is usually *temporary* if the underlying pathology can be corrected.

A pathologic contracture is considered a *permanent* muscle shortening caused by muscle spasm or weakness. It is associated with plentiful ATP and will occur in spite of a normal action potential. The most common form of contracture occurs in muscular dystrophy and central nervous system (CNS) injury. Contractures also may develop secondary to scar tissue contraction in the flexor tissues of a joint.

Stress-induced muscle tension has been associated with chronic anxiety, as well as a variety of stress-related muscular symptoms, including neck stiffness, back pain, and headache. The underlying pathophysiology is presumably caused by increased activity of *the reticular activating system* and increased *firing* of the efferent loop of the *gamma fibers*, which produce further muscle contraction and increased muscle tension.

Progressive relaxation training and biofeedback are possible ways to treat muscle tension. The hope is to enhance the individual's ability to relax specific muscle groups in order to relieve tension. This relief could reduce CNS and autonomic nervous system (ANS) arousal.

The term **disuse atrophy** describes the pathologic reduction in normal size of muscle fibers following inactivity or *immobility* because of bed rest, trauma, casting, or local nerve damage. Frequent forceful isometric muscle contractions and passive lengthening exercises may prevent atrophy.

6. Describe fibromyalgia.
Study pages 1008 and 1009; refer to Figures 37-24 and 37-25.

Fibromyalgia is a chronic musculoskeletal syndrome characterized by *increased sensitivity to touch, the absence of systemic or localized inflammation, fatigue, and sleep disturbances.* Because the symptoms are vague, clinicians have often misdiagnosed or completely dismissed fibromyalgia.

The etiology of fibromyalgia is likely *multifactorial.* The most common precipitating factors include viral illnesses, physical traumas, or emotional trauma. Certain rheumatic diseases, such as RA and systemic lupus erythematosus (SLE), may coexist if not initially present with fibromyalgia.

Most studies have demonstrated that increased muscle tenderness in fibromyalgia is a result of *generalized pain intolerance* that is possibly related to functional abnormalities within the CNS. The prominent symptom of fibromyalgia is *chronic pain.* The majority of individuals experience pain and fatigue during wakefulness. Fatigue is most notable when arising from sleep and during the midafternoon. Anxiety, particularly in regard to diagnosis and future, is almost universal. The only finding on examination is the presence of *multiple tender points.*

No one regimen of medication has proved successful for fibromyalgia. Aerobic exercise can reduce stress. Amitriptyline can significantly improve pain tolerance, morning stiffness, and sleep quality, but not tender points.

7. Distinguish among muscle membrane abnormalities.
Study page 1010.

The hyperexcitable membrane seen in myotonic disorders and the intermittently unresponsive membrane seen in the periodic paralyses are defects in the plasma membrane of the muscle fiber. **Myotonia** is a *delayed relaxation* after voluntary muscle contraction, such as gripes, eye closure, or muscle percussion. It is because of the *prolonged depolarization* of the muscle membrane. Myotonia occurs mostly in inherited disorders. Its symptoms are mild except in myotonic muscular dystrophy. Myotonia is treated with drugs that reduce muscle fiber excitability.

In **periodic paralysis,** the *muscle membrane is unresponsive to neural stimuli.* Periodic paralysis is triggered by exercise and any process or medication that alters serum potassium. The disorder is often inherited in an autosomal dominant pattern. Oral and intravenous potassium can relieve acute attacks. A low-salt diet and drugs are useful for long-term therapy.

8. Compare the metabolic, inflammatory, and toxic myopathies.
Study pages 1010-1013; refer to Figure 37-26.

Myopathies

Myopathy	Causes	Manifestations
Metabolic myopathy	Altered thyroid hormone levels change muscle protein synthesis and electrolyte balance	
	Thyrotoxicosis	Proximal weakness, paresis of extraocular muscles
	Hypothyroidism	Flabby and weak muscles, sluggish movements
McArdle disease	Absence of muscle phosphorylase, inability to catabolize glycogen or produce lactic acid	Exercise intolerance, fatigue, painful muscle cramps, muscle weakness and wasting
Acid maltase deficiency	Autosomal recessive; absence of acid maltase, accumulation of glycogen in lysosomes of muscle and other cells	Adult: similar to those of muscular dystrophy or polymyositis; severe respiratory muscle weakness
Pompe disease (infantile form of acid maltase deficiency)		Infant: hypotonia, areflexia enlarged heart, tongue, and liver; early death
Myoadenylate deaminase deficiency	Absence of myoadenylate deaminase, inability to form phosphocreatine and ATP during exercise	Exercise intolerance
Carnitine palmitoyl transferase (CPT) and carnitine deficiencies	Absence of CPT and carnitine; fatty acid byproducts and energy are not transported to myofibrils	CPT deficiency: mild muscular symptoms, episodes of renal failure because of myoglobinuria Carnitine deficiency: progressive muscle weakness
Inflammatory myopathy	Infectious	
	Tuberculosis and sarcoidosis	Granulomas in muscle and other tissues
	Trichinosis	Larvae from infected pork migrate to host lymphatics: pain, rash, and muscle stiffness
	Viral infections	Muscle pain and tenderness similar to symptoms of influenza
Polymyositis (generalized muscle inflammation) Dermatomyositis (polymyositis with skin lesions) Inclusion-body myositis (inclusions or granular material in muscle fibers)	Cell-mediated (cytotoxic T cells) and humoral (autoantibodies) immune factors, human leukocyte antigen (HLA) genetic markers	Necrosis of muscle fibers, malaise, fever, muscle swelling, pain, and tenderness, lethargy, symmetric proximal muscle weakness; in both diseases: dysphagia, vasculitis, Raynaud phenomenon, cardiomyopathy, fibrosis, coexisting pulmonary collagen disorders; dermatomyositis causes skin rash, calcinosis, and eyelid edema
Toxic myopathy	Alcohol abuse, lipid-lowering drugs; direct toxic effect and nutritional deficiency cause necrosis of muscle fibers	Benign cramps and pain, severe weakness, myoglobinuria and renal failure, generalized muscle weakness
	Sedatives and narcotics	Rhabdomyolysis
	Repeated therapeutic drug injection	Local muscle fiber necrosis, fibrotic bands

9. Classify bone tumors by tissue of origin, whether benign or malignant, and their pattern of bone destruction.
Study pages 1013-1015; refer to Figure 37-27 and Tables 37-7 and 37-8.

Bone tumors may originate from bone cells, cartilage, fibrous tissue, marrow, or vascular tissue. On the basis of mesodermal tissue of origin, bone tumors are classified as osteogenic, chondrogenic, collagenic, or myelogenic. The mesoderm contributes to primitive fibroblasts and reticulum cells. The fibroblast is the progenitor of the osteoblast, the chondroblast, and the fibrous connective tissue cell.

Benign bone tumors destroy small areas of bone, tend to be limited to the anatomic confines of the host bone, and have a well-demarcated border. Benign bone tumors push against neighboring tissue, have a symmetric, controlled growth pattern, and tend to compress and displace neighboring normal bone tissue, weakening the bone structure and leading to pathologic fracture.

The *geographic pattern*, the *moth-eaten* pattern, and the *permeative* pattern are patterns of bone destruction in bone tumors. Tumors exhibiting the *geographic pattern* have *well-defined margins* that can be easily separated from the surrounding normal bone. There is a uniform and well-defined lytic area in the bone of these *benign* lesions.

In the *moth-eaten pattern*, the cancerous lesion has a less defined or less demarcated margin that cannot be easily separated from normal bone. Areas of partially destroyed bone adjacent to completely lytic areas are found. This pattern of bone destruction is characteristic of rapidly growing, **malignant bone tumors**. An aggressive, malignant tumor causes the *permeative pattern* of bone destruction. The margins of the tumor are poorly demarcated, and abnormal bone merges with surrounding normal bone tissue. Malignant bone tumors tend to be large and aggressive in their bone destruction, to invade surrounding tissue, and to metastasize. (See the following flowchart.)

Origin of Benign and Malignant Bone Tumors

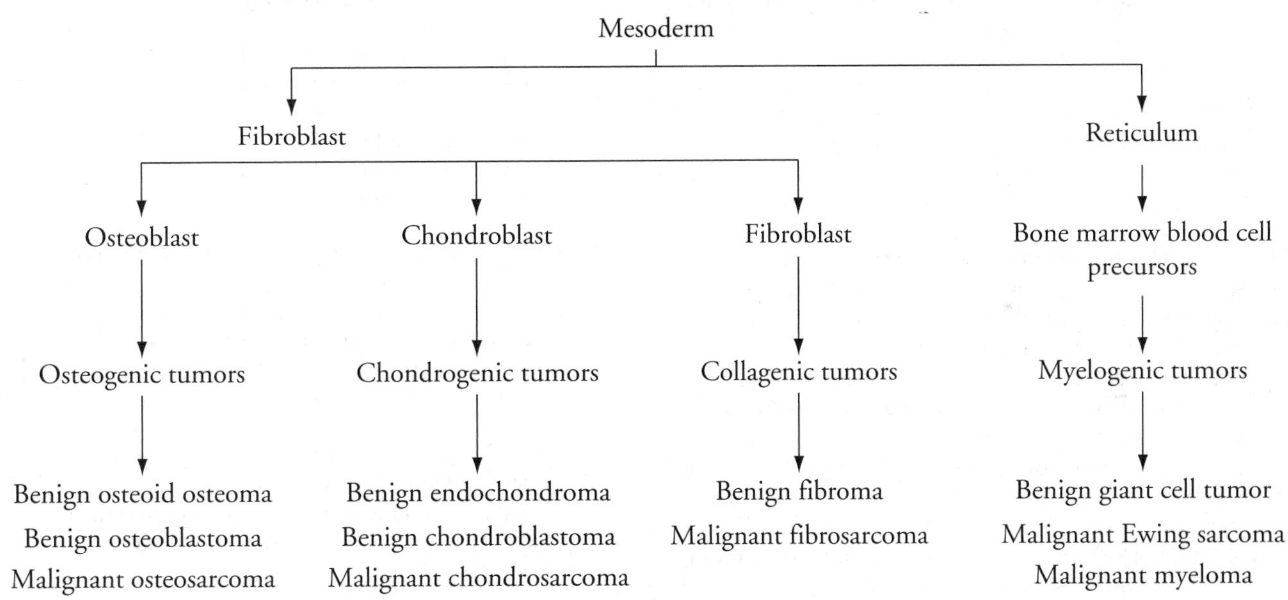

NOTE: Diagnosis depends on serum metabolite and enzyme levels, radiologic studies, CT scans, MRI, blood counts, and biopsy.

10. Characterize the common types of bone tumors.
Study pages 1015-1017; refer to Figure 37-28.

Osteosarcoma is a malignant bone-forming tumor that is large and destructive and most often is found in *bone marrow*; it has a moth-eaten pattern of bone destruction. Osteosarcomas always contain osteoid and callus and also may contain chondroid and fibrinoid tissue. The osteoid is deposited between the trabeculae of the callus. The "streamers" of osteoid infiltrate the normal compact bone, destroy it, and replace it with dense callus and masses of osteoid. The bone tissue never matures to compact bone. Ninety percent of osteosarcomas are located in the metaphyses of long bones. Fifty percent of osteosarcomas occur around the *knee area*. The tumor breaks through the cortex, lifts the periosteum, and forms a soft tissue mass that is not covered by new bone.

Common initial symptoms are pain and swelling; pain is usually worse at night. Systemic symptoms are uncommon. Preoperative chemotherapy has improved the treatment for localized osteosarcoma. Chemotherapy can be given both preoperatively and postoperatively. Combination treatment involves radiation therapy and surgery.

Chondrosarcoma, a chondrogenic tumor, is a large, ill-defined malignant tumor that *infiltrates trabeculae in spongy bone*. It occurs most often in the *metaphysis* or *diaphysis* of a long bone. The tumor contains large lobules of hyaline cartilage separated by bands of fibrous tissue and anaplastic cells. It expands and enlarges the contour of the bone, causes extensive erosion of the cortex, and expands into the soft tissues.

Symptoms associated with the chondrosarcoma have an insidious onset. Local swelling and pain are usual symptoms. At first, the pain is intermittent; then, it gradually intensifies and becomes constant. Surgical excision is generally regarded as the treatment of choice; however, individuals demonstrate recurrences, so amputation is considered.

Fibrosarcoma, a malignant collagenic tumor, is a *solitary tumor* that most often affects the *metaphyseal region of the femur or tibia*. The tumor is composed of a firm, fibrous mass of tissue containing collagen, malignant fibroblasts, and occasional osteoclast-like giant cells.

Pain and swelling are the usual symptoms and indicate that the tumor has broken through the cortex. Local tenderness, a palpable mass, limitation of motion, and a pathologic fracture are other symptoms and signs. Radical surgery and amputation are the treatments of choice for fibrosarcoma.

Giant cell tumors are common primary bone tumors. The giant cell tumor is a solitary, circumscribed tumor that causes extensive *bone resorption* because of its osteoclastic origin. The tumor is rich in osteoclast-like giant cells and anaplastic stromal cells and is found in the center of the *epiphysis* in the femur, tibia, radius, or humerus. The tumor has a slow, relentless growth rate and is usually contained within the original contour of the affected bone. It may extend into the articular cartilage. It has *recurrence rates* as high as 80%.

The most common symptoms associated with the giant cell tumor are pain, local swelling, and limitation of movement. Cryosurgery and resection of the tumor decrease recurrence and are more successful treatments than curettage and irradiation; amputation may be necessary.

11. Identify the incidence, manifestations, treatment, and prognosis of rhabdomyosarcoma.
Review page 1017.

The malignant tumor of *striated muscle* is a **rhabdomyosarcoma.** Rhabdomyosarcoma is extremely rare, but it is highly malignant because of its *rapid metastasis*. These tumors are located in the muscle tissue of the head, neck, and genitourinary tract 75% of the time. The rest are in the trunk and extremities.

The diagnosis of rhabdomyosarcoma is made by incisional biopsy and histologic examination of the specimen. Pleomorphic, embryonal, and alveolar types can be differentiated. The pleomorphic type is a highly malignant tumor of the extremities of adults.

Treatment consists of a combination of surgical excision, radiation therapy, and systemic chemotherapy. Cure in cases with distant metastasis is unlikely.

PRACTICE EXAMINATION

Multiple Choice

Circle the correct answer for each question:

1. In a complete fracture:
   a. the fracture crosses or involves the entire width or thickness of the bone.
   b. more than two bone fragments are present.
   c. separation of ligaments exists.
   d. posttraumatic infection is always present.
   e. the surface opposite the break is intact.

2. In an oblique fracture, the energy or force is:
   a. twisting with the distal part unable to move.
   b. compressive and at an angle.
   c. directly to an already weakened bone.
   d. directly to the distal fragment.

3. Which is a definite sign of a fracture?
   a. abrasion
   b. shock
   c. muscle spasm
   d. unnatural alignment
   e. All of the above are correct.

4. Secondary muscular dysfunctions:
   a. involve large compartments of hemorrhage.
   b. can display contractures.
   c. result from failure of calcium pump.
   d. are related to the muscle itself.
   e. Both b and c are correct.

5. The most common cause of osteomyelitis is:
   a. hematogenous spread of infection.
   b. rheumatoid disease.
   c. direct contamination of an open wound.
   d. deficiency of calcium.
   e. deficiency of vitamin D.

6. The pathogenesis of osteoporosis involves:
   a. inadequate mineralization.
   b. impaired synthesis of bone organic matrix.
   c. alteration in the OPG/RANKL/RANK system.
   d. formation of sclerotic bone.
   e. None of the above is correct.

7. Osteomalacia causes:
   a. loss of bone matrix.
   b. inadequate mineralization.
   c. radiolucency.
   d. All of the above are correct.
   e. Both b and c are correct.

8. Bone tumors may originate from all of the following *except:*
   a. epithelial tissue.
   b. cartilage.
   c. fibrous tissue.
   d. vascular tissue.
   e. mesoderm.

9. In benign bone tumors, there is:
   a. a uniform and well-defined lytic area.
   b. a moth-eaten pattern of bone destruction.
   c. abnormal bone merging with surrounding normal bone tissue.
   d. an area of partially destroyed bone adjacent to completely lytic areas.

10. An osteosarcoma is a(n):
   a. collagenic, malignant bone tumor.
   b. myelogenic, benign tumor.
   c. myelogenic, malignant tumor.
   d. osteogenic, benign bone tumor.
   e. osteogenic, malignant tumor.

11. A major symptom of bone cancer is:
   a. faltering gait.
   b. persistent pain that worsens at night.
   c. lack of sensation.
   d. general swelling over a bone.
   e. coolness over a bone.

12. Giant cell tumors:
   a. are collagenic tumors.
   b. are located in the diaphysis of a long bone.
   c. have extensive osteoblastic activity.
   d. have high recurrence rates.
   e. are multifocal.

13. Tendinopathy is:
   a. inflammation of a tendon where it attaches to bone.
   b. painful because of disorganized collagen fibers caused by repetitive stress on tendons.
   c. a torn tendon.
   d. a complete separation of a tendon.

14. RA begins with:
   a. destruction of the synovial membrane and subsynovial tissue.
   b. inflammation of ligaments.
   c. destruction of the articular cartilage.
   d. softening of the articular cartilage.
   e. destruction of the joint capsule.

15. The causes of OA include which of the following? (More than one answer may be correct.)
   a. enzymatic breakdown
   b. proteoglycan destruction
   c. rheumatoid factor
   d. circulating immune complexes
   e. infections

16. Ankylosing spondylitis: (More than one answer may be correct.)
   a. is a systemic immune inflammatory disease.
   b. is characterized by stiffening or fusion of the spine.
   c. causes instability of synovial joints.
   d. begins with inflammation of fibrocartilage.
   e. is manifested early by low back pain and stiffness.

17. In gout:
   a. the pathogenesis is formation of monosodium urate crystals in joints and tissues.
   b. purine metabolism is altered.
   c. affected individuals likely have an inherited enzyme defect.
   d. the hyperuricemia can be the result of acquired chronic disease or a drug.
   e. All of the above are correct.

18. A muscle contracture is:
   a. likely caused by increased activity in the reticular activating system and the gamma loop in the muscle fiber.
   b. muscle shortening possibly because of CNS injury.
   c. often helped by relaxation training and biofeedback.
   d. a consequence of reduced muscle protein synthesis.
   e. All of the above are correct.

19. Myotonia is all of the following *except:*
   a. delayed relaxation after voluntary muscle contractions.
   b. prolonged depolarization of the muscle membrane.
   c. mostly inherited.
   d. unresponsiveness to neural stimulation.
   e. progressive atrophy of skeletal muscle.

20. Rhabdomyosarcoma has:
   a. a poor prognosis.
   b. aggressive invasion.
   c. early, widespread dissemination.
   d. pleomorphic types.
   e. All of the above are correct.

Matching

Match the term with its characteristic:

_______ 21. Subluxation

_______ 22. Sprain

a. articular cartilages lose contact entirely
b. articular cartilages are partially separated
c. complete separation of a tendon or a ligament
d. a ligament tear

Match the myopathy with its cause:

_______ 23. McArdle disease

_______ 24. Acid maltase deficiency

_______ 25. Polymyositis

a. hypothyroidism
b. hyperparathyroidism
c. accumulation of glycogen in lysosomes
d. inability to catabolize glycogen
e. immune system abnormality

Fill in the Blank

Complete the following table differentiating the patterns of bone destruction caused by bone tumors:

Tumor Destructive Bone Patterns

Pattern	Feature	Type of Lesion
Geographic		
Moth-eaten		
Permeative	Poorly demarcated margin, imperceptible merging of normal with abnormal bone	Indicates an aggressive and very rapidly growing malignant lesion

CASE STUDY 1

Mrs. B. is a 52-year-old homemaker who complains of bilateral knee and hand pain. She states, "The pain has worsened over time. It is present during rest and limits my walking, climbing stairs, and it just hurts while I am standing." Her physical examination showed slight ulnar deviation of the digits and swelling of the metacarpal, phalangeal, and proximal interphalangeal joints with limited range of motion and some instability of both knees.

Laboratory studies revealed the following:
CBC = normal, except for mild anemia
Rheumatoid factor = high titer
Synovial fluid analysis = turbid appearance
Radiographic examination of knees = joint narrowing on both knees, thinning of the articular cartilage, cystic areas, and bony spurs

Which arthritis is Mrs. B. experiencing? Explain your answer.

CASE STUDY 2

Mrs. C.S. is a 64-year-old woman who complains of constant back pain that has lasted for 4 to 6 weeks and is aggravated by activity. A review of her history and activities reveals no previous injury to her back or bone fractures, and no relief of pain with changing positions; the history also notes that she has been postmenopausal since age 48 years. When asked whether she takes hormone replacement therapy, she replies, "No, I am afraid of getting breast cancer because my mother had it and my sister has it, but my last year's mammogram was normal." She adds that she is taking inhaled corticosteroids for chronic asthma; occasionally, an acute attack requires systemic corticosteroids therapy, and she takes no dietary supplements. Mrs. C.S. exercises little and drinks several caffeinated beverages daily.

The physical examination shows tenderness and decreased range of motion in the lumbar region and no kyphosis. A radiograph of the lumbosacral spine shows osteopenia (subnormal bone mineralization) and a fracture of L2. Blood chemistry results are normal with no rheumatoid factor present.

What likely caused the osteopenia, and what is your plan for treatment?

38 Alterations of Musculoskeletal Function in Children

LEARNING OBJECTIVES

After studying this chapter, the learner will be able to do the following:

1. Describe congenital musculoskeletal defects in children.
Study pages 1022, 1023, 1025 and 1026; refer to Figures 38-1 through 38-6 and Table 38-1.

Clubfoot, or congenital equinovarus, describes a deformity in which the forefoot is adducted and supinated and the heel is inwardly deviated or pointing down. The clubfoot deformity can be positional, idiopathic, or teratologic (because of another syndrome, such as spina bifida). Idiopathic clubfoot occurs in 1:1000 live births with males twice as likely as females to be affected. The deformity involves not only forefoot *adduction* and *supination,* but also hindfoot *equinus* (pointed downward) and *varus* (heel in toward the midline).

In the idiopathic clubfoot, manipulation and casting above the knee, begun soon after birth, can often correct the forefoot deformity. The hindfoot equinus may require lengthening of the Achilles tendon, which can be performed in a clinic with use of local anesthesia at about 8 to 9 weeks of age. Bracing may be required until age 3 years. Idiopathic clubfoot that is recalcitrant to these procedures requires a posteromedial release (PMR), a much larger surgical intervention. Teratologic clubfoot is usually stiffer, and a higher percentage of cases require PMR.

Developmental dysplasia of the hip (DDH) describes imperfect development of the hip that can affect the femoral head, the acetabulum, or both. Although most often present at birth, it may occur at any time in the newborn or infant period. Like clubfoot, DDH can be *idiopathic* or *teratologic.* Teratologic DDH is more difficult to treat and often needs operative intervention. In idiopathic DDH, 70% of cases are on the left, girls are more commonly affected, and certain antenatal events, such as breech position and oligohydramnios (low intracellular fluids), and presence of family history predispose to the disease. Variants of idiopathic DDH are **dislocated hip** (no contact between femoral head and acetabulum), **subluxated hip** (partial contact only), and **acetabular dysplasia** (the femoral head is located properly but the acetabulum is shallow).

Clinical examination is the mainstay of diagnosis. The examination must be performed in a relaxed infant for accuracy. The presence of *Ortolani sign* (hip out but reductive) or *Barlow sign* (hip in but dislocatable) is an absolute indication for treatment. Other indicators for further evaluation are imitation of abduction and apparent shortening of the femur, or *Galeazzi sign.*

Bracing with a Pavlik harness is successful in 95% to 98% of cases of DDH in children younger than 4 months. With advancing age, closed reduction of the hip and spica (body) casting under general anesthesia is required. The spica cast is worn for 3 months. Children older than 12 months require surgery on the joint, the femur, the acetabulum, or all three.

Osteogenesis imperfecta (OI) (brittle bone disease) is a spectrum of disease caused by *genetic mutation in the gene that encodes for type I collagen,* the main component of bone and blood vessels. Classification defines four types. Types I and IV are milder forms and inherited in an autosomal dominant pattern; Types II and III are more severe and inherited in a recessive pattern. Children with type II often die during infancy.

The classic clinical manifestations of OI are *osteopenia* (decreased bone mass) and an increased rate of *fractures.* With recurrent fractures, bone deformity (bowing) often occurs. Affected children are of short stature and have triangular faces, possibly *blue sclera,* and poor dentition.

Treatment is a combination of medical and surgical approaches. For fractures and deformity, intramedullary rodding of the bone is often utilized to help hold position and splint new fractures. Telescoping rods, which grow with the child, have been used, but mechanical failure limits their efficacy. Unfortunately, children with OI may undergo multiple surgical procedures and placement of additional rods with growth. The medical treatment, classically involving increased intake of calcium and vitamin D, is under study.

2. Describe bony infections.
Review pages 1026 and 1027; refer to Figures 38-7 and 38-8.

Osteomyelitis, or bone infection, is caused by either bacterial or granulomatous (i.e., tuberculosis) infective processes. **Acute hematogenous osteomyelitis** is the most common form in children.

Osteomyelitis usually begins as a *bloody abscess in the metaphysis* of the bone. The abscess may rupture under the periosteum and spread along the bone shaft. The periosteum separates and forms a shell of new bone around the infected portion of the shaft. The periosteum that maintains a blood supply generates new bone, or an **involucrum**.

Children often present with fever and elevations of the white blood cell (WBC) count, serum C-reactive protein (CRP) value, and erythrocyte sedimentation rate (ESR). Blood culture results are positive only 40% of cases.

Treatment consists of appropriate antibiotic coverage for 6 weeks. If there is no response to medication alone and blood culture results are negative, bone aspiration is required to identify the microorganism. With methicillin-resistant *Staphylococcus aureus* (MRSA), surgical débridement is required.

Septic arthritis can occur primarily or can be secondary to *osteomyelitis* at locations where the infection breaks out of the *metaphysis*. The most common sites for septic arthritis are knees, hips, ankles, and elbows. Children with septic arthritis present with severe joint pain, inability to bear weight or move the affected joint, and severe malaise. Anorexia, fever, and elevations of complete blood count (CBC), ESR, and CRP value are more common than in osteomyelitis. Plain radiographic findings are often normal, but a bone scan is helpful, especially with infected sites in the pelvis, scapula, or ankle.

S.aureus is the most common microorganism. MRSA is present in approximately 30% of cases. After definitive and essential surgical intervention, antibiotics are required for 2 to 3 weeks. Long-term follow-up to assess articular or physeal damage is required.

3. Describe the features of juvenile idiopathic rheumatoid arthritis (JIRA).
Study page 1027; refer to Table 38-2.

The basic pathophysiology of **JIRA** is the same as that of adult rheumatoid arthritis, but it differs in the following points:

a. Mode of onset has three distinct forms:
   - Arthritis in fewer than three joints (pauciarticular)
   - Arthritis in more than three joints (polyarthritis)
   - Systemic disease (Stills disease)
b. The large joints are predominantly affected.
c. Subluxation and ankylosis of the cervical spine are common.
d. Chronic uveitis is common.
e. JIRA continuing through adolescence can affect growth and adult morbidity.
f. Serologic tests seldom detect rheumatoid factor.

Treatment for children with JIRA is supportive, but not curative, the aims being to control inflammation and other clinical manifestations of the disease and to minimize deformity.

4. Describe the pathophysiology, evaluation, and treatment of the osteochondroses: Legg-Calvé-Perthes disease and Osgood-Schlatter disease.
Study pages 1027-1029; refer to Figures 38-9 through 38-11.

The **osteochondroses** are a series of childhood diseases involving areas of significant *tensile or compromise stress* (i.e., tibial tubercle, Achilles insertion, hip) that undergo partial, but insufficient, blood supply, death of bone (osseous necrosis), progressive bony weaknesses, and then micro-fracture. The *cause* of the decreased blood supply is controversial, but *could be trauma, change in clotting sensitivity, vascular injury, or a combination.* Reparative processes via neovascularization is the rule, although years may be required for full healing. Deformity from compression during osseous necrosis can persist.

Legg-Calvé-Perthes disease (LCP) is a process involving *interruption of the blood supply to the femoral head.* It commonly occurs between 3 and 10 years of age, with a peak incidence at 6 years of age. It is self-limiting in nature, running its course in 2 to 5 years. Interruption of blood flow to the femoral head results in necrosis of the femoral head. Inflammation and new bone formation follow over time, with a resultant flattening of the femoral head. In the first stage of LCP, the hip synovial membrane and joint capsule are swollen, edematous, and hyperemic. In the second or necrotic stage, the epiphysis dies, owing to lack of blood supply. In the third or regenerative healing stage, the dead bone in the femoral head is replaced by procallus and new bone is laid down. In the fourth or residual stage, remodeling occurs and newly formed bone is organized into live spongy bone.

Presentation of LCP disease may be fairly incipient, with the child complaining of lower extremity pain for months. A limp known as the *antalgic abductor lurch* then follows. The child often demonstrates pain when the hip is externally rotated while in extension.

Treatment is accomplished with anti-inflammatory medications. During episodes of synovitis, avoiding activities that stress the hip are helpful. Surgery may be required if the femoral head becomes subluxated or incongruent with the acetabulum.

Osgood-Schlatter disease consists of osteochondrosis of the *tubercle of the tibia* and, often, *tendinitis of the patella*. The mildest form of Osgood-Schlatter disease causes ischemic necrosis in the region of the bony tibial tubercle, with hypertrophic cartilage formation during the stages of repair. In more severe cases, the abnormality involves a true apophyseal separation of the tibial tubercle with avascular necrosis. The child complains of pain and swelling in the region around the patellar tendon and tibial tubercle, which becomes prominent and is tender to direct pressure. The pain is most severe after running or jumping.

The goal of treatment for Osgood-Schlatter disease is to decrease the stress at the tubercle. Often a period of 4 to 8 weeks of restriction from strenuous physical activity is sufficient. If pain is not relieved, a cast or knee immobilization is required, a situation that is particularly difficult if the condition is bilateral.

5. Describe scoliosis.
Study pages 1029 and 1030; refer to Figure 38-12.

There are three main types of scoliosis: idiopathic; congenital, resulting from a bony deformity such as hemivertebrae; and teratologic, resulting from another systemic syndrome such as cerebral palsy. Eighty percent of all cases of scoliosis are idiopathic and may have a genetic component. True structural scoliotic deformity involves not only a *side-to-side spinal curve* but *also rotation*; curves without rotation may be nonstructural or may result from another cause, such as limb length inequality.

Idiopathic curves progress while a child is growing, and the progression can be rapid during growth spurts. When idiopathic curves progress to 25 degrees or greater, the child is skeletally immature and bracing is required. Curves exceeding 50 degrees will progress after skeletal maturity, and spinal fusion is required to stop progression. Bracing is the only nonoperative measure known to slow scoliotic progression. Bracing is less successful in teratologic or congenital scoliosis, which unfortunately often requires surgical intervention.

6. Describe the pathophysiology, evaluation, and treatment of Duchenne muscular dystrophy (DMD).
Study pages 1030-1033; refer to Figures 38-13 and 38-14 and Table 38-3.

DMD is an *X-linked inherited disorder* that is caused by a deletion of a segment of DNA. This deletion results in an absence of *dystrophin*, which is found in normal muscle cells. The lack of dystrophin apparently causes loss of muscle bulk and fibers. In the late stages, interstitial connective tissue and fat may replace muscle fibers.

The disease is often diagnosed when parents of an affected child notice slow motor development, problems with coordination and walking, and generalized weakness. Weakness always begins in the pelvic girdle, and *hypertrophy* is present *in the calf muscles* of approximately 80% of affected children. *Gower sign*, a peculiar manner of standing up from a sitting position by "climbing up" the legs (walking the hands up the legs), is often evident. Later, the shoulder girdle muscle becomes involved, with constant progression of the illness. Pulmonary and cardiac failure may follow, and death usually results by the child's 20s.

Diagnosis is confirmed by serum enzyme studies and electromyelography. *The serum creatine phosphokinase (CPK)* value may be many times normal, histologic examination of *biopsied muscle* fibers has abnormal findings, and genetic mutations in the dystrophin or *myotonic muscular dystrophy (MMD)* gene can exist. Treatment is chiefly supportive, with the goal being to preserve function of remaining muscle groups for as long as possible. Steroid therapy can improve walking and life expectancy.

Becker muscular dystrophy (BMD) is caused by the same dystrophin gene as DMD. It is X- linked and has the same clinical spectrum as DMD. The children with BMD present later and have a longer life expectancy than those with DMD. **Fascioscapulohumeral (FSH) muscular dystrophy,** the most common of all muscular dystrophies, is an *autosomal dominant disease.* FSH muscular dystrophy usually occurs in late childhood and progresses slowly, with normal or near normal lifespan. It usually begins in the face and passes to the shoulders and legs. **MMD** is an *autosomal dominant multisystem disease* occurring because of mutations in two MMD genes. This entity affects brain, skeletal and smooth muscle, eye, the heart, and the endocrine system, manifesting as intellectual disability.

7. Characterize common benign bone tumors of childhood.
Study page 1033.

Osteochondromas (exostoses) can occur as solitary lesions or as an inherited syndrome of **hereditary multiple exostoses (HME)**. HME is an *autosomal dominant* condition. Osteochondromas appear as *bony protuberances.* They are most common near active growth plates of the proximal *humerus, distal femur,* and proximal tibia. The most common presentation is a palpable mass that is painful when traumatized. Rarely, the lesion may cause neurologic, vascular, or tendon excursion anomalies because of local compression on nearby structures. The lesions can lead to growth disturbance and mildly short stature. Knee valgus (knock knee), ankle valgus, and hip problems are common. Upper extremity lesions can lead to a pronounced deformity in the forearm with a very short ulna bone.

Treatment involves minimizing growth disturbance, local tissue compression, and pain by resection of symptomatic lesions. The regrowth rate is 30% when lesions are removed in early childhood; therefore, only symptomatic lesions should be surgically removed.

Nonossifying fibroma or fibrous cortical defect accounts for 50% of all benign bone tumors. Nonossifying fibromas are sharply demarcated, *cortically based lesions* of fibrocytes that have replaced normal bone. The lesions can occur in any bone, at any age. Nonossifying fibromas are discovered in 20% to 30% of all children as incidental findings.

Microscopically, these benign nonmetastasizing lesions appear as whorled bundles of fibroblasts and osteoclast-like giant cells. As such a tumor grows, lipids make the fibroblasts foamy in appearance, and they are known as foam cells.

Treatment is observational only. If these lesions grow too large, however, they will compromise the biomechanical strength of the bone, causing pathologic features. Curettage and bone grafting are suggested when fractures occur or are impending.

8. Characterize childhood osteosarcoma and Ewing sarcoma.
Study pages 1033-1035; refer to Figures 38-15 and 38-16.

Malignant bone tumors are uncommon in childhood, accounting for fewer than 5% of childhood malignancies and occurring mostly during adolescence. **Osteosarcoma** *originates in bone-producing mesenchymal cells.* It is found in *metaphyses* of long bone near active growth sites. It may extend beyond the bone into a soft bulky tissue mass and encircle the bone. Osteosarcoma can be induced by ionizing radiation or by therapeutic irradiation for other forms of cancer.

The most common complaint is pain; night pain is a foreboding sign. Symptoms also include cough, dyspnea, and chest pain when lung metastasis occurs.

Surgery and chemotherapy are the primary treatments for osteosarcoma. Chemotherapy is an important component of treatment because children treated with surgery alone eventually have metastatic disease. The tumor is resistant to irradiation.

Ewing sarcoma is the second most common and most lethal malignant bone tumor of childhood. It probably *originates from cells within the bone marrow space and does not involve bone-forming cells.* Cytogenic studies have shown a translocation of chromosomes 11 and 22. Its incidence is greatest in children between 5 and 15 years of age; the disease is rare after age 30 years. The most common site of this tumor is the *marrow of the femur,* followed by the marrow of the pelvis and then of the humerus.

The most common symptom is pain that increases in severity. A soft tissue mass is often present. Ewing sarcoma metastasizes early to nearly every organ. The most common sites are the lung, other bones, lymph nodes, liver, spleen, and central nervous system.

Treatment is preoperative chemotherapy followed by irradiation, surgical resection, or both and continued chemotherapy for 12 to 18 months afterward. Involved sites with the best prognosis are the extremities; tumors of the pelvis have the worst prognosis.

9. Note the characteristics of nonaccidental trauma.
Review pages 1035; refer to Figure 38-17.

Nonaccidental trauma must be considered whenever bone injury occurs in perambulatory children. The presence of soft tissue injury and multiple fractures at different stages of healing is suggestive of nonaccidental trauma or childhood abuse. All social strata are at risk and health care providers are legally responsible to report suspected trauma.

PRACTICE EXAMINATION

True/False

1. In clubfoot, the entire foot points upward.
2. Osteosarcoma is responsive to radiotherapy.
3. OI is a disease related to over-calcification of the bone that causes it to be brittle and easily broken.
4. Septic arthritis can involve sites where the metaphysis still is located within the joint capsule.
5. Osgood-Schlatter disease consists of osteochondrosis of the tubercle of the fibula and tendonitis of the patella.
6. Osteomyelitis is an infection of bone that can be spread to the site through the blood.
7. JIRA predominantly affects small joints.
8. True structural scoliosis involves spinal rotation.
9. Muscular dystrophies are characterized by defective creatine metabolism.
10. Nonossifying fibromas are caused by translocation of chromosomes 11 and 22.

Fill in the Blank

11. The process of Legg-Calvé-Perthes disease is presumably produced by interruption of the blood supply to the ______________head.
12. A risk factor in developmental dysplasia of the hip may be___________________ in utero.
13. DMD results from a lack of _________________ in muscle cells.
14. DDH in children younger than 4 months is treated by bracing the hips in a ______________.
15. Congenital equinovarus is also known as __________.

Matching

Match the outcome or circumstance with the alteration:

_______ 16. Fractures present at birth

_______ 17. Hypertrophied calf muscles

_______ 18. Chronic uveitis

_______ 19. Gower sign

_______ 20. Antalgic abductor lurch

_______ 21. Large joints affected

_______ 22. Pain in external rotation with affected limb

_______ 23. Long-term antibiotics required

_______ 24. Defect in collagen synthesis

_______ 25. Lateral curvature of the spine

a. scoliosis
b. OI
c. osteomyelitis
d. Legg-Calvé-Perthes disease
e. JIRA
f. DMD

Fill in the Blank

Complete the following table differentiating between childhood benign and malignant bone tumors:

Childhood Benign and Malignant Bone Tumors

Type	Site	Feature
Benign		
Osteochondroma	Near-active growth plates of proximal humerus or tibia and distal femur	
Nonossifying fibroma		
Malignant		
Osteosarcoma		When lung metastasis occurs, cough, dyspnea, and pain manifest
Ewing sarcoma		

CASE REVIEW

Bobby B. is a 3-year-old white boy visiting a pediatrician's office because of his mother's concern. She states, "Bobby is clumsy, frequently falls, and has difficulty climbing stairs." Physical examination reveals that Bobby B. tends to walk on his toes, exhibits Gower sign, and appears to have hypertrophy of calf muscles.

What disease is suspected? How could the diagnosis be confirmed?

39 Structure, Function, and Disorders of the Integument

FOUNDATIONAL OBJECTIVES

a. Describe the skin and its layers; note the dermal appendages.
Review pages 1038 and 1040; refer to Figures 39-1 and 39-2 Table 39-1.

MEMORY CHECK!

- The skin has two major layers: a superficial *epidermis* and a deeper layer, the *dermis*. The subcutaneous tissue, or *hypodermis,* is an underlying layer of connective tissue that contains macrophages, fibroblasts, and fat cells.
- The *dermal appendages* include the nails, hair, sebaceous glands, and the eccrine and apocrine sweat glands. The nails are protective keratinized plates that appear at the ends of fingers and toes. Hair follicles arise from the matrix, located deep in the dermis. Hair growth begins in the bulb, with cellular differentiation occurring as the hair progresses up the follicle. Hair is fully cornified by the time it emerges at the skin surface. The *sebaceous glands* open onto the surface of the skin through a canal and secrete sebum composed primarily of lipids, which oil the skin and hair and prevent drying.
- The eccrine sweat glands are distributed over the body and are important for cooling the body through evaporation. The apocrine sweat glands are fewer in number and are located in the axillae, scalp, face, abdomen, and genital area.
- The blood supply to the skin is through the papillary capillaries or plexus of the dermis. *Arteriovenous anastomoses* in the dermis facilitate the regulation of body temperature. Heat loss can be regulated by variation of the blood flow through the skin by opening or closing of the arteriovenous anastomoses to modify evaporative heat loss through sweat. The sympathetic nervous system regulates both vasoconstriction and vasodilation because there are *only adrenergic receptors in the skin.* The lymphatic vessels of the skin arise in the dermis and drain into larger subcutaneous trunks; these vessels remove cells, proteins, and immunologic mediators.

b. Identify the changes that occur in skin during aging.
Review page 1040.

MEMORY CHECK!

- The skin becomes thinner, dryer, and wrinkled, and pigmentation changes during aging. *Fewer melanocytes* decrease the protection against ultraviolet (UV) radiation. *Fewer Langerhans cells* decrease the skin's immune response during aging. The thickness of the dermis decreases, and the skin becomes translucent and assumes a paper-thin quality. *Loss of the rete pegs* gives the skin a smooth, shiny appearance. *Atrophy of eccrine, apocrine, and sebaceous glands* causes the skin to become drier with age. *Loss of elastin fibers* is associated with wrinkling. The collagen fibers become less flexible and reduce the skin's ability to stretch and regain shape. *Diminished cell generation and blood supply* delay wound healing in aging skin. Hair grays because of a loss of melanocytes. *Barrier function* of the stratum corneum *is reduced.* There is increased permeability and decreased clearance of substances from the dermis. The accumulation of such substances can irritate the skin. *Temperature regulation is less effective* in the elderly, and there is increased risk for both heatstroke and hypothermia. The pressure and touch receptors and free nerve endings all decrease in number, *reducing sensory perception.*

LEARNING OBJECTIVES

After studying this chapter, the learner will be able to do the following:

1. Distinguish among skin lesions.
Refer to Tables 39-2 and 39-3.

Basic Lesions of the Skin

Type	Characteristics	Example/Disease
Macule	A flat, circumscribed, discolored lesion of any size	Freckles, nevi, measles
Patch	A flat, irregular lesion larger than a macule	Vitiligo, port-wine stains, café au lait spots
Telangiectasia	Dilated, superficial blood vessels	Rosacea
Papule	A lesion 1 cm or less in diameter because of infiltration or hyperplasia of the dermis	Verrucae (warts), lichen planus, nevus
Plaque	A lesion with a large surface area, larger laterally than in height	Psoriasis, keratoses
Nodule	A palpable, circumscribed lesion 1 cm-2 cm in diameter located in the epidermis, dermis, or hypodermis; smooth to ulcerated	Benign or malignant tumors, erythema nodosum
Wheal	A transient lesion with well-defined and often changing borders caused by edema of the dermis	Insect bites, allergic responses
Vesicle (< 1 cm) and bulla (> 1 cm)	A fluid-filled, thin-walled lesion; a bulla is a vesicle more than 0.5 cm in diameter	Herpes zoster (shingles), varicella (chicken pox), second-degree burns
Pustule	A lesion containing a purulent exudate	Acne, impetigo
Keloid	Scar (collagen formation) beyond the wound border	Scar tissue following surgery
Scale	Accumulation of loose stratum corneum, flaky skin	Psoriasis
Lichenification	Thickening, toughening of the skin with accentuation of skin lines caused by scratching	Chronic dermatitis
Cyst	An encapsulated mass of dermis or subcutaneous layers (semisolid or fluid filled)	Sebaceous cyst, cystic acne
Tumor	A well-demarcated solid lesion more than 2 cm in diameter	Fibroma, lipoma, hemangioma
Scar	Thin or thick fibrous (collagenous) tissue	Healed laceration, burn, surgical incision
Atrophy	Thinning of the epidermis or dermis caused by decreased connective tissue	Thin facial skin of the elderly, striae of pregnancy
Ulcer	Loss of epidermis and dermis	Pressure sores
Excoriation	Loss of epidermis with exposed dermis	Scratches, scabies
Fissure	Linear crack or break exposing the dermis	Athlete's foot, cheilosis
Erosion	Moist, red break in epidermis; follows rupture of vesicle or bulla; larger than fissure	Chickenpox, diaper dermatitis

2. Describe pressure ulcers.
Study pages 1040, 1046 and 1047; refer to Figure 39-3.

Pressure ulcers are ischemic lesions resulting from unrelieved pressure, shearing forces, friction, and moisture. *Decubitus ulcers* develop when an individual lies in a recumbent position for long periods. Continuous pressure on tissue between bony prominences and resistant surface distorts capillaries and occludes the blood supply. If the pressure is shortly relieved, a brief hyperemia occurs. If the pressure remains, the endothelial cells become disrupted with platelet clumping and form *microthrombi that block blood flow and cause anoxic necrosis* of surrounding tissue.

Prevention is the primary goal. Superficial ulcers should be covered with hydrogel dressings. Large, deep lesions require necrotic tissue débridement and possible skin flap grafts with antibiotics and pain control.

3. Describe pruritus.
Study page 1047.

Pruritus, or itching, is associated with many primary skin disorders, such as eczema, psoriasis, and insect infestations. It can be a manifestation of chronic renal failure, cholestatic liver disease, thyroid disorders, iron deficiency, neuropathies, malignancy, or opiate drugs. *Peripheral itch mediators include histamine, serotonin, prostaglandins, bradykinins, neuropeptides, acetylcholine, and interleukin.* Small unmyelinated nerve fibers transmit itch sensations to the brain.

Topical therapy, oral histamine, and phototherapy with UV radiation can target pruritus in the skin. Antiepileptics, opioid antagonists, and antidepressants can block signals in the central nervous system.

4. Identify the causes and lesions of inflammatory and papulosquamous disorders of the skin.
Study pages 1048-1051; refer to Figures 39-5 through 39-13. (See following table on inflammatory and papulosquamous skin disorders in next page)

5. Compare pemphigus with erythema multiforme.
Study pages 1051-1053; refer to Figure 39-14.

Pemphigus is a rare, chronic, blister-forming disease of the skin and oral mucous membranes with several different types. An *autoimmune disease,* pemphigus is caused by circulating immunoglobulin G (IgG) autoantibodies and complement component C3, which react with the intracellular cement of substance that holds the epidermal cells together. The antibody reaction likely causes the intraepidermal blister formation and acantholysis, or loss of cohesion between epidermal cells.

Pemphigus vulgaris is the most common form, with acantholysis at the deeper suprabasal level. Oral lesions precede the onset of skin blistering, which is more prominent on the face, scalp, and axilla. The blisters rupture easily because of thin, fragile overlying epidermis. *Pemphigus vegetans* is a variant of pemphigus vulgaris, with large blisters occurring in the tissue folds of the axilla and groin. *Pemphigus foliaceus* is a milder form involving acantholysis at the more superficial, subcorneal level, with blistering, erosions, scaling, crusting, and erythema usually of the face and chest. Oral mucous membranes are rarely involved. *Pemphigus erythematosus is a subset* of pemphigus foliaceus often associated with systemic lupus erythematosus with the presence of serum antinuclear antibodies. The lesions are generally less widely distributed.

In the diagnosis of pemphigus, immunofluorescence demonstrates the presence of antibodies at the site of blister formation. The primary treatment for pemphigus is systemic corticosteroids, usually in high doses to suppress the immune response during acute episodes or when there is widespread involvement.

Erythema multiforme is an acute, recurring, inflammatory disorder of the skin and mucous membranes. It is associated with *allergic or immunologic reactions* to drugs or microorganisms. Immune complex formation and *deposition of C3, IgM, and fibrinogen* around the superficial dermal blood vessels, basement membrane, and keratinocytes can be observed in most individuals with erythema multiforme. The characteristic *"bull's eye" lesion* occurs on the skin surface, consisting of a central erythematous region surrounded by concentric rings or alternating edema and inflammation. A vesiculobullous form is characterized by mucous membrane lesions and erythematous plaques on the extensor surfaces of the extremities.

The most common form expressed in children and young adults is **Stevens-Johnson syndrome**, wherein there are numerous *erythematous, bullous lesions on both the skin and mucous membranes related to immune reactions to drugs.* The bullous lesions form erosions and crusts when they rupture. The mouth, air passages, esophagus, urethra, and conjunctiva may be involved. Mild forms of the disease require no treatment because they are self limiting; underlying infections should be treated.

Inflammatory and Papulosquamous Skin Disorders

Disorder	Cause	Lesion
Inflammatory Disorders		
Allergic contact dermatitis	Allergen binds to carrier protein to form a sensitizing antigen, T cell hypersensitivity, IgE	Pruritic (itching), vesicles
Irritant contact dermatitis	Nonimmunologic inflammation caused by chemicals	As above
Atopic dermatitis	Mast cells and IgE, T lymphocytes, and monocytes interact	Red, weeping crusts, lichenification
Stasis dermatitis	Venous stasis and edema	Initial erythema and pruritus' then scaling, petechiae, hyperpigmentation
Seborrheic dermatitis	Unknown	Scaly plaques with mild pruritus
Papulosquamous Disorders		
Psoriasis	Activated helper T cells, inflammatory cytokines	Thick, silvery, scaly, erythematous plaque surrounded by normal skin; rapid shedding of epidermis
Pityriasis rosea	Possible herpes-like virus	Pruritus, demarcated salmon-pink scale within a plaque
Lichen planus	Exposure to drugs or chemicals, abnormal T-cell response to epithelial cells recognized as foreign	Nonscaling, violet pruritic papules
Acne vulgaris	Increased activity of sebaceous glands or inability of sebum to escape through the narrow opening	Comedones
Acne rosacea	Unknown or altered immunity, associated with chronic flushing and sensitivity to sun	Erythema, papules, pustules, telangiectasis
Discoid (cutaneous) lupus erythematosus	Altered immune response to unknown antigen or UV wavelengths	Cutaneous manifestations of elevated red plaque with brown scale, hair loss, urticaria (hives), telangiectasis

6. **Identify the causes and lesions of cutaneous infections.**
Study pages 1053-1055; refer to Figures 39-15 through 39-19 and Tables 39-4 and 39-5.

Cutaneous infections

Infection	Cause	Lesion
Folliculitis	Bacterial infection of hair follicles usually by *Staphylococcus aureus*	Pustules with surrounding erythema
Furuncle	Infection from folliculitis spreading into dermis	Deep, red, firm, painful nodule changes to fluctuant and tender cystic nodule
Carbuncle	Collection of infected hair follicle	Erythematous, painful mass that drains through many openings
Cellulitis	Staphylococcal infection of dermis and subcutaneous tissue; extension from skin wound, ulcer, furuncle, or carbuncle	Erythematous, swollen, painful area
Erysipelas	Group A beta-hemolytic streptococci	Systemic manifestations; red spots progress to pruritic vesicles
Impetigo	Coagulase-positive staphylococci; beta-hemolytic streptococci	Serous and purulent vesicles that rupture and crust
Herpes simplex virus (HSV):		
HSV-1	Contact with infected saliva	Clusters of oral or nasal erythematous vesicles that become purulent and crusty ("cold sores" or "fever blisters")
HSV-2	Primary and secondary infection after sexual contact with infected person	Genital vesicles that progress to painful ulceration, pruritus, and weeping
Varicella (chickenpox) primary	Varicella-zoster virus (VZV)	Varicella: pink papules with reddened halo that is dry and crusty
Herpes zoster (shingles) secondary activation	VZV	Zoster: erythema followed by grouped vesicles along a unilateral dermatome that later crust
Warts (verrucae)	Human papillomavirus (HPV) transmitted by touch or sexual contact	Round, elevated with a rough, grayish surface, cauliflower-like lesions
Tinea capitis (scalp)	Dermatophytes (fungi) that invade and thrive on keratin	Scaling and erythema, vesicles and fissures
Tinea pedis (athlete's foot)		
Tinea corporis (ringworm)		
Candidiasis	*Candida albicans* (yeast-like fungus) changes from a skin and mucous membrane commensal to a pathogen because of immune deficits	Thin-walled pustule with inflammatory pruritic base

7. Differentiate among vasculitis, urticaria, and scleroderma.

Study pages 1055 and 1056; refer to Figure 39-20.

Vasculitis, or angiitis, is an inflammation of the blood vessels. *Cutaneous vasculitis* develops from the *deposit of immune complexes* in small blood vessels as a response to drugs, allergens, or streptococcal or viral infection. The deposit of immune complex likely activates complement, which is chemotactic for polymorphonuclear leukocytes. The lesions appear as palpable purpura and progress to hemorrhagic bullae with necrosis and ulceration because of occlusion of the vessel. Identifying and removing the antigen is the first step in treatment. Steroids may be used if symptoms are severe.

Urticarial lesions are most commonly associated with *type I hypersensitivity* reactions to drugs, certain foods, intestinal parasites, or physical agents. The lesions are mediated by histamine release, which causes the endothelial cells of skin blood vessels to contract and increase their permeability.

The fluid from the vessel appears as wheals, welts, or hives. Antihistamines usually reduce the hives and provide relief from itching. Corticosteroids may be required for treatment of severe attacks.

Scleroderma is *sclerosis* of the skin, which may remain localized to the skin or may affect the visceral organs. If systemic, scleroderma *involves the connective tissue* and affects the kidneys, gastrointestinal tract, and lungs. The cutaneous lesions can cover the entire skin, but are most often on the face and hands, the neck, and the upper chest.

The lesions exhibit massive deposits of collagen with fibrosis, inflammatory reactions, vascular changes in the capillary network with decreased capillary loops, and dilation of the remaining capillaries. Autoimmunity and an immune reaction to toxic substances are possible, initiating mechanisms of the disease. Autoantibodies often can be recovered from the skin and serum of individuals with scleroderma. Growth factors or failure of apoptosis of myofibroblasts may be causative mechanisms.

The skin is hard, hypopigmented, taut, and tightly connected to the underlying tissue. An immobile mask-like appearance with incomplete opening of the mouth results from the tightness of facial skin. The fingers become tapered and flexed and lose fingertips from atrophy. Calcium deposits develop in the subcutaneous tissue and erupt through the skin. When the condition progresses to body organs, death is caused by subsequent respiratory failure, renal failure, cardiac dysrhythmias, or obstructions or perforations of the esophagus or intestine. There is no specific treatment. Immunomodulation therapies with photopheresis, plasmapheresis, and stem cell treatment are in progress.

8. Identify diseases caused by insect bites.

Study page 1057.

Mosquitoes are responsible for malaria, yellow fever, dengue fever, filariasis, and St. Louis encephalitis. Mosquitoes can bite through thin, loose clothing and are attracted by warmth and perspiration. The edema, pruritus, and papular lesions are caused by insertion of a blood tube by a female mosquito. Irritating salivary secretions also contain anticoagulants. Reactions vary, depending on the sensitivity of the victim.

Several species of **flies** are bloodsuckers. The bite of a small female fly produces immediate pain, erythema, and vesicles. Itching and vesicular reactions may persist for weeks. The fiercest bloodsuckers are the larger types, such as the horseflies and deerflies. These produce painful, bleeding bites because of their large mouthparts. The bites produce urticaria that may be accompanied by weakness, dizziness, and wheezing.

Bees, wasps, hornets, and yellow jackets are **stinging insects**. The stinger is implanted in the skin with the release of venom. Reactions to venom can be localized or generalized (anaphylactic shock), depending on the individual's sensitivity.

9. Compare the benign tumors of the skin.

Study pages 1057 and 1058; refer to Figure 39-21.

Seborrheic keratosis is a benign proliferation *of basal cells* that produces elevated smooth or warty lesions. Multiple lesions appear on the chest, back, and face in older people. The color varies; it may be tan to waxy yellow, flesh colored, or dark brown-black, and the lesions are often oval and appear greasy with a *hyperkeratotic scale*. Lesion size varies from a few millimeters to several centimeters. Cryotherapy with liquid nitrogen or laser therapy is an effective treatment.

A **keratoacanthoma** is a benign, self-limiting tumor that *arises from hair follicles*. It usually occurs on sun-exposed surfaces and develops in elderly individuals. The lesion develops in stages. The proliferative stage produces a rapid-growing, dome-shaped nodule with a central crust. In the mature stage, the lesion is filled with whitish keratin. The mature lesion requires differentiation from squamous cell carcinoma. The involution stage usually occurs over a 3- to 4-month period as the lesion regresses. Although the lesion will resolve spontaneously, it can be removed surgically.

Actinic keratosis is a *premalignant lesion* found on skin surfaces exposed to UV radiation of the sun. The lesions can *progress to squamous cell carcinoma*. The prevalence is highest in individuals with unprotected, light-colored skin. The lesions appear as pigmented patches of rough, adherent scale, and surrounding areas may have telangiectasia. Freezing with liquid nitrogen provides quick, effective treatment. Excisions provide tissue for biopsy.

Nevi, or moles, are pigmented or nonpigmented lesions that form from *melanocytes*. During early development, the melanocytes accumulate at the junction of the dermis and epidermis and become macular lesions. Over time, the cells move into the dermis and become nodular and palpable. Nevi may appear anywhere on the skin singly or in groups and vary in size. Nevi can undergo transition to *malignant melanoma*; if irritated, they may be excised.

10. Describe malignant skin lesions.
Study pages 1058-1060; refer to Figures 39-22 through 39-25 and Table 39-6.

Cancerous Skin Lesions

Lesion	Cause	Growth Rate/ Metastasis	Appearance
Basal cell carcinoma	Sunlight-exposed skin; alterations in tumor supressor genes and DNA repair mechanisms	Slow growth; lesions rarely metastasize; invasive destruction	Smooth surface with rolled border, depressed center, telangiectasis
Squamous cell carcinoma	Sunlight-exposed skin; arise from premalignant lesions; activation of p53 mutations	Moderate growth; some lesions metastasize	Rough, firm nodule with an indurated base, ulceration, bleeding
Malignant melanoma	Protooncogenes, solar radiation, steroid hormones, precursor nevi	Fast growth; highly invasive, rapid metastasis	Nevi that change symmetry, color, size, or margins or grow rapidly; pruritus, bleeding nodule formation or ulceration
Kaposi sarcoma	Immunodeficient states; genetics and male gender—black, Jewish, or Italian males	Slow spread through skin; some aggressive change	Multifocal purplish, brown vascular macules that develop into plaques and nodules that may be painful and pruritic; may affect gastrointestinal and respiratory tract lymph nodes

Note: Treatment consists of surgery, electrodesiccation, radiation, or cryosurgery. For basal cell and squamous cell skin cancers, cure is virtually ensured with early detection and treatment. For malignant melanomas, wide and deep excisions and removal of lymph nodes are required. Early recognition of malignant melanomas affects the surgical cure of these lesions. Survival is poor for malignant melanoma because it metastasizes quickly. The general response to treatment of Kaposi sarcoma is poor.

11. Classify burns according to the extent of injury.
Study pages 1060 and 1062; refer to Figures 39-26 through 39-30, 39-32 and 39-33.

Burn Injuries

		Second-Degree		Third-Degree
Feature	First-Degree	Superficial Partial-Thickness	Deep Partial-Thickness	Full-Thickness
Morphology	Destruction of epidermis only	Destruction of epidermis and some dermis	Destruction of epidermis and dermis	Destruction of epidermis, dermis, and subcutaneous tissue
Skin function?	Yes	No	No	No

Burn Injuries—cont'd

		Second-Degree		Third-Degree
Feature	First-Degree	Superficial Partial-Thickness	Deep Partial-Thickness	Full-Thickness
Tactile and pain sensors?	Yes	Yes	Diminished	No
Blisters	Present after 24 hours	Present within minutes, fluid filled	May not appear; a flat dehydrated layer lifts off in sheets	Rare; a flat dehydrated layer lifts off easily
Appearance of wound after initial débridement	Skin peels after 24 to 48 hours; normal or slightly red	Red to pale ivory; moist surface	Mottled with areas of waxy white, dry surface	White, cherry red, or black; may contain visible thrombosed veins; dry, hard leathery surface
Healing time	3 to 5 days	21 to 28 days	30 days to many months; excision and grafting	Will not heal; may close from edges as secondary healing if wound is small; excision and grafting
Scarring	None	May be present; influenced by genetic predisposition	Highest incidence; influenced by genetic predisposition	Scarring minimized by early excision and grafting; influenced by genetic predisposition

12. Characterize the hypovolemic, cardiovascular, and cellular responses to burn injury.
Review pages 1063 and 1064; refer to Figure 39-31.

Hypovolemic shock develops quickly after major burn injury. Within minutes of a major burn injury, the capillary bed opens not only in the burn area but also *in the entire capillary system*. This *increased capillary permeability is the mechanism for fluid, electrolyte, and protein loss into the interstitium,* thus reducing circulating blood volume. The reduction leads to the ensuing hypovolemic shock and *massive edema*. The fluid and protein movement from the vascular compartment results in decreased cardiac contractility and output, elevated hematocrit and white blood cell (WBC) count, and hypoproteinemia. The diminished cardiac contractility decreases the function of all critical organs.

Reduced visceral perfusion decreases gut barrier protection, resulting in translocation of bacterial endotoxemia and sepsis. If the profound hypovolemic shock is not treated with fluid resuscitation, irreversible shock and death may occur within a few hours.

The **cellular response** to burn injury consists of a metabolic response and an immunologic response. Burn injury induces an immediate **hypermetabolic state.** Tachycardia, hypercapnia, and body wasting develop. Serum catecholamines, cortisol, glucagons, and insulin are elevated with a corresponding increase in gluconeogenesis, lipolysis, and proteolysis. Tissue hypoxia produces *lactic acidosis* with an increased rate of glycogenolysis.

In individuals surviving burn shock, **immunosuppression** and increased susceptibility to potentially fatal systemic burn wound sepsis develop. Phagocytosis is impaired, and cellular and humoral immunity is decreased. Burned individuals with altered immunocompetence are *at risk for distant organ failure and multiple-organ dysfunction syndrome.* With loss of the skin's ability to regulate *evaporative water loss,* there is volume deficit and shock.

13. Characterize frostbite.
Study pages 1064 and 1065.

Frostbite is an injury to the skin caused by exposure to extreme cold. It is related to direct cold injury to cells, indirect injury from ice crystal formation, and endothelial damage. The frozen skin becomes white or yellowish, is waxy, and has *no sensation of pain*. With mild frostbite during rewarming (immersion in a 40° to 42° C water bath), redness and discomfort are followed by a return to normal in a few hours. In more severe cases, *cyanosis* and mottling develop, followed by redness, swelling, and burning pain upon rewarming. The most severe cases result in gangrene and loss of the affected part. Frostbite may be classified according to depth of injury. Superficial frostbite includes partial skin freezing and is known as *first- degree* frostbite; full-thickness skin freezing is *second-degree* frostbite; full-thickness skin and subcutaneous freezing constitute *third-degree* frostbite; and deep tissue freezing is *fourth-degree* frostbite.

Pain during the rewarming, thawing period is severe and should be treated with potent analgesics. Antibiotics may be given. Débridement or amputation of necrotic tissue is delayed until a clear line of demarcation between it and healthy tissue appears.

14. Define terms used in disorders of the hair and nails; note possible treatments.
Review page 1065.

Male-pattern alopecia is an inherited form of irreversible baldness in which hair is lost in the central scalp and recession of the temporofrontal hairline occurs. **Female-pattern alopecia** is a thinning of the central hair of the scalp that begins in women at 20 to 30 years of age. **Alopecia areata** is patchy loss of hair usually associated with stress or metabolic diseases; it is usually reversible. Most treatments for alopecia are ineffective. **Hirsutism** is a male pattern of hair growth in women; it may be normal or the result of excessive secretion of androgenic hormones. Cosmetic removal of hair is possible.

Paronychia is an inflammation of the cuticle that can be acute or chronic and is usually caused by staphylococci, streptococci, or fungi. **Onychomycosis** is a fungal infection of the nail plate; the plate turns yellow or white and accumulates hyperkeratotic debris. Treatment is difficult because topical or systemic antifungal agents do not penetrate the tissues or the nail plate rapidly.

PRACTICAL EXAMINATION

Multiple Choice

Circle the correct answer for each question:

1. Which stratum of the epidermis contains dead keratinocytes?
   a. corneum
   b. lucidum
   c. granulosum
   d. spinosum
   e. germinativum

2. The dermis is composed of all of the following *except*:
   a. melanocytes.
   b. collagen.
   c. elastin.
   d. apocrine sweat glands.
   e. sebaceous glands.

3. Which does *not* occur as the skin ages?
   a. more melanocytes
   b. decreased Langerhans cells
   c. loss of rete pegs
   d. loss of elastin fibers
   e. depressed immune response

4. Arteriovenous anastomoses in the dermis:
   a. prevent skin drying.
   b. regulate vasoconstriction.
   c. oppose evaporative heat loss.
   d. facilitate the regulation of body temperature.
   e. None of the above is correct.

Matching

Match the lesion with its descriptor:

_______ 5. Macule
_______ 6. Nodule
_______ 7. Scale
_______ 8. Wheal

a. hardened, adherent
b. changed color; *not* raised not depressed
c. accentuated skin lines caused by scratching
d. palpable, elevated solid lesion
e. flaky, accumulated stratum corneum
f. ridge-like, reddened elevation caused by edema and congestion

Multiple Choice

Circle the correct answer for each question:

9. The cause of atopic dermatitis is:
   a. unknown.
   b. venous stasis.
   c. increased activity of sebaceous glands.
   d. mast cell degranulation, T-cell and monocyte interaction.
   e. nonimmunologic inflammation to chemicals.

10. The skin lesion of psoriasis is a(n):
    a. nonscaling, violet pruritic papule.
    b. comedo.
    c. pruritic vesicle.
    d. erythematous, butterfly-shaped rash.
    e. thick, scaly, erythematous plaque.

11. A circular, demarcated, salmon-pink scale within a plaque is characteristic of:
    a. psoriasis.
    b. seborrheic dermatitis.
    c. acne rosacea.
    d. pityriasis rosea.
    e. lichen planus.

12. Acantholysis is observed in:
    a. herpes simplex.
    b. pemphigus.
    c. erythema multiforme.
    d. Stevens-Johnson syndrome.
    e. Both c and d are correct.

13. The cause of impetigo in the adult is:
    a. *Streptococcus aureus.*
    b. group A streptococci.
    c. coagulase-positive staphylococci.
    d. beta-hemolytic streptococci.
    e. Both c and d are correct.

14. The usual manifestation of HSV is a:
    a. painful nodule.
    b. pustule.
    c. cold sore or fever blister.
    d. wheal.

15. Of the benign tumors of the skin, keratoacanthomas are characterized by:
    a. proliferation of basal cells.
    b. hyperkeratotic scales.
    c. origination from hair follicles.
    d. a proliferative stage that produces a nodule with a central crust.
    e. Both c and d are correct.

16. Which are most likely to undergo malignant transition?
    a. seborrheic keratosis and keratoacanthoma
    b. seborrheic keratosis and actinic keratosis
    c. nevi and keratoacanthoma
    d. nevi and actinic keratosis
    e. None of the above is correct.

17. The cause of Kaposi sarcoma likely is:
    a. solar radiation.
    b. steroidal hormones.
    c. precursor nevi.
    d. immunodeficiency.
    e. keratinization.

18. Squamous cell carcinoma of the skin is manifested as:
    a. irregular pigmentation.
    b. elevated, firm lesions.
    c. a smooth, pearly lesion with multiple telangiectasia.
    d. multifocal purplish, brown macules.

19. An untreated basal cell carcinoma:
    a. metastasizes frequently.
    b. often involves regional lymphatics.
    c. ulcerates and involves local tissue.
    d. grows rapidly.
    e. will eventually require removal of nearby lymph nodes.

20. Which malignant skin lesion metastasizes the earliest?
    a. basal cell carcinoma
    b. squamous cell carcinoma
    c. malignant melanoma
    d. Kaposi sarcoma

21. In which type of burn does skin function continue?
    a. first-degree
    b. superficial partial-thickness
    c. deep partial-thickness
    d. full-thickness

22. A burn that destroys the epidermis and dermis is a:
    a. first-degree burn.
    b. superficial partial-thickness burn.
    c. deep partial-thickness burn.
    d. full-thickness burn.

23. Hypovolemic shock in severely burned individuals is the result of:
    a. dilation of capillaries.
    b. increased capillary permeability.
    c. increased peripheral resistance.
    d. Both a and b are correct.
    e. a, b, and c are correct.

24. In individuals surviving burn shock, increased wound sepsis is caused by:
    a. released inflammatory cytokines.
    b. fewer opsonins.
    c. inability of phagocytes to migrate to the site of infection.
    d. All of the above are correct.
    e. Both b and c are correct.

25. Onychomycosis is:
    a. a fungal infection of the nail plate.
    b. caused by staphylococci or streptococci.
    c. an inflammation of the cuticle.
    d. None of the above is correct.

Fill in the Blank

Complete the following table identifying changes in skin integrity and their consequences:

Aging and Changes in the Skin

Change	Consequences
Fewer melanocytes	
Loss of rete pegs	
Loss of elastin	
Thinning of dermis	
Loss of collagen fiber flexibility	
Greater permeability with less ability to clear substances	
Atrophy of eccrine, apocrine, and sebaceous glands	
Fewer Langerhans cells	Less phagocytes and immune response
Decrease in free nerve endings	
Decreased blood flow and basal cell turnover	Decreased wound healing
Thinning of nail plates	

CASE STUDY

Mr. E. is a 26-year-old white man who sustained severe burns while welding an automobile gasoline tank that had been removed from a truck. Mr. E.'s friend, for whom the welding was being done, took him immediately to a regional burn center located 20 miles away. While traveling to the burn center, the friend said to Mr. E., "I am so sorry. One of us should have known not to light a flame where there could be gasoline fumes."

Initial assessment reveals that Mr. E. has received full-thickness burns on his face, to both arms and hands bilaterally and circumferentially, and to the anterior trunk.

What are the burn unit's immediate concerns? What other concerns would the burn unit have?

40 Alterations of the Integument in Children

LEARNING OBJECTIVES

After studying this chapter, the learner will be able to do the following:

1. Describe acne vulgaris.
Study pages 1070 and 1071; refer to Figure 40-1.

Acne vulgaris is the most common of the skin diseases, affecting 85% of the population between ages 12 and 25 years; age of onset is getting younger. The incidence of acne is the same in both genders; severe disease affects males more often. Genetics may determine the susceptibility and severity of the disease.

Acne develops primarily on the face and upper parts of the chest and back from *sebaceous follicles*. The follicles have many large sebaceous glands, a small vellus hair, and a dilated follicular canal that is visible on the skin surface as a pore. In **noninflammatory acne,** the comedones are open (blackheads) and closed (whiteheads) and the accumulated material causes follicular distention and thinning of follicular canal walls. **Inflammatory acne** develops in closed comedones when follicular walls rupture and expel sebum into the surrounding dermis and initiate inflammation.

The causes are abnormal keratinization of follicular epithelium, excessive sebum production, and proliferation of *Propionibacterium acnes* with release of inflammatory mediators. *Androgenic hormones increase the size and productivity of the sebaceous glands.* Sebum and bacterial accumulation produces inflammation of the dermis as the follicle ruptures.

Topical treatment, including retinoid and antimicrobial agents, is used because it is the least invasive. Use of systemic therapies, including antibiotics, sex hormones, and corticosteroids, may be limited because of side effects. Comedo extraction, intralesional steroids, and cryosurgery may be used. Dermabrasion, lasers, and resurfacing may be used in severe scarring.

2. Differentiate between atopic dermatitis and diaper dermatitis in infants and children.
Study pages 1071 and 1072; refer to Figures 40-2 and 40-3.

Atopic dermatitis, or eczema, is an inflammation of the skin of unknown etiology. There is an increased incidence of 75% to 80% in individuals who have allergies and a family history of asthma. Onset usually is in infancy, with 85% of cases occurring by 5 years of age. The disorder has a chronic course with frequent exacerbations. The cause involves an interrelationship of genetic predisposition, *filaggrin* gene mutations that alter keratin binding in the epidermis, reduced stratum corneum lipid levels, and altered immunity to allergens, irritants, and microbes.

Positive allergy tests, increased serum IgE levels, and eosinophilia are common findings. The face, scalp, trunk, and extensor surfaces of the extremities are commonly affected in younger children; the neck, hands, feet, and flexor surfaces are commonly affected in older children. The characteristic rash is erythematous with weeping and crusting lesions. Pruritus or itching develops.

Treatment includes avoidance of known irritants, hydration of the skin, and use of antihistamines to relieve pruritus and topical steroids to decrease inflammation. Antibiotics or antifungal agents may be necessary for secondary skin infections.

Diaper dermatitis is an inflammation of the skin in the diaper area that is caused by many factors, including lengthy exposure to wet and soiled diapers. Diaper dermatitis is characterized by an erythematous rash of varying severity and is often complicated by a secondary fungal infection caused by the microorganism *Candida albicans*. The characteristic rash of *C. albicans* is very erythematous and papular and is associated with *papulovesicular satellite lesions*.

The best treatment is preventive by keeping the perineal area clean and dry with frequent diaper changes and routine hygiene. If *C. albicans* is present, a topical antifungal agent should be included in the treatment.

3. Categorize and characterize the infectious processes of impetigo.
Review pages 1072 and 1073; refer to Figure 40-4.

Impetigo is a common bacterial skin infection in children and is either bullous or vesicular.

Impetigo

Feature	Bullous Impetigo	Vesicular Impetigo
Etiologic agent	*Staphylococcus aureus*	*Streptococcus pyogenes* or combined with staphylococci
Source	Other infected individuals or contaminated objects	Other infected individuals, contaminated objects, insect bites
Regional lymphadenitis	Uncommon	Common
Treatment	Systemic antibiotics	Systemic antibiotics
Potential complications	Uncommon	Acute glomerulonephritis

4. Describe the etiology and pathophysiology of staphylococcal scalded-skin syndrome.
Study page 1073; refer to Figure 40-5.

Staphylococcal scalded-skin syndrome is a serious infection caused by group II staphylococci. The primary site of infection often is in the throat or chest and is characterized by fever, rhinorrhea, and malaise. This severe infection is often seen in newborns because their immune systems are immature.

Skin manifestations are caused by an *epidermolytic toxin produced* by the staphylococcal microorganisms at the primary site of infection; the toxin circulates to the skin. The *toxin splits the epidermis away from the underlying layers*. The first sign of skin involvement is the acute onset of generalized erythema and tenderness over the entire body except the palms, soles, and mucous membranes. Blisters and bullae form over the next several days, which rupture and denude the skin, leaving the child at risk for dehydration and secondary infection. In severe cases, generalized skin sloughing may occur.

Diagnosis is confirmed by culture and histologic studies. Lesions are treated like severe burns, and the primary infection is treated with oral or parenteral antibiotics. Healing in uncomplicated cases usually requires 10 to 14 days.

5. Compare tinea capitis to tinea corporis; describe thrush.
Study pages 1073 and 1074; refer to Figure 40-6.

Comparison of Fungal Infections

	Tinea Capitis	Tinea Corporis
Etiologic agent	*Microsporum canis, Trichophyton tonsurans*	*Microsporum canis, Trichophyton mentagrophytes*
Source	*M. canis* from cats, dogs, or rodents; *T. tonsurans* from humans	*M. canis* and *T. mentagrophytes* from kittens or puppies
Lesion	Circular, slight erythema, scaling with raised border	Oval or round with scale, central clearing, mild erythema, or ringworm
Diagnostic test	KOH examination	KOH examination
Treatment	Oral antifungals (topicals do not penetrate hair bulb)	Topical antifungals

Thrush develops in the presence of *Candida albicans* in the mucous membranes in the mouths of infants and, less often, adults. This organism penetrates the epidermal barrier because of its *keratolytic proteases* and other enzymes. *C. albicans* attracts neutrophils to skin sites of invasion and generates inflammation by activating the complement system. Thrush is characterized by white plaques or spots in the mouth that lead to shallow ulcers. The underlying mucous membrane is red and tender and may bleed when the plaques are removed.

Treatment is with oral antifungal washes. Simultaneous treatment of nipple infection or vaginitis in the mother is helpful in reducing *C. albicans* surface colonization of the infant.

6. Describe the infections in children caused by poxviruses, papovaviruses, and herpes viruses.
Study pages 1074-1077; refer to Figures 40-7 through 40-9 and Table 40-1.

Molluscum contagiosum is a transmitted via *skin-to-skin contact* or by *contact with contaminated fabrics*. This viral (*poxvirus*) disease is characterized by a pearlescent, dome-shaped lesion that may appear anywhere on the body, but most often affects the face, trunk, and extremities. The lesions are filled with viral and cellular debris. No specific treatment is recommended because it is self-limiting, although recurrence is common.

Rubella, or 3-day measles, is a communicable disease of children and young adults caused by an *RNA virus* that enters the bloodstream through the *respiratory tract*. The incubation period is between 14 and 21 days. A faint-pink to red coalescing maculopapular rash develops on the face and spreads to the trunk and extremities 1 to 4 days after the prodromal symptoms. Women of childbearing age should be immunized if their antibody liters are low, and pregnancy should be avoided for 3 months after vaccination because the attenuated virus may remain for this time. *Congenital defects may develop in the fetus* of a pregnant woman who has rubella early in the first trimester. There is no specific, only supportive, treatment. Recovery is spontaneous.

Rubeola, or red measles, is a contagious disease of children transmitted by direct contact with *droplets from infected persons*. Rubeola is caused by an *RNA paramyxovirus* having an incubation period of 7 to 12 days. Prodromal symptoms are followed within 3 to 4 days by an erythematous maculopapular rash over the head that spreads distally over the trunk, extremities, hands, and feet. Early lesions blanch with pressure, but they do not do so as the rash fades. Pinpoint white spots surrounded by an erythematous ring develop over the buccal mucosa and are known as *Koplik spots*. Most children recover completely, but measles encephalitis occurs in about 1 in 800 cases. There is no specific treatment for measles.

Roseola likely is a viral infection; it occurs most often in infants between the ages of 6 months and 2 years. There is a sudden onset of fever that lasts for 3 to 5 days. After the fever, an erythematous macular rash develops primarily over the trunk and neck and lasts for about 24 hours. Usually, there is no treatment.

Chickenpox (varicella) is a highly contagious viral disease of early childhood that is primarily spread by *droplet transmission* from an infected person to others. Household infection rates approach 90% in susceptible individuals. The incubation period is approximately 14 days, with infected persons contagious for approximately 24 hours before the onset of the rash and for 5 to 6 days after the rash appears. Chickenpox is usually an illness of late winter or early spring. The first signs of illness are pruritus, or itching, and the appearance of vesicles. There may be no prodromal symptoms.

Characteristically, the rash undergoes a process of maturation, with lesions starting as *macules that progress to superficial papules and vesicles*, which then rupture and heal. The rash lasts for 4 to 5 days and may consist of up to 300 lesions distributed over the body. Complications from chickenpox are fairly rare, but may include pneumonia resulting from the varicella virus. Treatment is symptomatic and consists of cool baths, wet dressings, and oral antihistamines.

Herpes zoster (shingles) occurs mainly in adults, but approximately 5% of cases are in children younger than 15 years. *The chickenpox virus persists for life in sensory nerve ganglia and reactivates to cause herpes zoster.* The zoster consists of groups of vesicles situated on an inflammatory base that follows the course of a sensory nerve. The base of the lesion appears *hemorrhagic,* and some may become necrotic and ulcerative. In children, the thorax is the site of distribution of the lesions. Therapy is similar to that for chickenpox unless it is disseminated zoster or there is ophthalmic involvement, in which case antiviral agents are indicated.

7. Compare and contrast the infestations of scabies and lice; note other lesions from insects and parasites.
Study pages 1077 and 1078; refer to Figures 40-10 and 40-11.

Insect Infestations

Feature	Scabies (Mite)	Pediculosis (Lice)
Etiologic agent	*Sarcoptes scabiei*	*Pediculus capitis* (head)
		Pediculus corporis (body)
		Phthirus pubis (pubic)
Transmission	Contact with infested person	Contact with infested person or object (hat, clothing)
Symptoms	Burrows, papules, and vesicles; itching	Pruritus; ova (nits) may be seen on hair shafts; mature lice may be seen
Cause of symptoms	Sensitization to larva buried in the skin	Irritation from toxic saliva from louse bites
Treatment	Scabicide; wash and dry infested objects	Pediculicide; wash and dry infested objects

Note: Flea bites produce a pruritic wheal with a central puncture site and occur as clusters in areas of tight-fitting clothing. Lyme disease is a multisystem inflammatory disease caused by the spirochete *Borrelia burgdorferi* transmitted by tick bites. The disease occurs in stages. Soon after the bite, erythema migrans, myalgia, and fatigue occur. Nine months later, secondary erythema migrans, arthralgias, meningitis, neuritis, and carditis develop. Late persistent infection continues for years, manifesting as arthritis, encephalopathy, and polyneuropathy. Bedbugs are blood-sucking parasites that live in cracks of floors, furniture, or bedding and feed at night. They produce pruritic wheals and nodules.

8. Compare and contrast the congenital vascular disorders.
Study pages 1079 and 1080; refer to Figures 40-12 through 40-14.

Vascular Disorders

Feature	Strawberry Hemangioma	Cavernous Hemangioma	Salmon Patches	Port-Wine Stain
Description	Raised vesicular	Raised vesicular with larger mature vessels	Macular; most common	Flat; becomes popular and cavernous
Time of manifestation	At birth or in 3 to 5 weeks	At birth	At birth	At birth or in a few days
Color	Bright red (capillary projections)	Bluish, indistinct borders	Pink, distended dermal capillaries	Pink to dark reddish purple
Location	One lesion on head, neck, or trunk	Head, neck	Nape of neck, forehead, upper eyelid	Face and other body surfaces
Growth	Initially rapid; then at child's rate of growth	Rapid first 6 months; matures at 1 year	Fades in 1 year	Does not fade
Involution	Begins by 12 to 16 months, complete by 5 to 6 years	Begins by 6 to 12 months, complete by 9 years	N/A	N/A
Treatment	None	May require surgery, laser surgery, or liquid nitrogen, depending on location of lesion	None	Cryosurgery, laser surgery

PRACTICE EXAMINATION

True/False

1. Diaper dermatitis is caused by *Candida albicans*.
2. Impetigo is contracted only through human-to-human contact.
3. Molluscum contagiosum is a painful viral infection.
4. Atopic dermatitis is also called *eczema*.
5. Staphylococcal scalded-skin syndrome is a contagious disease of the skin.
6. Tinea capitis must be treated with systemic antifungal agents.
7. Lyme disease can exhibit symptoms for years.
8. Port-wine stains will involute by adulthood.
9. Acute glomerulonephritis is a complication of bullous impetigo.
10. The microorganism that causes bullous impetigo is *Streptococcus pyogenes*.

Matching

Match the description with the alteration:

_______ 11. Viral skin infection contracted during the first decade of life

_______ 12. Positive allergy tests, increased IgE, and eosinophilia

_______ 13. Erythematous lesions in the perineal area with secondary papulovesicular satellites

a. staphylococcal scalded-skin syndrome
b. tinea capitis
c. atopic dermatitis
d. pediculosis
e. diaper dermatitis complicated by Candida albicans
f. chickenpox
g. vascular disorders
h. impetigo

_______ 14. Raised, erythremic, scaling lesions on the scalp

_______ 15. Dome-shaped lesions ranging from 1 mm to 5 mm on the extremities without pruritus

_______ 16. Macules, fever, itching, papules, and rupturing and healing vesicles

_______ 17. Crusted lesion

_______ 18. Mite burrowing in the stratum corneum

_______ 19. Present at birth or shortly after birth

_______ 20. Entire skin sloughing

_______ 21. Nits on hair shaft

_______ 22. Chronic condition with acute exacerbations, pruritus

_______ 23. Oval or circular lesions, peripheral spreading, central clearing (ringworm)

_______ 24. Action of an epidermolytic toxin

_______ 25. Parasitic in nature, acquired by personal contact and sharing of combs or hairbrushes

i. molluscum contagiosum
j. scabies
k. tinea corporis

Fill in the Blank

Complete the following table differentiating among viral diseases that cause rashes:

Viral Diseases Causing Rashes

Disease	Incubation Period	Duration and Characteristics
Rubella (German measles)		
Rubeola (red measles)	7–12 days	3–5 days Koplik spots (buccal mucosa white pinpoint spots surrounded by an erythematous ring) precede a purple-red maculopapular rash on head, trunk, and extremities
Roseola (exanthema subitum)		
Varicella (chickenpox)		

CASE STUDY

Lance D. is a 5-year-old white boy who visits the nurse practitioner's office with a runny nose that started about one week earlier, but has not resolved. He has been blowing his nose frequently, and "sores" have developed on his face. His mother states, "His sores started as big blisters that ruptured; sometimes, a scab forms with a crust but they continue to weep and drain." She is worried because the lesions are now also on his forearm. Lance's past medical and family histories are normal. He has been febrile but is otherwise asymptomatic. The physical findings are unremarkable except for moderate, purulent rhinorrhea and weeping lesions 0.5 cm to 1 cm in diameter around the nose and mouth and on the radial surface of the right forearm. There is no regional lymphadenopathy.

What is the likely name and cause of these lesions? Why have these lesions spread to Lance's arm?

Answers to Practice Examinations

CHAPTER 1

1. c	6. a	11. b, d	16. c	21. e
2. a, c, e	7. d	12. d	17. d	22. f
3. a	8. d	13. a, b, c, d, e	18. h	23. j
4. e	9. e	14. a, b, c, d	19. b	24. b
5. d	10. b	15. b	20. g	25. c

Membrane Transport

Transport Mechanism	Description
Diffusion	A solute moves moves passively from an area of higher solute concentration to an area of lower solute concentration
Filtration	Water and solute move through a membrane because of greater hydrostatic pressure on one side of the membrane than on the other side
Osmosis	Water moves across a semipermeable membrane from lower solute concentration to higher solute concentration
Mediated transport	Two molecules move simultaneously in one direction (symport) or in opposite direction (antiport) or a single molecule moves in one direction (uniport)
Passive mediated transport/ facilitated diffusion	Does not require the expenditure of metabolic energy (ATP)
Active mediated transport	Requires the expenditure of metabolic energy (ATP)
Endocytosis	An active transport in which the substance transported is engulfed by the plasma membrane to form a vesicle that then moves into the cell
Pinocytosis	Endocytosis of fluids, and ingestion of solute molecules through vesicle formation
Phagocytosis	Endocytosis of larger substances, such as bacteria, which are ingested through vacuole formation

CHAPTER 2

1. a	6. b	11. d	16. f	21. h
2. b	7. b	12. d	17. h	22. d
3. d	8. a, b, c	13. b	18. g	23. f
4. c	9. c, e	14. c	19. i	24. g
5. d	10. a	15. a	20. b	25. c

Transmission Patterns for Genetic Diseases

	Single-Gene Diseases	Multifactorial Diseases
Inheritance pattern	The basic unit of heredity, DNA, is located on a specific locus on a chromosome; the recurrence risk for autosomal dominant disease is 50%; the recurrence risk for autosomal recessive disease is 25%; X-linked recessive diseases (most X-linked diseases) are mostly in males because males need only one copy of the gene to express the disease; recurrence risks remain the same for each offspring, regardless of the number of affected or nonaffected offspring	Traits from the combined effects of several genes are polygenic; when environmental factors also influence the trait, it is multifactorial; recurrence risks for multifactorial diseases become higher if more than one family member is affected or if the family member is severely affected; multifactorial disease risk decreases rapidly for more distant relatives

Case Study Analysis and Application

"Down syndrome occurs when the chromosomes fail to divide properly. An extra chromosome 21 is present (three instead of two). The risk of having a baby with Down syndrome for an older mother is greater than it is for younger mothers. The physical problems your son may have include heart chamber wall septal anomalies, respiratory infections, and kidney problems. Every child with Down syndrome has some mental retardation, but most are trainable. His increased susceptibility to leukemia may cause him to have a shorter life span."

CHAPTER 3

1. d
2. c, d
3. d
4. e
5. d
6. a
7. d
8. d
9. d
10. e
11. b
12. d
13. a
14. c
15. e
16. c
17. b
18. d
19. a
20. e
21. c
22. a
23. d
24. b
25. e

Cellular Necrosis

Type	Cause	Sites
Coagulative necrosis	Hypoxia by severe ischemia	Kidneys, heart, and adrenal glands
Liquefactive necrosis	Bacterial infections, ischemia	Brain neurons and glial cells
Caseous necrosis	Combined coagulative and liquefactive necrosis	Tubercular lesion in lungs
Fatty necrosis	Lipases break down triglycerides to fatty acids, which combine with ions to create soaps	Breast, pancreas, and abdominal structures
Gangrenous necrosis	Severe hypoxic injury subsequent to arteriosclerosis or blockage of major arteries followed by bacterial invasion	Connective tissue and cellular membranes, muscles

CHAPTER 4

1. e
2. b
3. d
4. c
5. d
6. b
7. b
8. c, e
9. d
10. d
11. a, b, e
12. b
13. e
14. c
15. e
16. b
17. b
18. b
19. a
20. d
21. a
22. e
23. b
24. a
25. b, c

Acid-Base Corrections

Buffer System	Mechanism	Time to Correct
Short term:		
Lungs	Regulates retention or elimination of CO_2 and thus H_2CO_3	Minutes to hours
Ionic shifts	Exchange of intracellular K^+ and Na^+ for hydrogen	2-4 hours
Long term:		
Kidneys	HCO_3^- reabsorption and regeneration, ammonia formation, phosphate buffering	Hours to days
Bone	Exchanges of calcium and phosphate and release of carbonate	Hours to days

Case Study Analysis and Application

Potassium and chloride levels are low. An emergency exists because of potassium depletion, which can cause cardiac arrhythmia. The patient should be admitted to the hospital for intravenous fluids with KCl and monitoring of blood pressure, pulse, and cardiac function.

CHAPTER 5

1. d
2. b
3. a
4. a
5. b
6. b
7. d
8. c
9. a
10. c
11. d
12. b
13. d
14. b
15. c
16. b
17. d
18. d
19. a
20. Neutrophils
21. Macrophages
22. Eosinophils
23. Natural killer cells
24. Resolution
25. Granulation tissue

Human Defenses

Characteristics	Barriers	Innate Immunity	Adaptive Immunity
Defensive level	First defensive line against infection and tissue injury	Second defensive line responding to infection or tissue injury	Third defensive line initiated when innate immune system signals the cells of adaptive immunity
Defensive timing	Constant	Immediate	Delay between first exposure to antigen and maximum response, immediate to second and subsequent antigenic exposure
Specificity	Broad, nonspecific	Broad, nonspecific	Specific response to antigen
Cells	Epithelial	Mast cells, granulocytes, monocytes, macrophages, natural killer cells, platelets, endothelial cells	T and B lymphocytes, macrophages, dendritic cells
Memory	None	None	Specific memory by T and B lymphocytes
Active molecules	Defensins, cathelicidins, lactoferrin, bacterial toxins	Complement, clotting factors, kinins, cytokines	Antibodies, complement, cytokines
Protection	Skin and mucous membranes, lysosomes, low pH of stomach and urine, ciliary activity	Vascular responses, neutrophils, basophils, macrophages, secretory molecules or cytokines, plasma protein systems	Activated T and B lymphocytes, antibodies, cytokines

CHAPTER 6

1. a
2. d
3. b
4. b
5. b
6. c
7. d
8. a
9. d
10. e
11. d
12. d
13. b
14. c
15. a
16. c
17. b
18. a
19. b
20. d
21. Helper T cells
22. anamnestic
23. Regulatory T cells
24. Superantigens
25. secretory immune system

Generation of Clonal Selection

Characteristic	Clonal Selection
Purpose	Select, expand, and differentiate clones of T and B cells against a specific antigen
Time of occurrence	Primarily after birth and throughout life
Site of occurrence	Peripheral lymphoid organs
Foreign antigen involvement	Yes; antigen determines cell clones selected
Cytokines involved	Many produced by T helper cells and APCs
Final products	Plasma cells to produce antibodies, effector T cells that help; kill targets; or regulate immune responses; memory B and T cells

CHAPTER 7

1. c
2. d
3. d
4. d
5. e
6. c
7. d
8. a
9. a
10. d
11. e
12. c
13. b
14. e
15. e
16. d
17. a
18. d
19. b
20. c
21. a
22. c
23. d
24. b
25. d

Primary and Secondary Immunodeficiencies

Primary Deficiencies		Secondary Deficiencies	
Cause	Example	Cause	Example
Lack of B cells	Burton agammaglobulinemia	Physiologic and psychologic stressors	Pregnancy, aging, emotional trauma, eating disorders
No IgA production	Selective IgA deficiency	Dietary deficiencies	Malnutrition, insufficient vitamins and minerals, hepatitis B, AIDS
Lack of T cells	DiGeorge syndrome	Malignancies	Lymphomas, leukemias, sarcomas, carcinomas
Lack of B cells, T cells, phagocytes	SCID	Physical trauma	Burns
Decreased IgM	Wiskott-Aldrich syndrome	Medical treatments	Surgery, immunotherapy, cancer therapy

Pathogen's Resistance to Immune Responses

	Mechanisms	Effect on Immunity
Bacteria	Produce endotoxins, exotoxins, hemolysins, leukocidins, coagulases, proteases, surface molecules that bind receptors and antibodies, surface antigens similar to self-antigens, and vasodilators that reduce blood pressure and oxygen delivery	Kill phagocytes, interfere with chemotaxis, promote bacterial attachment, prevent complement activation and antibody function, and antibodies are formed against self-antigens
Viruses	Invade host cell, mutate surface antigens, and activate genes that alter surface molecules	Failure to recognize new antigen so immune response is delayed, take over cell genetics so that host cell synthesis ceases, fuse host cells, attack host cell as if foreign, transform host cell into cancerous cell, and damage tissue so secondary bacterial infections develop

Case Study 1 Analysis and Application

A seasonal pattern to this patient's symptoms, a clear nasal discharge, itchy eyes, and high levels of allergen exposure as a teenager likely promoted humoral immunity. The probability of *allergic rhinitis* is high. Relief likely could be obtained by recommending oral antihistamines, steroid nasal sprays, or decongestants. A referral to an allergist to evaluate the allergens responsible for the symptoms is recommended. The initiation of hyposensitivity immunotherapy may be suggested to reduce the symptoms. If possible, known allergens should be avoided.

Case Study 2 Analysis and Application

A chest roentgenogram, sputum and blood cultures, a lymphocyte screen, and a test for antibody against HIV would be warranted. Laboratory tests would have the following results: The chest roentgenogram demonstrates diffuse infiltrates. The sputum and blood cultures would likely show presence of *Pneumocystis carinii,* which causes pneumonia in immunocompromised individuals. The lymphocyte screen would show reduced T helper cells. Circulating antibody against HIV would be present.

CHAPTER 8

1. a
2. b
3. c
4. b
5. d
6. c
7. c
8. c
9. a
10. a
11. a
12. a
13. a
14. c
15. d
16. corticoids
17. Stressors
18. stress response
19. exhaustion stage
20. alarm stage
21. IL-1
22. IL-2
23. NPY
24. IFN
25. Endorphins

Epinephrine Norepinephrine vs. Cortisol Actions

Effects	
Catecholamines (epinephrine and norepinephrine)	**Cortisol**
Epinephrine prepares the body to act; dilates blood vessels to increase cardiac output and blood flow to the heart, brain, and skeletal muscles; and dilates the airways to increase oxygen blood levels. Norepinephrine constricts peripheral blood vessels to aid in the shifting of blood to the dilated vessels and increases mental alertness	Mobilizes glucose and other substances to fuel the action; mobilizes glucose, amino acids, lipids, and fatty acids and delivers them to the bloodstream; low levels of cortisol increase adaptive immunity, may activate proinflammatory mediators, and decrease innate immunity; high levels of cortisol, including therapeutic levels, decrease both humoral and cellular immunity and are anti-inflammatory

CHAPTER 9

1. e
2. c
3. a
4. d
5. e
6. e
7. c
8. e
9. b
10. e
11. e
12. a
13. c
14. e
15. c
16. e
17. f
18. b
19. f
20. c
21. d
22. c
23. d
24. a
25. f

Common Benign and Malignant Tumor Origin Sites

Tissue	Benign Tumor	Malignant Tumor
Connective Tissue		
Fibrous	Fibroma	Fibrosarcoma
Cartilage	Chondroma	Chondrosarcoma
Bone	Osteoma	Osteosarcoma
Fat	Lipoma	Liposarcoma
Smooth muscle	Leiomyoma	Leiomyosarcoma
Striated muscle	Rhabdomyoma	Rhabdomyosarcoma
Blood vessels	Hemangioma	Hemangiosarcoma

(Continued)

Common Benign and Malignant Tumor Origin Sites—Cont'd

Tissue	Benign Tumor	Malignant Tumor
Hematopoietic		
Lymphoid tissue	Infectious mononucleosis	Lymphosarcoma (lymphoma)
Plasma cells		Multiple myeloma
Leukocytes		Leukemia
Nerve Tissue		
Nerve cell	Neuroma	
Nerve sheath	Neurilemmoma	Neurogenic sarcoma
Glial tissue		Glioma
Retina		Retinoblastoma
Epithelial Tissue		
Squamous epithelium	Papilloma	Squamous carcinoma
Glandular epithelium	Adenoma	Adenocarcinoma

CHAPTER 10

1. individual carcinogens
2. miRNAs
3. Developmental plasticity
4. Environmental tobacco smoke
5. Xenobiotics
6. meat
7. Hypomethylation
8. Adipose cells
9. mesothelioma
10. melanoma, basal cell carcinoma, and squamous cell carcinoma
11. benzol
12. genetic
13. bystander cells
14. TNF
15. phase I activators
16. endogenous androgen
17. BMI
18. Epigenetic
19. breast, endometrial
20. ionizing radiation
21. antioxidants, oxygen-degrading
22. Methylation
23. long latency
24. HPV-16
25. Radon

Possible Carcinogenic/Noncarcinogenic Foods

Increase Risk of Cancer	Decrease Risk of Cancer
Foods that contain fat, especially omega-6 fatty acids, and high-sugar carbohydrates, foods having excessive preservatives, alcohol, grilled and blackened foods, and fried foods	Foods that contain fiber and are low in sugar, fruits and vegetables like broccoli and cabbage, foods containing vitamins A, C, D, and E, and green tea

CHAPTER 11

1. False
2. False
3. True
4. True
5. False
6. True
7. True
8. False
9. True
10. True
11. e
12. f
13. a
14. d
15. b
16. c
17. True
18. False
19. False
20. True
21. True
22. False
23. False

Childhood Cancers and Their Associated Genes

Cancer	Oncogenes	Tumor-Suppressor Genes
Lymphoblastic leukemia	*BCR-abl, ATM*	
Neuroblastoma	*N-myc, c-myb, H/K-ras, N-ras*	
Leukemia, lymphoma, rhabdomyosarcoma	*N-myc, N/K-ras*	*NF1*
Wilms tumor		*WT1, WT2, WT3, FW,FWT1*
Retinoblastoma		*Rb1*
Sarcoma, osteosarcoma, brain tumors, leukemia	*Erb*	*p53, NF2*

CHAPTER 12

1. c
2. d
3. c
4. a
5. c
6. a
7. b
8. b, d
9. a
10. c
11. a
12. d
13. c
14. b
15. e
16. a
17. c
18. a
19. c
20. a
21. a
22. b
23. a
24. d
25. c

Responses of Selected Effector Organs to Automatic Nerve Impulses

Effector	Receptor	Adrenergic Response	Cholinergic Response
Eye:			
Radial muscle, iris	δ	Contraction	—
Sphincter muscle, iris	β_1	—	Contraction
Heart:			
SA node	β_1	Increases heart rate	Decreases heart rate
Ventricles	β_1	Increases contractility	—
Arterioles:			
Pulmonary	δ, β_2	Dilation predominates	—
Skeletal muscle	δ, β_2	Dilation predominates	—
Cerebral	δ	Constriction	—
Lung:			
Bronchial muscle	β_2	Relaxation	Contraction
Adrenal medulla	—	—	Secretion of epinephrine and norepinephrine

Note:

- Sympathetic *preganglionic* fibers, parasympathetic preganglionic fibers, and postganglionic fibers release *acetylcholine*. These fibers are characterized by cholinergic transmission. Most *postganglionic* sympathetic fibers release *norepinephrine* (adrenaline) and are considered to function by adrenergic transmission.
- Two types of adrenergic receptors exist, δ and β. Cells of effector organs may have only one or both types of these adrenergic receptors. δ_1 receptors are associated with excitation, whereas δ_2 receptors are associated with inhibition; β_1 receptors stimulate cardiac muscle and cause release of renin from the kidney, whereas β_2 receptors facilitate all other effects attributed to receptors.

CHAPTER 13

1. b	6. c	11. b	16. d	21. c
2. c	7. c	12. b	17. b	22. j
3. b	8. e	13. c	18. a	23. i
4. e	9. b	14. a	19. e	24. h
5. e	10. d	15. e	20. e	25. g

Comparison of Acute Pain and Chronic Pain

Characteristic	Acute Pain	Chronic Pain
Experience	An event	A situation or existing state
Onset	Usually sudden	Sudden or insidious
Duration	Transient, short time	Prolonged
Identification	Generally well defined	Differentiated areas less easily defined; sensations difficult to identify
Pattern	Self-limiting, readily corrected	Continuous or intermittent, intensity varies
Course	Suffering decreases over time	Suffering increases over time
Prognosis	Likelihood of eventual complete relief	Complete relief usually not possible

Case Study Analysis and Application

Mrs. D.'s history and response to medication were typical of *depression*. Depression causes sleep disturbances characterized by insomnia, early morning awakenings, or multiple awakenings during the night. The improvement in the quality of sleep following antidepressants often occurs before other appropriate behavioral changes are evident. It seems likely that her *insomnia* may return, and an appropriate course of action might involve seeking assistance from a sleep disorder center.

CHAPTER 14

1. b	6. d	11. c	16. e	21. l
2. a	7. b	12. a	17. d	22. b
3. b	8. a	13. e	18. c	23. e
4. c	9. c	14. c	19. j	24. f
5. e	10. c	15. e	20. k	25. g

Altered Levels of Consciousness

State	Definition
Confusion	Impaired thinking, judgment, decision making
Disorientation	Beginning loss of consciousness; disorientation to time, place, and person
Lethargy	Slow vocalization and decreased motor skills; easy arousal; may or may not be oriented to time, place or person
Obtundation	Awakens in response to stimulation; continuous stimulation needed for arousal
Stupor	Vocalization and spontaneous movement occur only with rigorous and repeated stimulation
Coma	No vocalization nor movement in response to any stimulus

Case Study 1 Analysis and Application

Normal serologic values and the normal CSF results likely exclude the possibility of an infection such as meningitis and other causes known to precipitate seizures. The skull radiograph ruled out the possibility of a skull fracture. A normal EEG tracing likely excludes intracranial pressure from brain masses. Because an EEG tracing may be normal between seizures, the episodic pattern and laboratory values suggest a *generalized grand mal seizure*. A judicious administration of anticonvulsant medications is indicated.

Case Study 2 Analysis and Application

The physician should conduct a focused history, with input from the son, looking for evidence of depression—an entity that overlaps dementia presentation; order a head CT scan to rule out any organic cause for the cognitive dysfunction; and order serum chemistry analysis to detect other organ disorders that can contribute to dementia. If the physician finds Alzheimer disease, cholinesterase inhibitors or drugs blocking the activity of glutamate can be used. Treatment of AD is also directed at compensation techniques, such as memory aids, maintaining cognition that is not impaired, and improving hygiene, nutrition, and health. Health care givers should help the patient avoid potential risks rather than teaching and reteaching.

CHAPTER 15

1. d	6. a	11. d	16. c	21. b
2. b	7. b	12. b	17. b	22. d
3. e	8. c	13. c	18. d	23. g
4. b	9. e	14. b	19. e	24. c
5. e	10. c	15. a, c	20. a	25. f

Focal and Diffuse Traumatic Brain Injuries

Type of Injury	Characteristics
Focal	
Contusion:	Small blood vessel tears and bleeding, possible loss of consciousness
Coup	Injury directly below impact
Contrecoup	Injury opposite the side of impact
Extradural hematoma	Arterial bleeding, immediate to delayed loss of consciousness, possible herniation
Subdural hematoma	Venous bleeding, delayed loss of consciousness, possible herniation
Delayed intracerebral hematoma	Sudden progression of unconsciousness, pupil dilation, altered breathing, herniation
Diffuse	
Mild concussion	Temporary axonal disturbance, consciousness not lost
Classic cerebral concussion	Axonal tears, unconsciousness lasting more than 6 hours
Mild DIA	Some decerebrate or decorticate posturing, disorientation, confusion
Moderate DIA	Axons tear in both hemispheres, unconsciousness lasting more than 24 hours
Severe DAI	Axonal tears in both hemispheres, diencephalon, and brain stem; sensory and cognitive deficits; increased intracranial pressure

Cerebrovascular Accidents

	Type				
	Thrombotic	Embolic	Hemorrhagic	Ischemic	Lacunar
Involved site(s)	Arteries supplying the brain or intracranial vessels	Small brain vessels at bifurcations or narrowings	Basal ganglia, thalamus, cortex, subcortex, pons, cerebellar hemispheres	Anywhere in cerebral vessels	Small and perforating arteries in the basal ganglia, internal capsule, and pons
Risk factors, causes	Arteritis, atheromatous plaques, dehydration, hypotension, vasoconstriction	Atrial fibrillation, myocardial infarction, endocarditis, rheumatic heart disease	Hypertension, ruptured aneurysms, bleeding disorders, head trauma	Diabetes, insulin resistance, polycythemia, atrial fibrillation	Smoking, hypertension, diabetes

Case Study Analysis and Application

Mrs. B. exhibits risk factors for a CVA. She smokes cigarettes, is overweight, and is hypertensive. Her mother and siblings have histories of diabetes, CVA, and hypertension; all of these indicate a family history that increases the risk for CVA.

Her symptoms and signs suggest a *thrombotic stroke* with ischemia rather than a hemorrhagic or embolic stroke. The absence of blood in the CSF rules out a hemorrhagic stroke. Because there was no fibrillation on the electrocardiogram, the heart was an unlikely source for emboli, thus ruling out an embolic stroke. Mrs. B.'s elevated blood pressure likely is caused by atherosclerosis, which can lead to a thrombus formation.

CHAPTER 16

1. False
2. False
3. False
4. True
5. False
6. True
7. True
8. True
9. False
10. False
11. False
12. Reye, hepatic
13. posterior
14. anterior
15. meningitis
16. Craniosynostosis
17. i
18. h
19. g
20. f
21. e
22. d
23. c
24. b
25. a

Common Brain Tumors in Children

Type	Frequency	Usual Site(s)
Astrocytoma	28%	Cerebellum, lateral hemispheres
Optic nerve glioma	6%	Optic chiasm or optic nerve
Medulloblastoma	18%	Cerebellum, extends into 4th ventricle spinal fluid pathway
Brain stem glioma	10%	Pons or myelencephalon
Ependymoma	19%	Ependymal cells lining ventricles
Craniopharyngioma	5%	Pituitary gland, optic chiasm, hypothalamus

Note: Astrocytomas and ependymomas may be either supratentorial or infratentorial.

Case Study Analysis and Application

Radiographs should reveal an absence of spinal processes on the vertebrae from L3 to L5. Then, MRI would be ordered and would show a *myelomeningocele* at the same level with tethering of the cord. A neurosurgical consultation would then be arranged, and surgery would be likely.

CHAPTER 17

1. a
2. e
3. c
4. b
5. d
6. e
7. a
8. c
9. d
10. d
11. e
12. c
13. d
14. d
15. e
16. c
17. b
18. b
19. d
20. e
21. a
22. c
23. a
24. d
25. e

Sites of Origin and Effects of Hormones

Site	Hormone	Effect
Hypothalamus	Releasing hormones	Act on anterior pituitary to stimulate release or inhibit synthesis and release of hormones
Posterior pituitary	Antidiuretic hormone (ADH)	Causes conservation of body water, reduces serum osmolality, may regulate CNS functions
	Oxytocin	Stimulates uterine contraction and lactation, has antidiuretic activity, may have a role in sperm mobility
Anterior pituitary	Adrenocorticotropic hormone (ACTH)	Stimulates production of glucocorticoids (gluconeogenesis, inhibits immunity, anti-inflammatory) by adrenal cortex
	Melanocyte-stimulating hormone (MSH)	Stimulates darkening of skin color

Sites of Origin and Effects of Hormones—Cont'd

Site	Hormone	Effect
	Growth hormone (GH)	Promotes growth of body tissues
	Thyroid-stimulating hormone (TSH)	Stimulates production and release of thyroid hormones (growth and maturation of tissues)
	Follicle-stimulating hormone (FSH)	Initiates maturation of ovarian follicles; stimulates spermatogenesis
	Prolactin	Stimulates secretion of breast milk
	Luteinizing hormone (LH)	Causes ovulation and stimulates ovary to produce estrogen and progesterone; stimulates androgen production by interstitial cells of testes
Thyroid	Thyroxine (T3, T4)	Increases rate of cellular metabolism
	Calcitonin	Osteoblastic—lowers serum calcium
Parathyroid	Parathyroid hormone (PTH)	Osteoclastic—raises serum calcium
Pancreatic islets of Langerhans	Insulin	Promotes utilization of glucose; lowers serum glucose
	Amylin	Delays nutrient uptake and suppresses glucagon after meals
	Glucagon	Promotes utilization of glycogen; raises serum glucose
Adrenal cortex	Glucocorticoids, mostly cortisol	Antagonize effects of insulin; inhibit inflammatory response and fibroblastic activity, protein catabolic
	Mineralocorticoids, mostly aldosterone	Promote retention of sodium by renal tubules
	Androgens and estrogens	Promote secondary sex characteristics
Adrenal medulla	Catecholamines (epinephrine and norepinephrine)	Regulate blood pressure through effects on vascular smooth muscle and heart
Pineal gland	Melatonin	Regulates circadian rhythms and reproductive systems

CHAPTER 18

1. c
2. a
3. a
4. d
5. b
6. a
7. d
8. a
9. a
10. d
11. a
12. b
13. b
14. b
15. c
16. c
17. a
18. e
19. c
20. e
21. a, b, c
22. c
23. e
24. d
25. b

SIADH vs. Diabetes Insipidus

	Cause	Manifestations
SIADH	ADH excess	Water retention, serum hyponatremia and hyposmolarity, concentrated urine, confusion, lethargy, muscle excitability
Diabetes insipidus	ADH deficiency, kidney unable to respond to ADH	Polyuria, polydipsia, nocturia, dilute urine, dry mucous membranes

Hypercortisolism vs. Hypercortisolism

Hypercortisolism	Hypocortisolism
Hypokalemia; hypernatremia; hypertension; hyperglycemia; increased truncal, facial, cervical adipose tissue; muscle wasting; osteoporosis; collagen loss (weakened skin, purple striae); and immunosuppression	Hyperkalemia; hyponatremia; hypotension; hypoglycemia; hypoaldosteronism; weakness; fatigue; gastrointestinal disturbances; and skin hyperpigmentation

Manifestations/Effects of Endocrine Disorders

Effect	Examples
Fluid and electrolyte imbalances	Addison disease, Cushing disease, Conn disease, diabetes insipidus, SIADH, hypoparathyroidism, hyperparathyroidism
Cardiovascular dysfunction	Addison disease, hyperthyroidism, pheochromocytoma, diabetes mellitus
General growth alterations	Dwarfism, giantism, acromegaly
Reproductive irregularities	Precocious puberty, adrenogenital syndrome, gynecomastia
Altered glucose metabolism	Addison disease, Cushing disease, diabetes mellitus
Metabolic rate abnormalities	Hyperthyroidism, hypothyroidism, cretinism, myxedema

Case Study 1 Analysis and Application

Scott's symptoms, signs, and laboratory values are classic for *diabetes ketoacidosis,* an acute complication of diabetes. The serum values indicate metabolic acidosis with some accompanying respiratory compensation. His elevated glycosylated hemoglobin shows that he has been hyperglycemic for several months. This diabetes is type 1 and will require insulin administration. Scott and his family must be provided with instructions regarding recognition of future signs and symptoms of hyperglycemia and hypoglycemia, blood glucose self-monitoring, insulin therapy, diet, and exercise.

Case Study 2 Analysis and Application

Initial laboratory tests are a random serum glucose measurement and a urine dipstick test. Subsequent laboratory tests could include a fasting glucose test, a glycosylated hemoglobin analysis, a fasting lipid profile, an electrocardiogram, and an electromyogram.

Repeat BP (152/100 mm Hg) is a hypertensive value. Random glucose value (262 mg/dl), fasting glucose value (171 mg/dl), and high quantities of glycosylated hemoglobin satisfy/exceed the criteria for a diagnosis of diabetes. Microalbuminuria indicates early nephropathy and an increased risk for renal and cardiovascular diseases. The fasting lipid profile indicates diabetic dyslipidemia with increased cardiovascular risk. Electrocardiogram tracing indicates left ventricular hypertrophy and suggests the existence of hypertension (HTN) for some time, and the presence of peripheral neuropathy is validated by the electromyogram.

The treatment of type 2 diabetes requires appropriate meal planning. Only oral hypoglycemic agents may be required if the pancreas can produce some insulin; otherwise, insulin may be required. Exercise is an important aspect in the treatment of type 2 diabetes. It reduces the after-meal blood glucose value and reduces insulin requirements. Increases in good, high-density lipoprotein (HDL) cholesterol and weight loss can be achieved by exercise.

CHAPTER 19

1. e	6. c	11. d	16. a	21. b
2. b	7. c	12. e	17. a	22. d
3. e	8. c	13. e	18. b	23. d
4. d	9. d	14. d	19. e	24. b
5. a	10. e	15. d	20. e	25. c

Cellular Components of the Blood

Cell	Normal Amounts	Function	Life Span
Leukocyte	5000-10,000/mm³	Bodily defense mechanisms	Variable (see below)
Lymphocyte	25%-36% of leukocytes	Immunity	Days or years
Natural killer cell (large granular lymphocyte)	5%-10% of circulating pool	Kills tumor cells and virus infected cells	Unknown
Monocyte and macrophage	3%-8% of leukocytes	Phagocytosis, mononuclear phagocyte system	Months or years
Eosinophil	1%-4% of leukocytes	Controls inflammation, phagocytosis, antibody-mediated defense against parasites, allergic reactions	Unknown
Neutrophil	54%-67% of leukocytes	Phagocytosis, particularly during early phase of inflammation/ infection	4 days
Basophil	0%-0.75% of leukocytes	Mast cell–like functions associated with allergic reactions and mechanical irritation	Unknown
Platelet	140,000-340,000/mm³	Hemostasis following vascular injury, normal coagulation and clot formation/reactions	8-11 days
Erythrocyte	4.2-6.2 million/mm³	Gas transport to and from tissue cell and lungs	80 to 120 days
Reticulocyte	0.5%-2 % of erythrocytes	Immature erythrocyte	

CHAPTER 20

1. e
2. d
3. d
4. a
5. b
6. b
7. e
8. c
9. d
10. c
11. e
12. c
13. b
14. a
15. d
16. e
17. a
18. b
19. a
20. b
21. b
22. c
23. a
24. a
25. b

Hematologic Values

Test	Disorder(s)*
	L: anemia
RBC count, Hgb, Hct	H: polycythemia
WBC count	L: irradiation, chemotherapy, anaphylactic shock, splenomegaly, immunosuppression, AIDS
	H: leukemia, allergy, bacterial and parasitic infections
Platelet count	L: hemorrhage, heparin administration, autoimmunity ITP, TTP
	H: myeloproliferative disorder (ET), splenectomy
Prothrombin time	L: (DIC)
	H: hemophilia, von Willebrand disease, impaired liver, DIC
Bleeding time	Similar to those listed for prothrombin time
Fibrin degradation products	Similar to those listed for prothrombin time

*L, low value; H, high value.

Case Study 1 Analysis and Application

Erythrocytes are microcytic and hypochromic in three anemias: iron deficiency anemia, sideroblastic anemia, and thalassemia. Ann's history has some factors that could contribute to anemia from blood loss. The menorrhagia causes more iron loss than is normal with each menstrual period, and excessive aspirin intake irritates the gastrointestinal mucosa and can precipitate chronic mucosal microhemorrhage.

Iron deficiency anemia is most likely and can be verified by providing oral iron replacement and checking her hemoglobin values in 1 month. If the hemoglobin deficit is corrected, it is likely that the correct diagnosis was made. The source of bleeding should be corrected. A substitute for aspirin should be used, as well as an iron supplementation for at least 1 year.

Ann's homeostatic mechanisms are trying to compensate in several ways, including shunting blood to more critical organs, increasing erythropoiesis as evidenced by the elevated erythrocyte count, raising the heart rate to handle improve venous return, and increasing the respiratory rate to make oxygen available to the remaining erythrocytes.

Case Study 2 Analysis and Application

The physician likely would conclude that L.L. has *acute lymphocytic leukemia*. The pale skin with petechiae and ecchymoses is abnormal, as is the gingival bleeding from minor trauma. Although abnormal values for RBC count, hemoglobin, total leukocyte count, and platelet count have many possible causes, the presence of leukocytic blasts in peripheral blood indicates a bone marrow dysfunction. At this time, the physician likely will refer L.L. to a pediatric oncologist for extensive diagnostic tests and treatment.

CHAPTER 21

1. False
2. True
3. True
4. False
5. True
6. False
7. False
8. a
9. b
10. e
11. d
12. c
13. e
14. d
15. e
16. b
17. e
18. e
19. a
20. b
21. e
22. c
23. d
24. c
25. d

Childhood Hemophilias

Type	Cause
Hemophilia A	Factor VIII deficiency, inherited as a X-linked recessive disorder
Hemophilia B (Christmas disease)	Factor IX deficiency, inherited as a X-linked recessive disorder (less severe than hemophilia A)
Hemophilia C	Factor XI deficiency, inherited as an autosomal recessive disease (less severe than either A or B)
von Willebrand disease	Factor VIII deficiency, inherited as an autosomal dominant disease

Case Study Analysis and Application

Steven has the typical manifestations of *idiopathic thrombocytopenic purpura* (ITP), although it has come to the attention of medical professionals in a circuitous manner.

CHAPTER 22

1. b
2. b
3. b
4. c
5. b, c
6. b
7. e
8. a
9. c
10. e
11. a
12. a
13. c
14. d
15. a
16. b, d, e
17. c
18. b
19. d
20. a
21. a
22. d
23. b
24. b
25. b

Cardiovascular Function in the Elderly

Determinant	Resting Performance	Exercise Performance
Heart rate	Slight decrease	Overall decrease
Cardiac output	Unchanged in male, slight decrease in female	Decreases as heart rate decreases
Contraction	Increased because of prolonged relaxation	Decreases with vigorous exercise

CHAPTER 23

1. d	6. b	11. e	16. b, d	21. b
2. e	7. d	12. a	17. a, b, c	22. b
3. c	8. e	13. b, d	18. d	23. c
4. b	9. c	14. c	19. e	24. e
5. a	10. b, d, e	15. a, c	20. c	25. f

Effects of Sustained Primary Hypertension

Injury Site	Injurious Mechanism	Pathology
Heart	Myocardial overload, coronary artery atherosclerosis	Left ventricular hypertrophy, myocardial ischemia
Kidneys	Reduced blood flow stimulates rennin and aldosterone secretion, reduced O_2 supply, increased renal arteriolar pressure	Sodium and H_2O retention, hypertension, compromised filtration, nephrosclerosis
Brain	Reduced blood flow and O_2, weakened vessel walls	TIAs, thrombosis, aneurysm, hemorrhage, infarction
Retina	Reduced blood flow, high arterial pressure	Vascular sclerosis, hemorrhage
Aorta	Weakened vessel wall	Dissecting aneurysm
Lower extremity arteries	Arterial high pressure	Intermittent claudication, possible gangrene

Case Study 1 Analysis and Application

Mr. T likely has HTN or is at risk for it. Appropriate questions are: How much fatty food and salt do you eat? Do you drink alcohol? Do you regularly exercise? Do you check your blood pressure regularly? Laboratory tests to confirm the presence of hypertension include blood chemistry analysis for BUN, creatinine, fasting glucose, calcium, and magnesium and a lipid profile with a CBC and an ECG.

The diagnosis of *stage 1 HTN* is confirmed by the initial and subsequent blood pressure measurements of mid-150s systolic over mid-90s diastolic. Laboratory results showed all blood chemistry values and CBC results normal, total cholesterol and LDL elevated, and HDL value low. The laboratory studies rule out secondary causes of HTN. Left ventricular hypertrophy observed on the ECG indicates long-standing HTN, adding to Mr T.'s risk for CHF. If conventional therapy is ineffective, specialized tests are required to determine the cause of secondary hypertension.

Case Study 2 Analysis and Application

Alterable myocardial infarction risk factors for W.S. are as follows: essential hypertension and cigarette smoking. Unalterable risk factors for W.S. include the following: advancing age, male sex, and family history of early cardiac death. Atherosclerosis in the anterior descending branch of the left coronary artery was the beginning process leading to this infarction. The precipitating event in this myocardial infarction was occlusion of the coronary artery.

Pulmonary thromboembolism is a common cause of death from myocardial infarction as emboli disseminate from debris or clots from the infarcted endocardium. Prophylactic heparin therapy is likely before W.S. is taken to the catheterization lab for definitive treatment, because it decreases the risk of pulmonary embolism. Coronary angiography can determine the anatomic extent of CAD. Thus, angiography evaluates for possible percutaneous coronary intervention (PCI) with stent placement or coronary artery bypass graph (CABG) surgery for W.S.

CHAPTER 24

1. False	7. left, right	12. first weeks	15. coarctation of	21. c
2. True	8. right, left	13. pulmonary	16. e	22. e
3. False	9. oxygenated,	stenosis the aorta	17. a	23. d
4. True	unoxygenated	14. afterload,	18. a	24. d
5. False	10. equal	congestive heart	19. b	25. a
6. shunt	11. left, right	failure	20. c	

Common Causes of Childhood Sustained Hypertension

Age Group	Causes
Newborn	Renal artery thrombosis and stenosis, congenital renal malformation, COA, bronchopulmonary dysplasia
< 6 yr	Renal parenchymal disease (RPD), COA, renal artery stenosis
6-10 yr	Renal artery stenosis, RPD, primary hypertension
> 10 yr	Primary hypertension, RPD

Case Study Analysis and Application

Following the consultation, David M.'s echocardiogram demonstrates a moderate *coarctation of the aorta* in the aortic arch. This discrepancy in the quality of upper and lower extremity pulses results from well-developed collateral circulation to the descending aorta; the femoral pulses decrease as blood fills the collateral vessels. Although this boy is currently asymptomatic, the coarctation will cause exertional dyspnea later in life.

CHAPTER 25

1. d	6. e	11. c	16. b	21. b
2. d	7. d	12. d	17. e	22. c
3. c	8. c	13. b	18. e	23. a
4. d	9. a	14. d	19. a	24. b
5. d	10. a	15. a	20. a	25. a

Pulmonary Defensive Mechanisms

Effector	Mechanism of Defense
Upper tract mucosa, nasal hairs, and turbinates	Humidifies and maintains temperature of gas entering lungs; traps and removes particles, bacteria, and noxious gases from inspired air
Mucus blanket	Protects lower tract from injury; traps and removes foreign particles that reach the lower airways
Cilia	Propel mucus blanket and entrapped particles toward the oropharynx, where they are either swallowed or expectorated
Alveolar macrophages	Phagocytosis; ingest and remove particles and bacteria from the alveoli
Irritant receptors in nares	Chemical or mechanical irritants trigger the sneeze reflex, resulting in rapid removal of irritants from the nasal passages
Irritant receptors in trachea and large airways	Chemical or mechanical irritants trigger the cough reflex resulting in removal of irritants from the lower airways

CHAPTER 26

1. c	6. a, b, c, d	11. a, b, d	16. g	21. d
2. e	7. e	12. d	17. c	22. e
3. d	8. b, c	13. e	18. h	23. f
4. e	9. b	14. b	19. l	24. j
5. a	10. a, b, d	15. a	20. i	25. m

Pathogenesis of Pulmonary Edema

Causes	Pathogenic Mechanism
Heart disease: Valvular dysfunction	Increased left atrial pressure, increased pulmonary capillary hydrostatic pressure
Left ventricular dysfunction	
Coronary artery disease	
Capillary endothelium injury	Increased capillary permeability and alveolar surfactant disruption, movement of fluid and plasma proteins from capillary to interstitial space and alveoli
Lymphatic vessel blockage	Inability to remove excess fluid from interstitial space, accumulation of fluid in interstitial space

Case Study 1 Analysis and Application

Necessary tests should begin with oximetry; if the oxygen saturation value falls below 90%, then arterial blood gas tensions should be measured. Blood gas analysis can show hypoxemia with early respiratory alkalosis or late respiratory acidosis. Peak flow measurement should be made to assess the severity of airway obstruction. Management of an acute asthma attack requires the immediate administration of oxygen and inhaled bronchodilators. Also, oral corticosteroids should be used. If the patient becomes more dyspneic, anxious, and confused accompanied by both inspiratory and expiratory wheezes, cyanosis, and cold and clammy extremities despite first-line therapy, hospitalization is required for careful monitoring and possible IV therapy.

Case Study 2 Analysis and Application

Mr. S. presents the classic symptoms and signs of *emphysema*. His long-term, extensive smoking is consistent with most cases of emphysema, as is his dyspnea on exertion progressing to dyspnea even at rest. Hyperinflation of lungs causes the anteroposterior chest diameter to increase. The chest radiograph is consistent with findings in emphysema. Prolonged forced expiratory volume, decreased tidal volume, and increased total lung capacity are also present in emphysema. These test results indicate that the walls of alveoli have been destroyed and the lungs have become more distended or less compliant and have less elastic recoil. Therefore, air is trapped and expiration flow is diminished.

CHAPTER 27

1. False	6. True	11. c	16. d	21. e
2. False	7. e	12. d	17. a	22. c
3. False	8. e	13. c	18. b	23. d
4. True	9. d	14. e	19. f	24. c
5. False	10. e	15. d	20. g	25. a

Common Types of Childhood Pneumonia

Type	Causal Agent	Age
Viral pneumonia	RSV, influenza, adenovirus, others	Infants for RSV, all ages for others
Pneumococcal pneumonia	*Streptococcus pneumoniae*	Usually 1-4 yr
Staphylococcal pneumonia	*Staphylococcus aureus*	1 wk to 2 yr
Streptococcal pneumonia	Group A beta-hemolytic streptococci	All ages
Mycoplasma and *Chlamydia* pneumonia	*Mycoplasma pneumoniae, Chlamydia pneumoniae*	School age and adolescents

Case Study Analysis and Application

Styler has classic manifestations of *bronchiolitis*. The most likely etiologic agent in his illness is respiratory syncytial virus, to which his parents likely exposed him during their "colds." He is displaying the classic signs of respiratory distress in an infant and is unable to feed because of this respiratory distress. His lethargy is probably the result of mild hypoxia and hypercapnia, and his general fatigue is from prolonged ventilatory effort. He may suffer respiratory failure if left untreated. Hospitalization for rehydration and assisted ventilation should support him through the worst of his illness, and he should improve within a few days.

CHAPTER 28

1. c	6. b	11. e	16. d	21. b
2. a	7. b	12. b	17. a	22. c
3. d	8. c	13. b	18. c, d, e	23. c
4. a	9. d	14. d	19. d	24. c
5. d	10. d	15. b	20. a	25. d

Glomerular Filtration Pressures

Pressures (mm Hg)		
Forces	Afferent Arteriole	Efferent Arteriole
Promoting filtration:		
Glomerular capillary hydrostatic pressure	47	45
Bowman capsule oncotic pressure	Negligible	Negligible
Total	47	45
Opposing filtration:		
Bowman capsule hydrostatic pressure	10	10
Glomerular capillary oncotic pressure	25	35
Total	35	45
Net filtration pressure	12	0

CHAPTER 29

1. d
2. b
3. a
4. a
5. e
6. d
7. a, b, c
8. b
9. b
10. b, c, d
11. d
12. e
13. d
14. d
15. a, e
16. b
17. d
18. c
19. a
20. d
21. c
22. b
23. d
24. a
25. e

Characteristics of Nephrotic Syndrome

Manifestations	Contributing Factors
Proteinuria	Increased glomerular permeability, decreased proximal tubule reabsorption
Hypoalbuminemia	Increased urinary loss of protein
Edema	Hypoalbuminemia, decreased plasma oncotic pressure, sodium and water retention, increased aldosterone and ADH secretion, unresponsiveness to atrial natriuretic peptides
Hyperlipidemia	Decreased serum albumin, increased hepatic synthesis of very LDLs, increased cholesterol, phospholipids, and triglycerides
Lipiduria	Sloughing of tubular cells containing fat, free fat from hyperlipidemia

Case Study 1 Analysis and Application

Ms. J. has either a recurrent UTI (cystitis) or pyelonephritis. All of the historical evidence, the physical examination, and the laboratory results support a final diagnosis of a lower tract UTI *(cystitis)* rather than an upper tract UTI (pyelonephritis) because she does not have a fever or any atypical symptoms or signs. The antibiotic therapy used should be effective against *E. coli*.

Case Study 2 Analysis and Application

Eddie's history of sore throat and back pain and his laboratory values suggest *poststreptococcal glomerulonephritis*. Proteinuria is a sensitive indicator of glomerular dysfunction. In glomerulonephritis, the glomerulus is injured and its permeability is increased enough to permit protein to enter into the filtrate and urine. Blood and RBC casts also occur in glomerulonephritis. BUN and creatinine are excreted entirely by the kidneys and therefore are directly related to renal excretion. Eddie's pediatrician most likely will start him on penicillin therapy and may prescribe an antihypertensive medication and monitor his blood pressure, electrolyte balance, and BUN and creatinine levels.

CHAPTER 30

1. False
2. True
3. False
4. False
5. True
6. False
7. d
8. a
9. d
10. c
11. e
12. d
13. d
14. d
15. d
16. d
17. e
18. e
19. d
20. f
21. b
22. c
23. c
24. a
25. e

Childhood Urinary Structural Abnormalities

Type	Characteristics
Hypospadias	The urethral meatus is located on the ventral surface of the penis or midline of the scrotum or perineum
Epispadias and exstrophy of the bladder	In epispadias, the urethra opens on the dorsal side of the penis; exstrophy of the bladder, which occurs in both males and females, occurs when the bladder opens directly on the abdominal wall and the pelvis remains open
Bladder outlet obstruction	Thin membranes of tissue occlude the urethral lumen and obstruct urinary flow in males; prostate urethral polyps cause severe obstruction that may impair renal embryogenesis
Ureteropelvic junction disorder	The renal pelvis transitions into the ureter; uteropelvic junction disorder is the most common cause of hydronephrosis in neonates
Hypoplastic/dysplastic kidney	The hypoplastic kidney is small but normal; the dysplastic kidney is an abnormal differentiation of renal tissues
Renal agenesis	The failure of the kidney to develop or grow
Polycystic kidneys	Inherited disorder that results in large, fluid-filled cysts within the kidneys

Case Study Analysis and Application

The laboratory values reveal an anemia and thrombocytopenia; the child is losing red blood cells and platelets. Because she has not voided any urine, acute renal failure is likely. These results suggest the diagnosis of *hemolytic-uremic syndrome*. She will require hospitalization for blood transfusions with packed red blood cells, fluid and electrolyte balance must be maintained, and hypertension and seizures must be controlled.

CHAPTER 31

1. b, d
2. a
3. e
4. d
5. c
6. d
7. a
8. b
9. e
10. b
11. a
12. e
13. b
14. c
15. a, c
16. c
17. e
18. c
19. e
20. a
21. a
22. c
23. c
24. e
25. a

Effects of Estrogen and Progesterone

Structure	Estrogen Effects	Progesterone Effects
Breasts	Growth of ducts, promotes prolactin effects	Growth of lobules and alveoli, inhibits prolactin effects
Vaginal mucosa	Squamous epithelium proliferation, increases glycogen content of cells, cellular cornification	Squamous epithelium thinning, cellular decornification
Cervical mucosa	Produces secretions flavoring survival, enhances sperm motility	Produces secretions tending to plug the cervical os
Fallopian tube	Increases motility and ciliary action	Decreases motility and ciliary action
Uterine muscle	Increases blood flow; increases contractile proteins, uterine muscle, and myometrial excitability and action potential; increases sensitivity to oxytocin	Relaxes myometrium; decreases sensitivity to oxytocin
Endometrium	Stimulates growth, increases number of progesterone receptors	Activates glands and blood vessels, decreases number of estrogen receptors

CHAPTER 32

1. d	6. b	11. d	16. d	21. c
2. c	7. d	12. d	17. b	22. e
3. e	8. a	13. d	18. a	23. f
4. d	9. e	14. a	19. b	24. h
5. e	10. b	15. d	20. b	25. i

BPH vs. Prostatic Cancer

Characteristics	BPH	Prostatic Cancer
Involved site	Periurethral gland	Posterior periphery of gland
Causes	Altered testosterone/dihydrotestosterone, estradiol, IGFs/receptor ratios	Same as BPH, genetics, chronic inflammation, possible high fat diet, low calcium intake
Symptoms	Remitting: slow urinary stream, hesitancy, incomplete emptying, frequency, nocturia	Progressive worsening of BPH symptoms without temporary remissions
Subsequent course	Bladder distention, urine retention, urethral obstruction, bladder or kidney infection	Metastasis to bones (lumbar spine, pelvis, ribs) with pain, lower extremity edema, lymphadenopathy,

Case Study 1 Analysis and Application

A transabdominal and transvaginal pelvic ultrasound is necessary.

Result: *Indistinct right ovary-grossly normal; 7.6 × 9.0 × 3.3–cm left adnexal mass; ill-defined left ovary*

Next, a MRI of the pelvis with contrast is required.

Result: *Left adnexal mass; no free pelvic fluid; no significant adenopathy; right ovary—grossly normal; sigmoid colon—diverticulosis*

These diagnostic test results dictated a diagnostic laparoscopy with excision of the mass with frozen cytologic examination of any suspicious lesions. *Frozen sections—malignancy*. The presence of malignancy requires a total abdominal hysterectomy and a bilateral salpingo-oophorectomy and staging of the extent of the malignancy. The surgery and staging were completed. Specimens, including a resected section of the descending colon, were submitted for cytologic evaluation. The *final diagnosis = Papillary carcinoma consistent with serous carcinoma of uterine tube (favored) or serous carcinoma of both ovaries and metastatic papillary carcinoma of descending colon.*

The standard treatment protocol for this ovarian cancer is chemotherapy; then, complete debulking surgery followed by more chemotherapy.

Case Study 2 Analysis and Application

Mrs. B.'s history and examination indicate *breast cancer* in her left breast. A positive familial history of breast cancer has a strong causal link to breast cancer. A chromosome 13 and 17 defect has been implicated as a genetic causal factor in breast cancer as well. Other associated risk factors for breast cancer that Mrs. B. exhibits include late age at first delivery, early menarche, birth control pills, and benign breast tumors.

The cardinal manifestation of breast cancer was a hard, fixed mass palpable in Mrs. B.'s left breast. The freely movable, soft masses of the right breast are likely benign, because they display fluctuating patterns of tissue proliferation different from those of the left breast. The palpation of the left axillary lymph node indicates that cancer cells have metastasized through the lymphatic channels surrounding the breast.

CHAPTER 33

1. d	6. d	11. d	16. d	21. b
2. d	7. d	12. b	17. a	22. c
3. b	8. a	13. a	18. b	23. e
4. e	9. d	14. c	19. a	24. c
5. e	10. b	15. c	20. c	25. a

Digestive Enzyme Actions and Food Absorption Routes

Food Type	Enzymes	Products	Absorption Routes
Starch	Salivary amylase	Polysaccharides	
Polysaccharides	Pancreatic amylase	Lactose, maltose, sucrose	
Lactose, maltose, sucrose	Small intestinal lactase, maltase, sucrose	Galactose, glucose, fructose	Through small intestine capillary villi and then transported by hepatic portal vein to liver
Proteins	Stomach pepsin in presence of HCl	Peptones, proteoses	
Peptones, proteoses	Pancreatic enzymes (trypsin, chymotrypsin, carboxypeptidase) within the small intestine	Small polypeptides, dipeptides	
Small polypeptides, dipeptides	Small intestinal aminopeptidases and dipeptidases	Amino acids	Same as the above; carbohydrates
Unemulsified fats	Emulsifying agents (bile acids, fatty acids, monoglycerides, lecithin, cholesterol, and protein) and pancreatic lipases with the small intestine	Monoglycerides, glycerol, and fatty acids	Monoglycerides an fatty acids: Lacteals in small intestinal villi, then transported to liver via the systemic circulation, which receives thoracic duct lymph, or via the hepatic portal vein; Glycerol and fatty acids: capillaries in villi, then transported by the hepatic portal vein to the liver

CHAPTER 34

1. b	6. d	11. b	16. d	21. b
2. d	7. c	12. e	17. e	22. e
3. a	8. e	13. b	18. e	23. d
4. e	9. a	14. a	19. a, b, c, d	24. a
5. e	10. b	15. c	20. a	25. d

Manifestations of Gastrointestinal Bleeding

Manifestations	Characteristics
Acute bleeding:	
Hematemesis	Fresh or bright red bloody vomitus or dark grainy digested blood appearing as "coffee grounds"
Melena	Black, sticky, tarry, foul-smelling stools caused by digestion of blood in the GI tract
Hematochezia	Fresh, bright red blood passed by the rectum
Occult bleeding	Traces of blood in normal appearing stools or gastric secretions, requires a guaiac test to detect

Case Study 1 Analysis and Application

A *gastric ulcer* is likely. Factors associated with these ulcers include smoking, stress, and use of aspirin or other ulcerogenic drugs. Although the clinical manifestations of gastric ulcers are similar to those of duodenal ulcers, the pain of gastric ulcers is more likely to occur immediately after eating. Also, gastric ulcers tend to be chronic rather than to alternate between periods of remission and exacerbation. An upper gastrointestinal study using barium sulfate as a contrasting medium and endoscopy can detect the location of the ulcer and confirm that Dr. R. has a gastric ulcer.

Case Study 2 Analysis and Application

Laboratory values should include a CBC with a differential count for evidence of infection; liver function tests to assess the liver's metabolism, storage, filtration, and excretion;

blood chemistry analysis to evaluate renal function; and serologic analysis to reveal the presence or absence of HBsAg, anti-HAV, anti-HCV, and anti-HIV. D.K. is at risk for HIV as well as hepatitis because of possible sharing of contaminated needles with other IV drug users.

D.K.'s history by itself does little to suggest a particular diagnosis. The absence of ascites, occult or rectal blood, and confusion during the physical examination tend to rule out hepatic failure. An elevated WBC count with increased lymphocytes indicates a viral infection. Normal coagulation and albumin values indicate insignificant hepatic and renal dysfunction. Unremarkable increases in bilirubin and alkaline phosphatase tend to exclude biliary disease. The serologic analysis of antigen and antibodies implicates HBV but not HAV, HCV, or HIV. D.K. has *hepatitis B*.

CHAPTER 35

1. False
2. True
3. False
4. False
5. False
6. True
7. True
8. False
9. True
10. False
11. True
12. Gastroesophageal reflux
13. diarrhea
14. decrease
15. nasal, oral
16. pancreatic insufficiency
17. a
18. c
19. b
20. a
21. e
22. e
23. d
24. c
25. c

Cystic Fibrosis Characteristics

Involved Organ	Secretory Dysfunction	Manifestations	Complications
Sweat glands	Elevated levels of Na and Cl in the sweat	Hyponatremia, hypochloremia	Heat prostration, shock
Pancreas	Pancreatic enzyme deficiency	Fatty, bulky stools	Hypoproteinemia and iron deficiency anemia; decreased absorption of vitamins A,D,E, and K; rectal prolapse; diabetes mellitus
Lungs	Overproduction of viscid mucus in bronchi and bronchioles	Obstruction of bronchioles causing bronchiolectasis, bronchiectasis, and lung infection	Hemoptysis, pneumothorax, cor pulmonale, respiratory failure

Case Study Analysis and Application

A *pyloric stenosis* is diagnosed on the basis of clinical manifestations. The standard and usual treatment is a pyloromyotomy to separate the muscles of the pylorus.

CHAPTER 36

1. a, c, d
2. d
3. b
4. b
5. d
6. b
7. b
8. d
9. d
10. a
11. a
12. b
13. d
14. b
15. c
16. e
17. e
18. e
19. c
20. d
21. e
22. b
23. c
24. a
25. d

Bone Remodeling and Repair

Stage	Process
Remodeling (Minor Injuries)	
Phase 1	A stimulus activates bone cell precursors to become to become osteoclasts
Phase 2	Osteoclasts resorb bone leaving a resorption cavity
Phase 3	Osteoblasts lining the resorption cavity lay down new or secondary bone by forming a new haversian cavity in compact bone or new trabeculae in spongy bone

Bone Remodeling and Repair—Cont'd

Stage	Process
Repair (Fracture and Surgery)	
Hematoma formation	Blood leaks from torn blood vessel across the fracture line, causing a hematoma
Procallus formation	Infiltrating new capillaries into the hematoma organize into granulation tissue
Callus formation	Osteogenic cells convert the granulation tissue into fibrocartilage
Callus replacement	Osteoblasts replace the callus with either lamellar or trabecular bone
Remodeling	Periosteal and endosteal surfaces are remodeled to the size and shape of the bone before injury

CHAPTER 37

1. a	6. c	11. b	16. a, b, d, e	21. b
2. b	7. e	12. d	17. e	22. d
3. d	8. a	13. e	18. b	23. d
4. e	9. a	14. a	19. d	24. c
5. c	10. e	15. a, b	20. e	25. e

Tumor Destructive Bone Patterns

Pattern	Feature	Type of Lesion
Geographic	Well-defined smooth or irregular margin with a narrow zone between normal and abnormal bone, uniform and well-defined lytic bone area	Usually indicates a less aggressive, slow-growing, or benign lesion
Moth-eaten	Less defined or less well demarcated margin, lytic area not easily separated from normal bone	Indicates a more aggressive, rapidly growing, or malignant lesion
Permeative	Poorly demarcated margin, imperceptible merging of normal with abnormal bone	Indicates an aggressive and very rapidly growing malignant lesion

Case Study 1 Analysis and Application

Mrs. B.'s presenting symptoms are compatible with either osteoarthritis or rheumatoid arthritis. The laboratory results support a diagnosis of *rheumatoid arthritis*. The presence of rheumatoid factor is helpful in the diagnosis of rheumatoid arthritis. It is present in about 80% of individuals who have rheumatoid arthritis. Although other diseases may cause a positive result of the rheumatoid factor test, osteoarthritis does not. Demonstration of inflammatory exudates by synovial fluid analysis satisfies the diagnostic criteria for rheumatoid arthritis. The radiograph is more representative of rheumatoid arthritis than osteoarthritis. In osteoarthritis, deformity of articular cartilage, bone sclerosis, cystic areas, and bony spurs would be likely observations.

Case Study 2 Analysis and Application

The osteopenia is the result of *menopausal osteoporosis*. The fracture must be stabilized with a back brace, and then the goal is to prevent future fractures and disability. Management requires regular, moderate weight-bearing exercise; dietary supplements of calcium, vitamin D, and magnesium; selective estrogen receptor modulators; intranasal calcitonin; and bisphosphonates to encourage osteocyte survival.

CHAPTER 38

1. False	6. True	11. femoral	16. b	21. e
2. False	7. False	12. breech position	17. f	22. d
3. False	8. True	13. dystrophin	18. e	23. c
4. True	9. True	14. Pavlik harness	19. f	24. b
5. False	10. False	15. clubfoot	20. d	25. a

Childhood Benign and Malignant Bone Tumors

Type	Site	Feature
Benign		
Osteochondroma	Near-active growth plates of proximal humerus or tibia and distal femur	Occur as a solitary lesion or as multiple lesions throughout the body; palpable mass that is painful if traumatized
Nonossifying fibroma	Any bone at any age in cortical bone	Whorled bundles of fibroblasts and osteoclast-like giant cells
Malignant		
Osteosarcoma	Metaphyses of long bones near site of active physeal growth	When lung metastasis occurs, cough, dyspnea, and pain manifest
Ewing sarcoma	Cells in bone marrow of femur, pelvis, and humerus	Does not involve bone-forming cells, metastasizes early to every organ

Case Study Analysis and Application

Bobby B. displays the clinical manifestations of *Duchenne muscular dystrophy*. The diagnosis can be confirmed by measurement of serum creatine phosphokinase (CPK) levels, electromyography, and muscle biopsy. The CPK level in Duchenne muscular dystrophy will increase more than 10 times normal. Histologic examination of the biopsy will show muscle degeneration, with fat and connective tissue replacing muscle fibers.

CHAPTER 39

1. a	6. d	11. d	16. d	21. a
2. a	7. e	12. b	17. d	22. c
3. a	8. f	13. e	18. b	23. d
4. d	9. d	14. c	19. c	24. d
5. b	10. e	15. e	20. c	25. a

Aging and Changes in the Skin

Change	Consequence(s)
Fewer melanocytes	Decreased protection from UV radiation, graying of hair
Loss of rete pegs	Smooth and shiny appearance
Loss of elastin	Wrinkling
Dermis thins	Translucency
Collagen fibers lose flexibility	Less ability to stretch and return to shape
More permeable and less able to clear substances	Substances accumulate and irritate
Eccrine, apocrine, and sebaceous glands atrophy	Dry skin, less sweat, and possible heat stroke
Fewer Langerhans cells	Less phagocytes and immune response
Free nerve endings decrease	Reduced sensory response
Decreased blood flow and basal cell turnover	Decreased wound healing
Thinning nail plates	Brittle nails

Case Study Analysis and Application

Adults with burns involving large surface areas require cardiovascular support through intravenous fluid because *hypovolemic shock* develops quickly following major burn injury. Within minutes of a major burn injury, the capillary bed not only at the site of the burn but throughout the entire body becomes more permeable to water, sodium, and proteins. This leads to fluid loss from the intravascular spaces into the interstitial spaces and massive edema; the blood volume and cardiac output diminish. The infusion of intravenous fluid or burn-shock resuscitation for the first 24 hours must be faster than the rate of loss of circulatory volume. To determine adequate levels of infusion, urine output must be measured, so Mr. E. must undergo placement of a catheter into his bladder.

Although hypovolemic shock is the immediate concern for major burn patients, other alterations are important; monitoring and maintenance of electrolytes are required. The hypermetabolic rate of burned individuals requires adequate nutrition. Finally, early excision and grafting procedures are likely required.

CHAPTER 40

1. False
2. False
3. False
4. True
5. False
6. True
7. True
8. False
9. False
10. False
11. f
12. c
13. e
14. b
15. i
16. f
17. h
18. j
19. g
20. a
21. d
22. c
23. k
24. a
25. d

Viral Diseases Causing Rashes

Disease	Incubation Period	Duration/Characteristics
Rubella (German measles)	14-21 days	1-3 days/Face and trunk pink-red maculopapular rash
Rubeola (red measles)	7-12 days	3-5 days/Koplik spots (buccal mucosa white pinpoint spots surrounded by an erythematous ring) precede a head, trunk, and extremities purple-red maculopapular rash
Roseola (exanthema subitum)	5-15 days	1-3 days/Head and trunk red macular rash
Varicella (chickenpox)	11-20 days	7-14 days/Face, scalp, trunk, and extremities red papules, vesicles, pustules in clusters

Case Study Analysis and Application

This is a fairly classic case of *bullous impetigo* caused by a *Staphylococcus aureus* infection in Lance's nasopharynx. Abrasion from blowing and wiping his nose frequently has opened the skin and allowed the bacteria to enter the skin and cause the lesions. The infection spread to his arm because he has been wiping his nose on his arm.